Nanomaterials for Wound Regeneration & Dressings

This book provides a comprehensive overview of the role of nanomaterials in wound regeneration and the development of advanced wound dressings. It presents their recent advances; explains their materials, properties, and manufacture; and describes promising solutions for improving patient outcomes.

Nanomaterials for Wound Regeneration & Dressings: Advanced Applications is divided into two sections: wound regeneration and wound dressings, respectively. It first discusses nanomaterials, the wound-healing process, and the limitations of traditional wound care methods. Following this, it addresses the use of nanomaterials in wound regeneration and the selection and manufacture of nanomaterial-based wound dressings. Section I discusses biocompatibility and toxicity issues, regulatory and ethical considerations, and manufacturing and scalability challenges. Section II explains the technologies and applications of advanced wound dressings incorporating nanomaterials and their benefits for wound care. It also addresses advanced wound dressings for both chronic and acute wounds to ensure a comprehensive understanding. The book concludes with a discussion of current challenges in the field, particularly the rise of AI, and outlines future research directions and potential innovations to improve patient outcomes by shortening healing times and reducing the risk of infection. Throughout the book, contributors provide case studies and clinical trial results that demonstrate the efficacy of these dressings, giving readers a comprehensive understanding of the materials, mechanisms, and appropriate applications of different nanomaterials that they will be able to apply experimentally and practically in both laboratory and clinical settings.

This book provides vital knowledge to upper undergraduate and postgraduate students in fields such as biomaterials science and engineering, medicine, textile engineering, nursing, and biochemistry, as well as research scientists and industry experts working in the fields of life sciences and nanomaterials.

Nanomaterials for Wound Regeneration & Dressings
Advanced Applications

Edited by
Muhammad Qamar Khan and Ick Soo Kim

CRC Press
Taylor & Francis Group
Boca Raton London New York

CRC Press is an imprint of the
Taylor & Francis Group, an **informa** business

Designed cover image: Shutterstock

First edition published 2027
by CRC Press
2385 NW Executive Center Drive, Suite 320, Boca Raton FL 33431

and by CRC Press
4 Park Square, Milton Park, Abingdon, Oxon, OX14 4RN

CRC Press is an imprint of Taylor & Francis Group, LLC

ISBN: 9781041018711 (hbk)
ISBN: 9781041018735 (pbk)
ISBN: 9781003616726 (ebk)

DOI: 10.1201/9781003616726

Typeset in Times
by codeMantra

Contents

About the Editors

Muhammad Qamar Khan is the Chair of the Department of Clothing at the National Textile University in Faisalabad, Pakistan. He obtained his B.S. from the National Textile University in Faisalabad, Pakistan in 2013; his M.Phil. from Mehran UET in Jamshoro, Pakistan in 2016; and his Dr. Eng. from Shinshu University in Nagano, Japan in 2019.

Ick Soo Kim is the Director of the Institute of Fiber Engineering at Shinshu University in Japan. He received his Ph.D. from Nagoya University in Japan in 2000.

Contributors

Maleeha Akram is a B.S. Textile Engineering student in the Department of Textile Engineering at the National Textile University in Faisalabad.

Muhammad Abbas Haider Alvi is a Garment Manufacturing Graduate in the Department of Clothing at the National Textile University in Faisalabad He currently serves as an Assistant Manager of the Garments Wet Processing Department at Sapphire Diamond Denim.

Muhammad Ayyoob is working as the Chairman of the Department of Textile & Clothing at the National Textile University Karachi Campus in Karachi.

Syeda Rubab Batool is a postdoctoral researcher at the School of Engineering and Technology at the National Textile University in Faisalabad, Pakistan. She did her Ph.D. in Biomedical Studies from Koç University, Istanbul, Turkey.

Aleeza Fatima is a B.S. Textile Engineering student at the National Textile University in Faisalabad.

Rubab Fatima is a research officer at the National Textile University in Faisalabad, Pakistan.

Sehrish Iftikhar is a B.S. Textile Engineering student at the National Textile University in Faisalabad.

Tooba Jabri is currently a postdoctoral researcher at the University of Leeds, UK. She obtained her Ph.D. in Biotechnology from Husein Ebrahim Jamal Research Institute of Chemistry, Husein Ebrahim Jamal Research Institute of Chemistry (HEJ) Pakistan.

Muhammad Tauseef Khawar is an Assistant Professor at the National Textile University in Faisalabad. He completed his Ph.D. in Materials from the University of Manchester, UK, and later served as a Research Fellow in Sustainable Textile Manufacturing at the University of Leeds. He holds an M.Sc. in Textile Engineering (Nonwovens) from National Textile University (NTU) and a B.Sc. in Textile Engineering (Garment Manufacturing) from Bahauddin Zakria University (BZU, Multan. With over four years of industry experience in garment and socks manufacturing, his research interests include sustainable textiles, nonwovens, nanocomposites, and garment technology.

Ji Ha Lee is an Associate Professor in the Faculty of Textile Science and Technology at Shinshu University.

Simeng Liu is a Ph.D. student in Ji Ha Lee's lab at Shinshu University.

Rashid Masood, Rector of the National Textile University in Faisalabad, holds a Ph.D. in Biomedical Textiles and an M.Sc. in Textile Studies from the University of Bolton, UK. With extensive academic and administrative experience, including serving as the Chairman of NTU and the Director of the National Textile Research Centre, his research interests span medical and healthcare textiles, thermoregulating fabrics, drug delivery systems, and protective textiles. He has published several research papers and led funded projects on multifunctional dressings and thermoregulating fabrics.

Gopiraman Mayakrishnan is a Specially Appointed Associate Professor in the Faculty of Textile Science and Technology at Shinshu University.

Zohra Naseem is pursuing a Ph.D. in the Department of Clothing at the National Textile University in Faisalabad. She completed her M.Phil. in Advanced Fashion and Clothing from NTU, with research interests in apparel manufacturing and innovative fashion technologies.

Muhammad Anwaar Nazeer Assistant Professor in the Department of Clothing at the National Textile University in Faisalabad, holds a B.Sc. in Textile Engineering (Gold Medalist, NTU), a Ph.D. in Biomedical Sciences & Engineering, and a Postdoctoral Fellowship in Chemical & Biological Engineering from Koç University in Turkey. With 19 journal publications, 18 conference papers, and awards including the NTU Gold Medal (2011) and EVER Young Investigators Innovation Award (2019), his research focuses on polymer synthesis, biomaterials, scaffolding, tissue engineering, and regenerative medicine.

Duy-Nam Phan graduated as an engineer from Hanoi University of Science and Technology in 2010. He graduated from the combined master's and doctoral program in Bioscience and Textile Technology at Shinshu University in Japan in 2020. Since 2020, he has been a lecturer at Hanoi University of Science and Technology and holds the position of Deputy Head of the Department of Garment Technology and Fashion Design. He is currently a member of the Standing Committee of the Youth Union at Hanoi University of Science and Technology.

Maham Raza is pursuing a Ph.D. in Apparel Manufacturing in the Department of Clothing at the National Textile University in Faisalabad, where she is also a Research Assistant in Smart Textiles. She holds an M.S. in Advanced Fashion and Clothing (Gold Medalist) from NTU and a B.S. in Textiles and Clothing from Punjab University. Her research focuses on apparel manufacturing, smart textiles, and advanced fashion technologies.

Sadia Razzaq is a postdoctoral researcher on the project of GCF-63 funded by Higher Education Commission (HEC) Pakistan.

Shagufta Riaz Assistant Professor in the Department of Textile Engineering at the National Textile University in Faisalabad, holds a Ph.D. in Textile Engineering and an M.S. in Advanced Materials Engineering.

Abdul Salam is a graduate student at North Dakota State University, USA.

Muhammad Nauman Sarwar is a postdoctoral researcher in the Faculty of Textile Science and Technology at Shinshu University.

Hina Shafique is a B.S. Textile Engineering student at the National Textile University in Faisalabad.

Thi Ngat Tran is a Faculty Member at Hanoi University of Science and Technology and holds the position of Deputy Head of the Department of Garment Technology and Fashion Design. He is currently a member of the Standing Committee of the Youth Union at Hanoi University of Science and Technology.

Azeem Ullah is an Assistant Professor in the Faculty of Textile Science and Technology at Shinshu University in Japan.

Muhammad Umar obtained undergraduate and master's degrees in Textile Engineering from the National Textile University and a Ph.D. in Materials from the University of Manchester. He is now an Application Scientist at Henry Royce Institute for sustainable materials with research experience in hydrogels, fiber-based composites, 2D materials especially Graphene and MoS2, textile-related technologies, and materials characterization techniques. He has a breadth of experience in developing sustainable products, materials, and commercializing lab research. He also had working experience as Materials Scientist and Lab Manager of AEH labs at the Graphene Engineering Innovation Centre. His scientific work has been published in several high-impact journals, and he has also won four bursaries to present his work at prestigious international events. He is also experienced in formulation of gels for agricultural and biomedical applications. His other research areas of interest are fiber spinning, fibrous or nonwoven wound dressings, membranes, and polymer composites. He is also a peer reviewer of many high-impact journals and performs duties as mentor and assessor for the Leadership in Education Awards Program (LEAP). He was awarded the status of Fellow from the Higher Education Academy in 2020, and he has been endorsed as Global Talent by The Royal Society in 2022.

Ling Wang is affiliated with Shinshu University.

Gul I. Zahra is the M.S. student at the Department of Clothing, School of Engineering and Technology at National Textile University in Faisalabad, Pakistan.

Iqra Zainab is pursuing a Ph.D. in the Department of Clothing at the National Textile University in Faisalabad. She completed her M.Phil. in Advanced Fashion and Clothing from NTU, with research interests in apparel manufacturing and innovative fashion technologies.

1 Introduction to Nanomaterials

Thi Ngat Tran and Duy-Nam Phan

POLYMERS AND SOLVENTS FOR ELECTROSPINNING

Electrospinning generates nanofibers from various materials, including polymers, small molecules, colloidal particles, and composites. Polymers in the electrospinning process can be utilized as either solutions or melts, with organic polymers being the most commonly used (Xue et al. 2019). Organic polymers that can be dissolved in suitable solvents or melted without degradation can be directly used in electrospinning, either by the solution or melt electrospinning method. Over 100 types of organic polymers, both natural and synthetic, have been successfully used in solution electrospinning to produce nanofibers directly. For electrospinning to be successful and yield the desired results, it is essential to utilize a polymer that possesses a high molecular weight (Xue et al. 2019). Additionally, selecting an appropriate solvent that is capable of effectively dissolving this polymer is also crucial to the process. The commonly used solvents include alcohols, dichloromethane (DCM), chloroform (CF), N,N-dimethylformamide (DMF), tetrahydrofuran (THF), acetone, dimethyl sulfoxide (DMSO), 1,1,1,3,3,3-hexafluoroisopropanol (HFIP), and 2,2,2-trifluoroethanol (TFE) (Xue et al. 2019). Water is not considered an ideal solvent for the process of electrospinning primarily because of its high dielectric constant. This property leads to a reduction in electrostatic repulsion during the electrospinning process, which is crucial for producing fine fibers (Xue et al. 2019). By carefully selecting and optimizing the solvent blend, it is possible to enhance the electrospinning outcomes and improve the quality of the resulting nanofibers (Xue et al. 2019).

Synthetic polymers, such as polystyrene (PS) and polyvinyl chloride (PVC), were widely employed in the electrospinning process owing to their low cost, ease of production, and high mechanical properties. In one study, the PS solutions (20 wt%) were prepared by dissolving PS in various solvents such as DMF, THF, N-methyl-2-pyrrolidone (NMP), toluene, and CF. The resulting electrospun PS fibers averaged 808, 2,854, 1,671, 972, and 1,845 nm in diameter with varying membrane morphologies (Rezaei et al. 2018). PVC nanofiber materials with average diameters of 121 and 253 nm were obtained from 12 and 14 wt% solutions using a 1:1 (w/w) DMF/THF solvent mixture during electrospinning (Tarus et al. 2020).

Biocompatible and biodegradable synthetic polymers such as polycaprolactone (PCL), poly lactic acid (PLA), and poly lactic-co-glycolic acid (PLGA) can be used in the electrospinning method for nanofibers. Environmental and sustainable issues have grown in importance. Synthetic polymers pose significant long-term health and ecological risks due to their non-biodegradable and toxic properties. Consequently,

DOI: 10.1201/9781003616726-1

minimizing waste generation by maximizing material use or opting for recyclable and biodegradable materials is essential (Benelli et al. 2017). Researchers in both industry and academia are increasingly focusing on green polymers for nanofiber synthesis. In a study, PCL (10% w/v) was dissolved in a co-solvent of 9:1 (v/v) CF:DMF to obtain electrospun nanofibers (Yew et al. 2018). The commonly used solvents for electrospinning of PLA-based solutions are DCM, CF ($CHCl_3$), DMF, HFIP, and TFE (Maleki et al. 2022). An effective and optimal solution for the creation of PLGA electrospun nanofibers is formulated using a mixture that consists of 50% DCM and 50% DMF, combined with 20% PLGA by weight (Uyanik et al. 2022).

Natural biopolymers include chitosan (CS) and its derivatives, cellulose and its derivatives, DNA, silk fibroin (SF), fibrinogens, dextran, chitin, alginate, collagen, and gelatin (GT). Electrospun CS nanofibers were produced using a TFA/DCM solvent mixture (70:30 v/v), resulting in smooth fibers with an average diameter of 126 ± 20 nm and no beads (Sun and Li 2011). Most CS derivatives are soluble in water and various common organic solvents, significantly enhancing their spinnability (Sun and Li 2011). Direct solvents for cellulose, such as N-methyl-morpholine N-oxide/water (NMMO/H_2O) and lithium chloride/dimethyl acetamide (LiCl/DMAc), along with ionic liquids, have been identified for use in electrospinning. However, successfully electrospinning cellulose from these solvents necessitates innovative approaches in system design (Frey 2008). Cellulose derivatives such as cellulose acetate, hydroxypropyl cellulose, and ethyl cellulose have garnered interest for electrospinning into nanofibers. This process is advantageous due to the solubility of these derivatives in common solvents, such as THF and DMAc, which can enhance the ability of electrospinning for cellulose (Frey 2008). Electrospinning solutions were prepared by mixing stock bacteriophage DNA with the fluorescent dye YOYO-1, resulting in a fiber diameter of approximately 27 nm (Bellan, Strychalski, and Craighead 2007). An aqueous solution of silk/polyethylene oxide (PEO) (4:1 ratio) was prepared by adding PEO to a 5.8 wt% SF aqueous solution ($CaCl_2$, H_2O, and ethanol in a molar ratio of 1:8:2) for fabricating 3D electrospun SF scaffolds (Park et al. 2016). Fibrinogen solutions at concentrations of 10, 11, and 12 wt% were prepared in HFIP with DMEM (9/1 v/v), formic acid, and formic acid/acetic acid (FA/AA) in ratios of 75/25, 50/50, and 25/75 (v/v), resulting in electrospun nanofiber diameters ranging from 184 to 241 nm (Mirzaei-Parsa et al. 2018).

Functional polymers, such as conductive polymers (polyaniline (PANI), polypyrrole (PPy), and poly vinylidene fluoride (PVDF)), were investigated to fabricate nanofiber via electrospinning method. Pure PPy electrospun nanofibers were produced by dissolving [(PPy3)C (DEHS)K]x in DMF, achieving an average diameter of about 70 nm. To enhance PPy's processability, 1.5 wt% PEO was added to the solution for electrospinning ultrafine fibers (Chronakis, Grapenson, and Jakob 2006). PANI nanofibers with an average diameter of around 139 nm were created by electrospinning 20 wt% PANI solution in 98% formic acid (MacDiarmid et al. 2001). However, PANI has restricted solubility and decreased dispersion in typical organic solvents. To create a spinnable polymer blend for easy electrospinning, polymer PEO was added to the PANI structure (Yanılmaz and Sarac 2014). 15 wt% of PVDF in the solvent mixture DMF and acetone with a volume ratio of 70/30 was prepared to fabricate the PVDF electrospun nanofibers (Cozza et al. 2013).

Certain polymers might not be appropriate to electrospin out of their solution. Therefore, electrospun composite nanofibers have been developed through the process of blending different polymers together, which has resulted in a substantial enhancement of their overall properties and characteristics (Robinson et al. 2021). This innovative approach to nanofiber production allows for a significant improvement in performance metrics, enabling a wider range of applications and functionalities (Wang et al., 2009).

The outcome of electrospinning a polymer solution and the shape and structure of the resultant polymer nanofibers are generally influenced by a variety of elements, including the polymers, solvents, polymer solution, processing settings, and ambient conditions. The electrical characteristics and rheological behaviors of a solution are significantly influenced by the molecular weight of the polymer. The solubility of the solvent parameter is a significant factor in the creation of a homogenous polymer (Beachley and Wen 2009; Jacobs, Anandjiwala, and Maaza 2010).

STRUCTURE AND MORPHOLOGIES OF ELECTROSPUN NANOFIBERS MEMBRANE

Electrospinning is a sophisticated processing technique that involves the application of a high electric voltage to a carefully prepared polymer solution, leading to the creation of submicron fibers. The process begins when the voltage reaches a level that exceeds the liquid's surface tension, resulting in the formation of jets of the polymer solution jet toward the collector surface. Fibers that are formed are usually in diameters of several hundred nanometers. This unique formation results in a fibrous mat that has a wide array of potential applications due to its distinctive properties and high surface area. Collectors or a modified electrospinning method can make a variety of fiber assemblies. The most basic type of membrane that can be formed is a nonwoven fiber mesh without any specific alignment. Besides, different kinds of membranes can be formed due to the desire such as random three-dimensional structures and aligned and patterned fiber mesh.

High surface-area-to-volume ratio, micro-scaled interstitial space, high porosity and interconnectivity, good morphological stability, and variable mesh thickness are some of the structural characteristics of the electrospun nonwoven fiber mesh. Because of these characteristics—particularly the high surface-area-to-volume ratio brought forth by the polymer fiber's tiny diameter—the electrospun nonwoven fiber mesh is a good choice for affinity membranes. It is already known that electrospun nonwoven polymer fiber can be used as a protective cloth to keep small aerosols out of the air or as a gas filtration membrane. Because of its large surface area, fiber mesh effectively removes airborne particles by physical adsorption as well as physical trapping (Ma, Kotaki, and Ramakrishna 2006).

Aligned fiber arrays can be assembled using several electrospinning techniques. Centrifugal electrospinning, a combination of electrospinning and force spinning technologies, can be used to do this through electrostatic and centrifugal forces. Electrospinning with the assistance of a magnetic field is another method for creating this purported fiber mesh. Post-drawing can also be viewed as a way to turn randomly aligned meshes into well-aligned structures. By combining stretching force and thermal annealing, this post-fabrication fiber alignment enables an enhanced degree of orientation to transform poorly oriented fibers into highly oriented meshes. The process is typically performed using a tensile stretching device that has been specially fitted with a heating chamber. Nevertheless, because of fiber physical constraints and alignment degradation over time, this may make it more difficult to create large materials (both in terms of area and thickness) (Robinson et al. 2021).

A growing number of 3D nanostructures with notable thickness are being studied in comparison to their 2D counterparts for applications needing a third dimension/direction. Some disciplines, such as tissue engineering, filtration, and energy materials, could benefit from the use of these 3D structures due to their huge surface area, pore size, and inter-pore channels, which set them apart from 2D mats. The method for 3D structures is sequential electrospinning or multilayering electrospinning. This will result in an electrospun fiber membrane of a specific thickness that can grow to hundreds of microns and form a 3D fibrous structure; however, the process may take a while (for example, 20 minutes to 20 hours) to reach a sufficient 3D structure. An alternative method involves post-processing the electrospun fibers by removing the thin film from the collector and subsequently bending, folding, or stacking the fiber layers to create a three-dimensional fibrous structure similar to a thick mass or pipe. Furthermore, it is possible to successfully produce 3D fiber structures by altering the collector; for instance, a 3D collecting template can be used in place of the traditional 2D flat collector. Other techniques have also been documented, such as collecting liquid and eliminating microparticles trapped between nanofibers; however, these usually require a second step to dry the 3D structures once they are made. Furthermore, without the need for extra help (such as fibrous yarns or spongiform fiber stacks), a rapid growth (or self-assembly) of 3D fibrous structures has been achieved by controlling some parameters during the electrospinning process (e.g., the solution concentration/viscosity, electrostatic field, and ambient humidity). Potential applications of the 3D structure through the electrospinning method may lie in catalyst supports, micro-containers, sensors, drug delivery, and sound absorption (Robinson et al. 2021).

APPLICATIONS IN THE ENVIRONMENTAL FIELD

Purification of Air

Air pollution has long-term harmful effects on human health, especially when it comes to particulate matter (PM)-induced haze, where PM is a mixture of liquid droplets and solids suspended in air (Lv et al. 2018). Fine particle pollutants found in the air include carbon and coal, powdered minerals, vehicular exhaust, regular combustion, and smoke from forest fires. Moreover, there is a chance that ultrafine and nanoscale particles could have a negative short- and long-term impact on human health. Air filtration remains the most promising technique for reducing the contamination of nanoparticles and hazardous chemicals in the atmosphere. Electrospun nanofiber membranes have a great surface-to-volume ratio, high porosity, good interconnectivity, and micrometer-sized interstitial space, which makes them excellent materials for air purification (Lv et al. 2018).

There are two stages to the air filtering process: the steady state (the first state) and the non-steady state (the second state). The initial stage's particle capture efficiency and filtration pressure drop through the filter material are determined exclusively by the air filter medium's intrinsic qualities, the type of particles, and the airflow velocity. These values are unchangeable throughout time. As particles build up on the filter, the second state's filtration effectiveness and flow resistance gradually alter. Because of the typically low particle concentration in air, particle deposition from the air will not appreciably alter the thickness of the electrospun nanofiber membranes during the working duration. Consequently, it is possible to think of the electrospun fibrous air filtration membrane as operating in a steady filtering stage. The stable stage of fiber filtration can be further categorized into the following five trapping mechanisms based on classical filtration theory: Brownian diffusion, interception, inertial impaction, electrostatic effect, and gravity influence (Lv et al. 2018).

An extensive collection of polymers was used in electrospun membrane for air purification such as PAN (Canalli Bortolassi et al. 2019), PVA (Bian et al. 2018), PET (Zhou et al. 2024), polyamide (Bonfim et al. 2021), CS (Wang, Zhang et al. 2016), and cellulose acetate (Nicosia et al. 2016). For single-polymer nanofiber prepared by electrospinning, the performance of the filtering membrane is mainly dependent on the performance of the material itself and the characteristics of nano-grade materials (Zhou et al. 2022). The filter membrane, which had an average diameter of about 400 nm and was created by electrospinning PAN polymer dissolved in DMF solvent, had a PM2.5 removal efficiency of 92.03% with the quality factor of 0.1264 (Kim et al. 2018). The process of filtration capacity can be improved even more by reducing the fiber diameter, which will concurrently increase the material's specific surface area and allow for the removal of PMs and other impurities with smaller sizes. The relationship between the fiber diameter and the quality factor of filtration performance was reported, with thinner fiber diameters having higher filtration. However, single polymer-based air filter membranes typically lack additional important features including mechanical flexibility as well as excellent filtration performance (such as filtration efficacy, pressure drop, and air permeability). They are either unable to satisfy human needs or the demands of a complicated surrounding area. Consequently, research into composite nanofibers—which are made by blending various polymers, blending polymer with inorganic nanoparticles—has been done to create filters that have a high purification efficiency and can introduce new functions by employing the mutually beneficial relationship between various components (Zhou et al. 2022).

Treatment of Water

Due to its capacity to both separate and break down contaminants in wastewater at the same time, nonwoven materials made of electrospun nanofibers have been thoroughly investigated as water treatment filters. Nanofiber-based filters are capable of effectively filtering out particles ranging in size from micrometers to nanometers from water without causing a noticeable decrease in flow rate. Hazardous chemicals, heavy metals in increasing demand, and their remnants were disposed of in water on a daily basis, which decreased the quality of water (Aldalbahi et al. 2021). Electrospun nanofibers also offer an alternative approach to the removal of toxic ions (heavy metal ions) from wastewater.

The removal of toxins from water (either daily water or wastewater) can be accomplished by functionalizing the surface electrospun nanofiber membrane with active groups. Pre-electrospinning or post-electrospinning modification technologies can obtain functionalized electrospun nanofiber membranes (Chen et al. 2020). The mechanism can be the adsorption of such toxicants on their surface, which exhibits different adsorption behaviors based on the nature of functional groups on their surface. A high adsorption capacity and a large number of adsorption sites are directly correlated with a large specific surface area of the nanofiber-based filter. Nanofibers for separation or water treatment have great performance capacity thanks to the membrane's selectivity and flux. Due to its non-toxic and non-hazardous characteristics, CS has become a highly sought-after adsorbent material. Functional itself can remove metal ions when they are present in the 2-amino-2-deoxy-d-glucose (glucosamine) unit. This is mostly because amino groups and hydroxyl groups are abundant in this compound (Habiba et al. 2017). The CS electrospun nanofiber layer with an average diameter of 75 nm using 5 wt% CS as the spinning solution was cross-linked to remove Cr (VI) from water by static adsorption. Both amino and hydroxyl groups of CS were engaged in the adsorption. The maximum adsorption capacity of the nanofibers was 131.58 $mg{\cdot}g^{-1}$ (Li et al. 2015). The incorporation of PAN/CS nanofibers with UiO-66-NH2 MOF for the purpose of adsorption and filtering Pb (II), Cd (II), and Cr (VI) ions from aqueous solutions was investigated. With Pb (II), Cd (II), and Cr (VI) reaching 441.2, 415.6, and 372.6 $mg{\cdot}g^{-1}$, respectively, the membrane showed good adsorption performance. The synthesized PVDF/PAN/CS/UiO-66-NH2 10 wt% nanofibrous membrane filtered for a long time without significantly altering the water flow or the removal of metal ions. Adsorption kinetics revealed that metal ion adsorption was greatly aided by amine complexation, indicating that chemisorption was the main process underlying the electrospun nanofiber membrane (Jamshidifard et al. 2019).

In the textile, leather, paper, cosmetics, plastics, printing, and other industries, dyes and pigments are frequently utilized (Zollinger 2003). These industries release complex organic contaminants that are not biodegradable into the water, endangering aquatic life as well as human health. Electrostatic attraction is the primary physical factor behind the adsorption of dyes on nanofiber membranes (Chen et al. 2022). This is so because the solution's pH has an impact on the dye's level of ionization and the charge on the electrospun nanofiber membrane's surface (Li et al. 2012). In addition to cationic and anionic dyes, the produced PVDF@PDA@PPY composite nanofiber membranes through electrospinning technology may absorb heavy metal ions such as chromium ions. Methylene Blue and Congo Red have maximal adsorption capabilities of 370.4 and 384.6 mg/g, respectively. A higher pH value in the solution promotes the adsorption of MB, whereas a lower pH value makes it easier for CR to bind. The composite nanofibers demonstrate exceptional efficacy in eliminating heavy metal ions, with Cr(VI) having an adsorption capacity of 126.7 mg/g (Ma et al. 2018).

In our daily lives, drinkable water must be purified before consumption. Appropriate technology should be able to filter out unwanted elements from the water supply, including sand, organic suspended particles, parasites, giardia lamblia, cryptosporidium, bacteria, algae, viruses, and fungus (Matilainen and Sillanpää 2010). Since the majority of aquatic bacteria have diameters greater than 0.2 µm, electrospun nanofiber membranes with lower hole sizes can serve as an excellent filter platform for the purification of water (Wang and Hsiao 2016). The PAN/PET membrane via electrospinning method with a total thickness of 200 ± 10 m and an average fiber diameter of 100 ± 20 nm demonstrated an optimized small pore size (maximum pore size of 0.62 ± 0.03 m and mean flow pore size of 0.22 ± 0.01 m) and high effective porosity (up to 80%). In terms of flow, this membrane outperformed the Millipore GSWP 0.22 m membranes by a factor of 2–3 (Wang et al. 2012).

APPLICATIONS IN THE ENERGY FIELD

Electrospun nanofibers were seen to be an excellent material as catalyst for organic transformations. Electrospun polyethyleneimine/polyvinyl alcohol (PEI/PVA) nanofibers via electrospinning with a mean diameter of 490 nm were immobilized with gold nanoparticles. These nanofiber membranes were utilized in a reduction reaction. When used on PEI/PVA nanofibers, gold nanoparticles measuring 11.8 nm showed excellent catalytic activity and reusability in the conversion of 4-nitrophenol to 4-aminophenol (Fang et al. 2011).

The properties of the electrode have a major impact on how well energy storage systems operate. To provide a long cycle life, the electrode, which is often made of a composite material, must preserve the structural integrity of its constituent parts throughout a number of cycles. To enable the simultaneous movement of free electrons and alkali metal ions, the electrode also needs to have the appropriate porosity structure. Electrospinning produces nanofiber materials with a porous or mesh-like structure, offering benefits that enhance battery performance (Li et al. 2021). Electrospun Lithium Lanthanum Titanate Oxide/Polyacrylonitrile (LLTO/PAN) nanofiber separators demonstrate increased ionic conductivity, decreased interfacial resistance with lithium, and high electrolyte absorption. These characteristics increase lithium-ion batteries' capacity and cycling stability. This suggests that a viable technique for producing high-performing nanofiber separators, cathodes, and anodes that could replace the materials used in current lithium-ion batteries is electrospinning (Xiangwu et al. 2011).

Innovative innovations such as wearable electronics (Stoppa and Chiolerio 2014), smart clothes (Cho, Lee, and Cho 2009), implantable medical devices (Khan et al. 2014), and electronic skin (Wang et al. 2015) have been made possible by the quick development of flexible electronics. There is an obvious need for integrated flexible power sources because of these wearable, portable, and flexible electronic gadgets. Finding the right electrode/electrolyte materials and refining device layouts and structures have been the main goals of numerous studies in an effort to achieve high energy and power density, long cycling stability, good mechanical qualities, and device safety. Because of their high surface-to-volume ratios, exceptional mechanical qualities, and adaptability in constructing different energy storage device components, nanofibers have been recognized as outstanding alternatives. Fibers made from a variety of materials can be fabricated with special advantages thanks to electrospinning, which also gives superior control over microstructure and size. The mechanical and electrochemical performance of electrospun fibers is significantly influenced by their composition and shape.

APPLICATIONS IN THE BIOMEDICAL FIELD

Through their huge specific surface area, high loading capacity, and increased catalyst surface area, nanofibers have a comprehensive effect on enzymes and the biological catalyst field (Wang et al. 2009). There are a few different techniques to add enzymes to electrospun nanofibers, such as grafting enzymes onto the fiber's surface, physical adsorption, and adding enzymes through the electrospinning process that is followed by the crosslinking reaction. Nanofibers should only include at least one reactive polymer to bind with the enzyme before adding biological catalysts or enzymes (Nadaf et al. 2022). Model enzyme R-chymotrypsin was chemically attached to bioactive PS nanofibers, which had an average diameter of 120 nm. This resulted in a 27.4% monolayer coverage of the nanofibers' exterior. When compared to other types of immobilized enzymes, the nanofibrous enzyme's apparent hydrolytic activity in aqueous solutions was more than 65% of the natural enzyme's, demonstrating a high catalytic efficiency. Compared to the natural enzyme, the nanofibrous enzyme had an 18-fold longer half-life in methanol (Jia et al. 2002).

The advantages of electrospinning for drug delivery are its high loading capacity, high encapsulation efficiency, the ability to deliver many medicines at once, cost-effectiveness, and ease of usage (Shahriar et al. 2019). Electrospun fibers have been modified to contain various pharmaceuticals, such as proteins, aptamer, DNA, RNA, and anticancer chemicals. CS's polycationic composition mostly explains its strong anticancer action. It is well known that quaternized CS derivatives exhibit strong in vitro anticancer activity against HeLa, Hep3B, and SW480 cells (Toshkova et al. 2010). With the use of nanofibers, two easy drug delivery mechanisms are drug loading and drug release. Typically, drug loading refers to the trapping of a drug into nanofibers to regulate the drug's release and give it site-specificity. It is known that the drug release mechanism involves in vivo fiber breakdown, diffusion of fibers through solid-state, and demagnetization from the fiber surface (Fang et al. 2008). For local antibiotic medication administration, a transdermal patch made of hydrophilic biodegradable PVA and sodium alginate (NaAlg) electrospun composite nanofiber was created. In the PVA/NaAlg composites nanofiber patch, the maximal 98.7% of drug release occurs in 7 hours. A control release pattern is noticed after 7 hours and up to 24 hours (Kataria et al. 2014). Due to issues with appropriate functionality, regulating capacity, toxicity, and large-scale production restrictions, the therapeutic application of nanofibers for drug or gene administration is restricted. But the field of nanofiber-based delivery system development is expanding quickly, and several of these systems have demonstrated exceptional qualities for use in therapeutic delivery in the future (Shahriar et al. 2019). Electrospun nanofibers have been utilized extensively recently to improve the solubility of anticancer medications. The anticancer drugs in this system can be encircled and crystallized within the drug-loaded nanofibers, improving the pace at which the agents dissolve in the biological system (Shahriar et al. 2019).

The skin, the largest organ in the body, functions as the main defense system to keep disease from entering the body (Sanford and Gallo 2013). An injury known as a wound occurs when there is damage to the dermis due to abrasion (White 1999), puncture (Racz, Ramanujam, and Zgonis 2010), or avulsion (Boettcher-Haberzeth and Schiestl 2013). Consequently, the development of wound dressings and wound healing is crucial for quick healing of the afflicted area and for providing defense against microbial infection (Thenmozhi et al. 2017). The combination of inflammation, proliferation, remodeling phase, and epithelization results in the intentional process of wound healing. A pore size of 500–1,000 nm is typically required for wound dressings to adequately shield the wound from the external environment and bacteria (Fang et al. 2008). For many years, SF, a complexly structured protein, has been utilized in textile and sewing applications. Because of its exceptional mechanical qualities, biocompatibility, biodegradability, flexibility, water vapor permeability, and mild antibacterial qualities, SF derived from silkworm cocoons is employed in the field of biomedicine. It has emerged as a strong contender, particularly for applications involving wound dressings (Liu et al. 2021; Patil, Reagan, and Bohara 2020). SF/GT nanofiber dressing was prepared by electrospinning nanotechnology and loaded with astragaloside IV (AS) on acute trauma (Zhang et al. 2019). The novel natural spider silk (SS) embedded on an electrospun nanofiber membrane PVA/NaAlg proved to be an excellent candidate material for rapid wound healing of skin scar (Öksüz et al. 2021). SF/zinc oxide (ZnO) is used as the core and hyaluronic acid (HA) is used as the sheath spinning solution to create nanofibers with a core-sheath structure for use as a wound dressing. The results of rats' burn wound healing showed that the dressing had a specific burn therapy effect (Hadisi et al. 2020). The ability to load a range of biologically active materials to create functionalized products is a significant benefit of using electrospinning to prepare nanofiber wound dressings. Antibiotic medications, inorganic nanoparticles, natural substances (honey, essential oils, CS), and growth factors are frequently utilized active ingredients to improve the antibacterial characteristics of dressings, which is one of the major aspects for wound healing (Liu et al. 2021).

Tissue engineering, a key focus of integrative research in regenerative medicine, encompasses diverse and impactful applications. It includes biomimicking extracellular matrix (ECM), enzymes, blood vessels, genes, and pharmaceuticals to restore skin, cartilage, and nerves (van Blitterswijk and De Boer 2022). This field excels in various procedures, addressing biocompatibility, mechanical properties, permeability, and degeneration within the human body (Rahmati et al. 2021). Mimicking the ECM while ensuring oxygen and nutrient circulation and removing metabolic wastes is crucial for tissue engineering during regeneration. Creating advanced three-dimensional scaffolds is an effective solution. Electrospinning can produce fibers ranging from micro- to nanometer scales with a large surface area, leading to significant advancements in designing and utilizing electrospun nanofibrous scaffolds for various tissues (Rahmati et al. 2021). Nanofibers electrospinning reveals its wide application over the medical surgical field related to tissue engineering such as cell migration, stem cell differentiation, peripheral nerve repair, cardiac tissue regeneration, and vascular tissue regeneration. The nanofibers in electrospun nanofibrous scaffolds can be modified with various additives to provide special properties, allowing them to properly function as ECM in tissue. Nanofibers can be directly electrospun from a broad variety of synthetic and natural polymers, and nanoparticle integration with the nanofibers is likewise a simple process. An ECM substitute can be produced by combining synthetic and natural polymers at the right proportion ratio to provide the desirable mechanical strength and biodegradability for the scaffolds (Wise et al. 2011).

Nanomaterials, which typically have at least one dimension between 1 and 100 nm, can be modified to give sensors unique characteristics by altering the transduction surface (Kwon et al. 2018). These materials are beneficial for stabilizing the platform used for sensing biological molecules due to their high reactivity, increased surface area, and biocompatibility (Kyriakides et al. 2021). However, because of their small size, they exhibit significant differences from their bulk counterparts in terms of electrical conductivity and optical properties. This makes nanofibers suitable for use as sensors, particularly in the detection or recognition of glucose, cancer, and cardiovascular disease, to ensure prompt and accurate treatment (Iftikhar et al. 2023). Sensors based on nanofiber electrospinning come in various types and are used in healthcare diagnosis. For example, electrochemical biosensors (DNA biosensors) are used to detect proteins, glucose, and genes, while gas sensors are used for diagnosing lung cancer (Liu et al. 2020; Chen et al. 2016). Polymers in electrospinning process, including PANI and poly(3,4-ethylene dioxythiophene):poly(styrene sulfonate) (PEDOT: PSS), were used in sensors for detecting health problems (Wang, Yap et al. 2016). In a study, PANI nanofibers were created using electrospinning and then incorporated into interdigitated gold electrodes. Next, COX-2 antibodies were immobilized on the surface of PANI nanofibers that were functionalized with dithiobis sulfosuccinimidyl propionate (DTSSP). The nanofibers, with a diameter of 256 nm, achieved a low detection limit of 0.01 pg/mL, which was 10,000 times better than the biosensor using plain interdigitated electrodes. This biosensor demonstrated high selectivity against human protein albumin and exhibited only a 10% reduction in response when detecting COX-2 antigen in human serum samples (Asmatulu et al. 2019). An additional method to improve anti-fouling surface treatments is by adding polyethylene glycol (PEG) to the surface of PANI NFs. Subsequently, DNA probes can be attached to the PANI/PEG nanofibers for the breast cancer susceptibility gene (BRCA1) detection. The biosensor exhibited high sensitivity to the target BRCA1 in a linear range from 0.01 pM to 1 nM. The biosensor displayed acceptable selectivity and retained good performance at 92.4% after 10 days (Hui et al. 2017).

Membranes fabricated by electrospinning have a wide range of applications in cosmetic applications including facial masks, deodorants, and antiperspirants. The feasibility of incorporating active ingredients into electrospun nanofibers also makes this spinning process suitable for cosmetic applications. Adding different ingredients imparts various medicinal properties for different types of skin treatments. Fabricated membranes were investigated using a PVA fibrous matrix to contain volatile fragrance via emulsion electrospinning. The study indicated that encapsulated (R)-(+)-limonene was released over 15 days under ambient temperatures and has potential application in cosmetics (Camerlo et al. 2013).

APPLICATIONS IN THE DEFENSE FIELD

Protective clothing shields the human body from extreme weather conditions such as heat, cold, and rain, as well as ensures safety in various work environments such as health, agriculture, and military settings (Zhou, Reddy, and Yang 2005). It also fulfills the requirements of defense systems, sports, and industrial applications. In the textile industry, protective clothing includes bulletproof gear as well as garments designed to protect against chemical or biological agents, fire, cold, and heat. A variety of materials, including single-use nonwoven personal protective equipment and impermeable polymeric suits, are used to minimize exposure to biological and chemical hazards (Karim et al. 2020). The development of nanofibrous membranes for protective clothing offers promise due to their lightweight nature, ultrafine fiber, and pore size, highly open porous structure, and high surface-area-to-volume ratio. One noteworthy aspect of electrospinning for protective clothing is the potential for directly applying them to garment systems, which would streamline manufacturing processes and address seam-sealing issues (Raza et al. 2014). Additionally, functioned nanofibers can be directly electrospun to create fibrous membranes that resist the permeation of organic molecules while remaining permeable to air and water vapor. This makes them suitable for protective clothing against chemicals while maintaining breathability and moisture transfer. The electrospun membrane's nano-sized pores enable moisture transport while blocking water and wind. Utilizing an inherently hydrophobic polymer in the electrospinning process results in nanofiber materials that exhibit excellent waterproofing and breathability (Baji, Agarwal, and Sruthi 2020).

Waterproof, breathable, chemical-protective, antibacterial, and UV radiation-protective clothing have attracted a lot of interest over the years. The electrospun polyurethane membranes have excellent hydrolytic stability, abrasion resistance, and elastomericity, making them ideal for creating waterproof and breathable apparel. However, the waterproof property of these membranes was previously lower than the practical limit of 5 kPa. Using electrospinning of a novel fluorinated PU (FPU), the hydrophilic PU membranes have been transformed into superhydrophobic membranes with a water contact angle of 156 degrees, good air permeability (8.46 L $m^{-2}s^{-1}$), and water vapor transmittance (0.384 kg $m^{-2}h^{-1}$; Jianfeng et al. 2013). It is commonly known that exposure to ultraviolet (UV) radiation and sunlight can cause serious skin damage. Specifically, it has been shown that aging symptoms arise from exposure to UV light in the 315–400 nm wavelength range, while skin cancer is brought on by exposure to UV light with wavelengths between 280 and 315 nm (Li et al. 2014). When mixing TiO_2 nanoparticles with a 20% nylon-6 solution prepared in a 4:1 ratio by weight of formic acid and acetic acid to create a spinning solution for electrospinning, it resulted in a membrane with an average fiber diameter ranging from 110 to 172 nm. The composite material absorbs UV light by TiO_2 NPs, which means the membrane can be used for UV blocking (Pant et al. 2011). Polymer cellulose with a polymerization degree above 10,000 was electrospun into nanofibers and functionalized with cerium dioxide, demonstrating excellent UV protection. The interface and electrostatic interactions between the nanoparticles and nanofibers effectively attached the nanoparticles to the nanofiber surface (Li et al. 2013). Antibacterial agents have been incorporated into electrospun nanofibers to enhance the protective properties of textiles. A spinning solution of polyvinylpyrrolidone (PVP) and silver was electrospun to produce antimicrobial fibers. The efficacy of silver-loaded PVP fibers against *Escherichia coli* and *Staphylococcus aureus* was investigated, revealing a significant reduction in metabolic activity and cell viability. The fibers clearly inhibited the microorganisms in contact with them (Quirós et al. 2015).

REFERENCES

Aldalbahi, Ali, Mehrez E El-Naggar, Mohamed H El-Newehy, Mostafizur Rahaman, Mohammad Rafe Hatshan, and Tawfik A Khattab. 2021. "Effects of technical textiles and synthetic nanofibers on environmental pollution." *Polymers* 13 (1):155.

Asmatulu, Ramazan, Zeinab Veisi, Md Nizam Uddin, and Anil Mahapatro. 2019. "Highly sensitive and reliable electrospun polyaniline nanofiber based biosensor as a robust platform for COX-2 enzyme detections." *Fibers and Polymers* 20:966–974.

Baji, Avinash, Komal Agarwal, and Venugopal Oopath Sruthi. 2020. "Emerging developments in the use of electrospun fibers and membranes for protective clothing applications." *Polymers* 12 (2):492.

Beachley, Vince, and Xuejun Wen. 2009. "Effect of electrospinning parameters on the nanofiber diameter and length." *Materials Science and Engineering:* C 29 (3):663–668.

Bellan, Leon M, Elizabeth A Strychalski, and Harold G Craighead. 2007. "Electrospun DNA nanofibers." *Journal of Vacuum Science & Technology B: Microelectronics and Nanometer Structures Processing, Measurement, and Phenomena* 25 (6):2255–2257.

Benelli, Giovanni, Roman Pavela, Filippo Maggi, Riccardo Petrelli, and Marcello Nicoletti. 2017. "Commentary: Making green pesticides greener? The potential of plant products for nanosynthesis and pest control." *Journal of Cluster Science* 28:3–10.

Bian, Ye, Rutao Wang, Sin Hang Ting, Chun Chen, and Li Zhang. 2018. "Electrospun SF/PVA nanofiber filters for highly efficient PM $_{2.5}$ capture." *IEEE Transactions on Nanotechnology* 17 (5):934–939.

Boettcher-Haberzeth, Sophie, and Clemens Schiestl. 2013. "Management of avulsion injuries." *European Journal of Pediatric Surgery* 23 (05):359–364.

Bonfim, Daniela PF, Fabiana GS Cruz, Rosario ES Bretas, Vádila G Guerra, and Mônica Lopes Aguiar. 2021. "A sustainable recycling alternative: Electrospun PET-membranes for air nanofiltration." *Polymers* 13 (7):1166.

Camerlo, Agathe, Corinne Vebert-Nardin, René M Rossi, and Ana-M Popa. 2013. "Fragrance encapsulation in polymeric matrices by emulsion electrospinning." *European Polymer Journal* 49 (12):3806–3813.

Canalli Bortolassi, Ana Cláudia, Vádila Giovana Guerra, Mônica Lopes Aguiar, Laurence Soussan, David Cornu, Philippe Miele, and Mikhael Bechelany. 2019. "Composites based on nanoparticle and pan electrospun nanofiber membranes for air filtration and bacterial removal." *Nanomaterials* 9 (12):1740.

Chen, Haisheng, Manhong Huang, Yanbiao Liu, Lijun Meng, and Mengdie Ma. 2020. "Functionalized electrospun nanofiber membranes for water treatment: A review." *Science of the Total Environment* 739:139944.

Chen, Yue-Sheng, Chien Wei Ooi, Pau Loke Show, Boon Chin Hoe, Wai Siong Chai, Chen-Yaw Chiu, Steven S-S Wang, and Yu-Kaung Chang. 2022. "Removal of ionic dyes by nanofiber membrane functionalized with chitosan and egg white proteins: Membrane preparation and adsorption efficiency." *Membranes* 12 (1):63.

Chen, Zhou, Zhaofeng Chen, Aili Zhang, Jiaming Hu, Xinmei Wang, and Zhaogang Yang. 2016. "Electrospun nanofibers for cancer diagnosis and therapy." *Biomaterials Science* 4 (6):922–932.

Cho, Gilsoo, Seungsin Lee, and Jayoung Cho. 2009. "Review and reappraisal of smart clothing." *International Journal of Human-Computer Interaction* 25 (6):582–617.

Chronakis, Ioannis S, Sven Grapenson, and Alexandra Jakob. 2006. "Conductive polypyrrole nanofibers via electrospinning: Electrical and morphological properties." *Polymer* 47 (5):1597–1603.

Cozza, Erika Simona, Orietta Monticelli, Enrico Marsano, and Peggy Cebe. 2013. "On the electrospinning of PVDF: Influence of the experimental conditions on the nanofiber properties." *Polymer International* 62 (1):41–48.

Fang, Jian, HaiTao Niu, Tong Lin, and XunGai Wang. 2008. "Applications of electrospun nanofibers." *Chinese Science Bulletin* 53:2265–2286.

Fang, Xu, Hui Ma, Shili Xiao, Mingwu Shen, Rui Guo, Xueyan Cao, and Xiangyang Shi. 2011. "Facile immobilization of gold nanoparticles into electrospun polyethyleneimine/polyvinyl alcohol nanofibers for catalytic applications." *Journal of Materials Chemistry* 21 (12):4493–4501.

Frey, Margaret W. 2008. "Electrospinning cellulose and cellulose derivatives." *Polymer Reviews* 48 (2):378–391.

Habiba, Umma, Amalina M Afifi, Areisman Salleh, and Bee Chin Ang. 2017. "Chitosan/(polyvinyl alcohol)/zeolite electrospun composite nanofibrous membrane for adsorption of Cr^{6+}, Fe^{3+} and Ni^{2+}." *Journal of Hazardous Materials* 322:182–194.

Hadisi, Zhina, Mehdi Farokhi, Hamid Reza Bakhsheshi-Rad, Maryam Jahanshahi, Sadegh Hasanpour, Erik Pagan, Alireza Dolatshahi-Pirouz, Yu Shrike Zhang, Subhas C Kundu, and Mohsen Akbari. 2020. "Hyaluronic acid (HA)-based silk fibroin/zinc oxide core–shell electrospun dressing for burn wound management." *Macromolecular Bioscience* 20 (4):1900328.

Hui, Ni, Xiaotian Sun, Shuyan Niu, and Xiliang Luo. 2017. "PEGylated polyaniline nanofibers: Antifouling and conducting biomaterial for electrochemical DNA sensing." *ACS Applied Materials & Interfaces* 9 (3):2914–2923.

Iftikhar, Faiza Jan, Afzal Shah, Qamar Wali, and Tayyaba Kokab. 2023. "Advancements in nanofiber-based electrochemical biosensors for diagnostic applications." *Biosensors* 13 (4):416.

Jacobs, Valencia, Rajesh D Anandjiwala, and Malik Maaza. 2010. "The influence of electrospinning parameters on the structural morphology and diameter of electrospun nanofibers." *Journal of Applied Polymer Science* 115 (5):3130–3136.

Jamshidifard, Sana, Shahnaz Koushkbaghi, Seyedehgolshan Hosseini, Sina Rezaei, Alireza Karamipour, and Mohammad Irani. 2019. "Incorporation of UiO-66-NH_2 MOF into the PAN/chitosan nanofibers for adsorption and membrane filtration of Pb (II), Cd (II) and Cr (VI) ions from aqueous solutions." *Journal of Hazardous Materials* 368:10–20.

Jia, Hongfei, Guangyu Zhu, Bradley Vugrinovich, Woraphon Kataphinan, Darrell H Reneker, and Ping Wang. 2002. "Enzyme-carrying polymeric nanofibers prepared via electrospinning for use as unique biocatalysts." *Biotechnology Progress* 18 (5):1027–1032.

Jianfeng, Ge, Yang Si, Fen Fu, Jialin Wang, Jianmao Yang, Lingxiao Cui, Bin Ding, Jianyong Yu, and Gang Sun. 2013. "Amphiphobic fluorinated polyurethane composite microfibrous membranes with robust waterproof and breathable performances." *RSC Advances* 3 (7):2248–2255.

Karim, Nazmul, Shaila Afroj, Kate Lloyd, Laura Clarke Oaten, Daria V Andreeva, Chris Carr, Andrew D Farmery, Il-Doo Kim, and Kostya S Novoselov. 2020. "Sustainable personal protective clothing for healthcare applications: A review." *ACS Nano* 14 (10):12313–12340.

Kataria, K, A Gupta, G Rath, RB Mathur, and SR Dhakate. 2014. "In vivo wound healing performance of drug loaded electrospun composite nanofibers transdermal patch." *International Journal of Pharmaceutics* 469 (1):102–110.

Khan, Wahid, Eameema Muntimadugu, Michael Jaffe, and Abraham J Domb. 2014. "Implantable medical devices." In: *Focal Controlled Drug Delivery*, edited by Abraham Joshua Domb and Wahid Khan, 33–59. Springer.

Kim, Han-Jung, Seon Joo Park, Chul Soon Park, Thanh-Hai Le, Sang Hun Lee, Tai Hwan Ha, Hyoung-Il Kim, Jinyeong Kim, Chang-Soo Lee, and Hyeonseok Yoon. 2018. "Surface-modified polymer nanofiber membrane for high-efficiency microdust capturing." *Chemical Engineering Journal* 339:204–213.

Kwon, Oh Seok, Hyun Seok Song, Tai Hyun Park, and Jyongsik Jang. 2018. "Conducting nanomaterial sensor using natural receptors." *Chemical Reviews* 119 (1):36–93.

Kyriakides, Themis R, Arindam Raj, Tiffany H Tseng, Hugh Xiao, Ryan Nguyen, Farrah S Mohammed, Saiti Halder, Mengqing Xu, Michelle J Wu, and Shuozhen Bao. 2021. "Biocompatibility of nanomaterials and their immunological properties." *Biomedical Materials* 16 (4):042005.

Li, Chaorong, Shunxin Shu, Rui Chen, Benyong Chen, and Wenjun Dong. 2013. "Functionalization of electrospun nanofibers of natural cotton cellulose by cerium dioxide nanoparticles for ultraviolet protection." *Journal of Applied Polymer Science* 130 (3):1524–1529.

Li, Chaorong, Yong Xie, Qiuyan Liu, Yingying Zheng, Xiaobo Zhang, and Wenjun Dong. 2014. "The formation and UV-blocking property of flower-like ZnO nanorod on electrospun natural cotton cellulose nanofibers." *Fibers and Polymers* 15:281–285.

Li, Lei, Yanxiang Li, Lixia Cao, and Chuanfang Yang. 2015. "Enhanced chromium (VI) adsorption using nanosized chitosan fibers tailored by electrospinning." *Carbohydrate Polymers* 125:206–213.

Li, Minxia, Hongtao Wang, Shengju Wu, Fengting Li, and Pengdan Zhi. 2012. "Adsorption of hazardous dyes indigo carmine and acid red on nanofiber membranes." *RSC Advances* 2 (3):900–907.

Li, Xiaoyan, Weichen Chen, Qingrong Qian, Haitao Huang, Yuming Chen, Ziqiang Wang, Qinghua Chen, Jing Yang, Ju Li, and Yiu-Wing Mai. 2021. "Electrospinning-based strategies for battery materials." *Advanced Energy Materials* 11 (2):2000845.

Liu, Xinkuan, Haixia Xu, Mingxin Zhang, and Deng-Guang Yu. 2021. "Electrospun medicated nanofibers for wound healing." *Membranes* 11 (10):770.

Liu, Yanbo, Ming Hao, Zhijun Chen, Lingling Liu, Yao Liu, Wenxiu Yang, and Seeram Ramakrishna. 2020. "A review on recent advances in application of electrospun nanofiber materials as biosensors." *Current Opinion in Biomedical Engineering* 13:174–189.

Lv, Dan, Miaomiao Zhu, Zhicheng Jiang, Shaohua Jiang, Qilu Zhang, Ranhua Xiong, and Chaobo Huang. 2018. "Green electrospun nanofibers and their application in air filtration." *Macromolecular Materials and Engineering* 303 (12):1800336.

Ma, Fang-Fang, Di Zhang, Nan Zhang, Ting Huang, and Yong Wang. 2018. "Polydopamine-assisted deposition of polypyrrole on electrospun poly (vinylidene fluoride) nanofibers for bidirectional removal of cation and anion dyes." *Chemical Engineering Journal* 354:432–444.

Ma, Zuwei, M Kotaki, and S Ramakrishna. 2006. "Surface modified nonwoven polysulphone (PSU) fiber mesh by electrospinning: A novel affinity membrane." *Journal of Membrane Science* 272 (1–2):179–187.

MacDiarmid, AG, WE Jones Jr, ID Norris, Junbo Gao, AT Johnson Jr, NJ Pinto, J Hone, B Han, FK Ko, and H Okuzaki. 2001. "Electrostatically-generated nanofibers of electronic polymers." *Synthetic Metals* 119 (1–3):27–30.

Maleki, Homa, Bahareh Azimi, Saeed Ismaeilimoghadam, and Serena Danti. 2022. "Poly (lactic acid)-based electrospun fibrous structures for biomedical applications." *Applied Sciences* 12 (6):3192.

Matilainen, Anu, and Mika Sillanpää. 2010. "Removal of natural organic matter from drinking water by advanced oxidation processes." *Chemosphere* 80 (4):351–365.

Mirzaei-Parsa, Mohamad Javad, Amin Ghanizadeh, Malihe TK Ebadi, and Reza Faridi-Majidi. 2018. "An alternative solvent for electrospinning of fibrinogen nanofibers." *Bio-Medical Materials and Engineering* 29 (3):279–287.

Nadaf, Arif, Akash Gupta, Nazeer Hasan, Shadaan Ahmad, Prashant Kesharwani, and Farhan J Ahmad. 2022. "Recent update on electrospinning and electrospun nanofibers: Current trends and their applications." *RSC Advances* 12 (37):23808–23828.

Nicosia, A, T Keppler, FA Müller, B Vazquez, F Ravegnani, P Monticelli, and F Belosi. 2016. "Cellulose acetate nanofiber electrospun on nylon substrate as novel composite matrix for efficient, heat-resistant, air filters." *Chemical Engineering Science* 153:284–294.

Öksüz, Kerim Emre, Nese Kurt Özkaya, Zeynep Deniz Şahin İnan, and Ali Özer. 2021. "Novel natural spider silk embedded electrospun nanofiber mats for wound healing." *Materials Today Communications* 26:101942.

Pant, Hem Raj, Madhab Prasad Bajgai, Ki Taek Nam, Yun A Seo, Dipendra Raj Pandeya, Seong Tshool Hong, and Hak Yong Kim. 2011. "Electrospun nylon-6 spider-net like nanofiber mat containing TiO2 nanoparticles: A multifunctional nanocomposite textile material." *Journal of Hazardous Materials* 185 (1):124–130.

Park, Ye Ri, Hyung Woo Ju, Jung Min Lee, Dong-Kyu Kim, Ok Joo Lee, Bo Mi Moon, Hyun Jung Park, Ju Yeon Jeong, Yeung Kyu Yeon, and Chan Hum Park. 2016. "Three-dimensional electrospun silk-fibroin nanofiber for skin tissue engineering." *International Journal of Biological Macromolecules* 93:1567–1574.

Patil, Priyanka P, Michaela R Reagan, and Raghvendra A Bohara. 2020. "Silk fibroin and silk-based biomaterial derivatives for ideal wound dressings." *International Journal of Biological Macromolecules* 164:4613–4627.

Quirós, Jennifer, João P Borges, Karina Boltes, Ismael Rodea-Palomares, and Roberto Rosal. 2015. "Antimicrobial electrospun silver-, copper-and zinc-doped polyvinylpyrrolidone nanofibers." *Journal of Hazardous Materials* 299:298–305.

Racz, Roger S, Crystal L Ramanujam, and Thomas Zgonis. 2010. "Puncture wounds of the foot." *Clinics in Podiatric Medicine and Surgery* 27 (4):523–534.

Rahmati, Maryam, David K Mills, Aleksandra M Urbanska, Mohammad Reza Saeb, Jayarama Reddy Venugopal, Seeram Ramakrishna, and Masoud Mozafari. 2021. "Electrospinning for tissue engineering applications." *Progress in Materials Science* 117:100721.

Raza, Aikifa, Yang Li, Junlu Sheng, Jianyong Yu, and Bin Ding. 2014. "Protective clothing based on electrospun nanofibrous membranes." In: *Electrospun Nanofibers for Energy and Environmental* Applications, edited by Bin Ding and Jianyong Yu, 355–369. Springer.

Rezaei, Babak, Ahmad Mousavi Shoushtari, Mohammad Rabiee, Lokman Uzun, Anthony PF Turner, and Wing Cheung Mak. 2018. "Multifactorial modeling and optimization of solution and electrospinning parameters to generate superfine polystyrene nanofibers." *Advances in Polymer Technology* 37 (8):2743–2755.

Robinson, Andrew J, Alejandra Pérez-Nava, Shan C Ali, J Betzabe González-Campos, Julianne L Holloway, and Elizabeth M Cosgriff-Hernandez. 2021. "Comparative analysis of fiber alignment methods in electrospinning." *Matter* 4 (3):821–844.

Sanford, James A, and Richard L Gallo. 2013. "Functions of the skin microbiota in health and disease." *Seminars in Immunology* 25 (5):370–377.

Shahriar, SM Shatil, Jagannath Mondal, Mohammad Nazmul Hasan, Vishnu Revuri, Dong Yun Lee, and Yong-Kyu Lee. 2019. "Electrospinning nanofibers for therapeutics delivery." *Nanomaterials* 9 (4):532.

Stoppa, Matteo, and Alessandro Chiolerio. 2014. "Wearable electronics and smart textiles: A critical review." *Sensors* 14 (7):11957–11992.

Sun, K, and ZH Li. 2011. "Preparations, properties and applications of chitosan based nanofibers fabricated by electrospinning." *Express Polymer Letters* 5 (4):342–361.

Tarus, Bethwel K, Nermin Fadel, Affaf Al-Oufy, and Magdi El-Messiry. 2020. "Investigation of mechanical properties of electrospun poly (vinyl chloride) polymer nanoengineered composite." *Journal of Engineered Fibers and Fabrics* 15:1558925020982569.

Thenmozhi, S, N Dharmaraj, K Kadirvelu, and Hak Yong Kim. 2017. "Electrospun nanofibers: New generation materials for advanced applications." *Materials Science and Engineering:* B 217:36–48.

Toshkova, R, N Manolova, E Gardeva, M Ignatova, L Yossifova, I Rashkov, and M Alexandrov. 2010. "Antitumor activity of quaternized chitosan-based electrospun implants against Graffi myeloid tumor." *International Journal of Pharmaceutics* 400 (1–2):221–233.

Uyanik, Orkun, Kubra Cigdem Pekkoc-Uyanik, Siddika Findik, Ahmet Avci, and Zeynep Altuntas. 2022. "Prevention of peritendinous adhesions with electrospun poly (lactic acid-co-glycolic acid)(PLGA) bioabsorbable nanofiber: An experimental study." *Colloids and Surfaces B: Biointerfaces* 209:112181.

van Blitterswijk, Clemens, and Jan De Boer. 2022. *Tissue Engineering*. Academic Press.

Wang, Hai-Sheng, Guo-Dong Fu, and Xin-Song Li. 2009. "Functional polymeric nanofibers from electrospinning." *Recent Patents on Nanotechnology* 3 (1):21–31.

Wang, Lei, Changbo Zhang, Feng Gao, and Gang Pan. 2016. "Needleless electrospinning for scaled-up production of ultrafine chitosan hybrid nanofibers used for air filtration." *RSC Advances* 6 (107):105988–105995.

Wang, Ran, Yang Liu, Brandon Li, Benjamin S Hsiao, and Benjamin Chu. 2012. "Electrospun nanofibrous membranes for high flux microfiltration." *Journal of Membrane Science* 392:167–174.

Wang, Su-Xi, Chin Chong Yap, Jiating He, Chao Chen, Siew Yee Wong, and Xu Li. 2016. "Electrospinning: A facile technique for fabricating functional nanofibers for environmental applications." *Nanotechnology Reviews* 5 (1):51–73.

Wang, Xiandi, Lin Dong, Hanlu Zhang, Ruomeng Yu, Caofeng Pan, and Zhong Lin Wang. 2015. "Recent progress in electronic skin." *Advanced Science* 2 (10):1500169.

Wang, Xuefen, and Benjamin S Hsiao. 2016. "Electrospun nanofiber membranes." *Current Opinion in Chemical Engineering* 12:62–81.

Wang, Zhen-Gang, Ling-Shu Wan, Zhen-Mei Liu, Xiao-Jun Huang, and Zhi-Kang Xu. 2009. "Enzyme immobilization on electrospun polymer nanofibers: An overview." *Journal of Molecular Catalysis B: Enzymatic* 56 (4):189–195.

White, Richard AS. 1999. "The aetiology and classification of wounds and skin deficits." In: *Manual of Canine and Feline Wound Management and Reconstruction,* edited by David Fowler and John M. Williams, 5–12. Iowa State University Press/British Small Animal Veterinary Association.

Wise, Steven G, Michael J Byrom, Anna Waterhouse, Paul G Bannon, Martin KC Ng, and Anthony S Weiss. 2011. "A multilayered synthetic human elastin/polycaprolactone hybrid vascular graft with tailored mechanical properties." *Acta Biomaterialia* 7 (1):295–303.

Xiangwu, Zhang, Liwen Ji, Ozan Toprakci, Yinzheng Liang, and Mataz Alcoutlabi. 2011. "Electrospun nanofiber-based anodes, cathodes, and separators for advanced lithium-ion batteries." *Polymer Reviews* 51 (3):239–264.

Xue, Jiajia, Tong Wu, Yunqian Dai, and Younan Xia. 2019. "Electrospinning and electrospun nanofibers: Methods, materials, and applications." *Chemical Reviews* 119 (8):5298–5415.

Yanılmaz, Meltem, and A Sezai Sarac. 2014. "A review: Effect of conductive polymers on the conductivities of electrospun mats." *Textile Research Journal* 84 (12):1325–1342.

Yew, Chee Hong Takahiro, Pedram Azari, Jane Ru Choi, Farina Muhamad, and Belinda Pingguan-Murphy. 2018. "Electrospun polycaprolactone nanofibers as a reaction membrane for lateral flow assay." *Polymers* 10 (12):1387.

Yonghui, Yan, Xiangye Liu, Jing Yan, Cao Guan, and John Wang. 2021. "Electrospun nanofibers for new generation flexible energy storage." *Energy & Environmental Materials* 4 (4):502–521.

Zhang, Danping, Longjian Li, Yinghui Shan, Jie Xiong, Zhongjie Hu, Yan Zhang, and Jianqing Gao. 2019. "In vivo study of silk fibroin/gelatin electrospun nanofiber dressing loaded with astragaloside IV on the effect of promoting wound healing and relieving scar." *Journal of Drug Delivery Science and Technology* 52:272–281.

Zhou, Gang, Zhuo Xu, Yongliang Zhang, Jianguo Liu, Liwei Jiang, Rulin Liu, and Yongmei Wang. 2024. "Effect of different antibacterial agents doping in PET-based electrospun nanofibrous membranes on air filtration and antibacterial performance." *Environmental Research* 243:117877.

Zhou, Wenlong, Narendra Reddy, and Yiqi Yang. 2005. "Overview of protective clothing." In *Textiles for Protection*, edited by Richard A. Scott, 3–30. Woodhead Publishing/CRC Press.

Zhou, Yangjian, Yanan Liu, Mingxin Zhang, Zhangbin Feng, Deng-Guang Yu, and Ke Wang. 2022. "Electrospun nanofiber membranes for air filtration: A review." *Nanomaterials* 12 (7):1077.

Zollinger, Heinrich. 2003. *Color Chemistry: Syntheses, Properties, and Applications of Organic Dyes and Pigments*. John Wiley & Sons.

Section I

Wound Regeneration

2 Introduction to Wound Dressing

Muhammad Ayyoob and Muhammad Umar

INTRODUCTION

Over the course of millions of years, humans have evolved and so has our skin. Human skin is a highly adaptive and multifunctional body organ. It is the first line of defense against a wide range of external exposures, including physical harm, chemical exposure, and hazardous radiation. Other functionalities of the skin include temperature regulation, sensory reception, and immune response. One of the functions of the skin is to protect the internal organs from injury. However, due to external abrasion or injury, the skin in the human body can be damaged, and its recovery process is called wound healing. Wound healing is a natural process to regenerate the tissues at the site of injury. It is a natural physiological reaction of the body to injury. In other words, we can say it is a self-healing mechanism. However, wound healing is a complex phenomenon involving multiple layers of different types of cells, such as cytokines, mediators, the vascular system, and a multiphase process. The human wound healing process was initially considered as a three-phase process. Early researchers presented the concept of three phases, namely inflammatory, fibroblastic, and maturation [1]. Some authors also denoted these three phases as inflammatory, proliferation, and remodeling [2]. However, more recent studies suggest a four-phase concept, including the hemostasis phase, the inflammatory phase, the proliferation phase, and the remodeling phase. In the three-phase concept, the hemostasis phase is included within the inflammatory phase.

Wound care has evolved since ancient civilization, such as Egypt, where resin or honey-soaked gauze was applied as a wound dressing for healing. However, the traditional bandages or gauze dressings cause trauma and pain when dry out and stick on the wound. Therefore, different methodologies have been adopted to keep them moist as well as providing a healing environment while keeping safe from germs attack. Bioactive dressings, enhanced with agents like honey, collagen, and chitosan, further improve healing by managing moisture, pH, and bacterial growth. Advanced innovations include electrospun biodegradable scaffolds infused with herbal medicines and nanoparticles for controlled drug release and better wound penetration. These have shown improved healing in both animal and clinical studies. Smart wound dressings now incorporate sensors for real-time monitoring of wound conditions like moisture, temperature, and biochemical markers. Coupled with AI technology, these systems support early diagnosis, outcome prediction, and improved chronic wound management. The integration of wearable electronics and human–machine interfaces represents a promising future in personalized wound care. Current wound healing practices are the result of thousands

DOI: 10.1201/9781003616726-3

of years of evolution—from primitive methods to modern evidence-based approaches. Early wound care involved natural remedies and continuous observation of the healing process. With the development of civilization, more sophisticated wound care techniques emerged, including the use of antiseptics, cleanliness, bandaging, and surgical interventions when needed. The development of germ theory in the 19th and 20th centuries and the introduction of specialized antiseptics significantly transformed traditional wound care practices, although alcohol had previously been used for this purpose. Early humans applied honey, mud, and natural herbs to facilitate wound healing. A clay tablet from the Sumerian civilization (2100 BC) suggests three wound healing gestures, including washing, applying herbal mixtures, and bandaging. Egyptians used bandages, honey, grease, and lint for wound dressing. Vinegar and wine were also used for cleaning and as antibacterial agents, as suggested by the early Roman and ancient Greek civilizations. In the subcontinent, a mixture of herbs and plants was used for wound dressing and wound care.

Wound cleanliness and wound protection from germs remained crucial in wound healing. For that purpose, wound dressings have evolved. The main purpose of wound dressing initially was to protect the wound from the attack of external germs and bacteria. Initially, they were used to provide a barrier against bacteria. However, the barrier is not the only function of wound dressing today; they not only provide a barrier but also promote wound healing by providing a suitable healing environment and facilitating tissue regeneration, keeping the wound moist, and helping to manage exudate. Dressings also provide facilitation in debridement, pain relief, comfort, and provide fast and efficient healing. Proper care and wound dressing lead to healthy wound healing. In case of improper care, wounds can be infected with bacteria or any sort of secondary infection. Therefore, wound dressings are crucial in proper wound care.

In this chapter, the evolution of wound dressing and wound care is reviewed comprehensively. It provides insights into the evaluation of wound dressings and the treatment of wounds, and discusses the various phases of wound healing. Furthermore, it highlights the role of wound dressings in wound care management and the treatment of patients with wounds.

Early Practices and Traditional Wound Care

In ancient times, medicine was not practiced in a clinical or scientific manner; however, empirical observations were adopted by medical practitioners to use products associated with scientific improvements to provide health benefits and more efficient and effective treatments. In the early history of medicine, many therapies were used that today seem absurd. Early reports suggest several such treatments were employed. For example, one such treatment was to rub a frog warmed in oil on a hot surface or inflammation, as reported in the Papyrus of Ebers (Eb), dating back to about 1500 BC. Another such treatment was the use of excrement as a potential material to treat injuries [3–5].

Ancient civilizations were scattered in different parts of the globe; however, medical care is said to have developed in the following four major areas: Far East, India, Mesopotamia and Mediterranean, South America and Polynesia. Early history suggests that there was definitely a certain level of communication through different channels; for example, Indian medicine might have reached in Greece through the conquests of Alexander the great. The origin of Chinese medicine also expands to prehistoric times. Surgery was flourished in India, and it is said that it was transmitted to Polynesia. The oldest civilization known for scientific and artistic work is the Egyptian civilization. The Egyptian civilization was also the most advanced in the science of health care, with no exception in wound management. They are considered masters in wound care, with a unique style of applying bandages while considering signs of infection and inflammation. Wound dressing and wound management are reported as early as the Egyptian civilization. In Mesopotamia and Mediterranean (now Iraq and Egypt), wounds were washed with milk or water, dressed with honey or wood resin, and covered with wool or linen bandages [6]. Some minerals were also initially used by Egyptians for wound treatment such as green copper and mercury compounds.

From ancient Indian history, surgery and wound care were highly skilled branches of Ayurvedic medicine dating back to the Vedic Period (1500–500 BC). Various types of wound treatments and guided healing practices existed in ancient Indian culture, as documented in classical texts. The Vedas, and later the *Sushruta Samhita*, emphasized herbal treatments for wounds with a strong surgical focus. Practices such as *Vrana Shodhana* (wound purification) and *Vrana Ropana* (wound healing) described the different stages of wound healing, including septic, clean, healing, and healed stages [5].

Since prehistoric and early historic times, particular attention has been given to wound care and healing—especially during times of war, when injuries were frequent and potentially fatal if left untreated. However, the understanding of managing fresh wounds, particularly controlling bleeding (hemostasis), was limited in ancient civilizations. The concept of stopping blood loss gained importance much later, especially with the advent of firearms, which caused more severe and frequent injuries. Interestingly, the Smith Papyrus, one of the oldest known medical texts from ancient Egypt, does not mention methods for stopping bleeding. It is in the Ebers Papyrus (circa 1500 BCE) where the first documented guidance appears, suggesting that if a wound continues to bleed, it should be cauterized (burned with fire), highlighting an early awareness that excessive blood loss was dangerous [6].

Ancient texts described various surgical procedures collectively known as "Ashtavidha Shastra Karma"—eight types of techniques used to treat diseases requiring surgical intervention at the time. Sushruta emphasized that any foreign matter—such as fragments of metal, fractured bone, nails, spikes, blood clots, or hair—must be removed before wound closure through suturing. All types of wounds were to be cleaned aseptically, using water boiled with various medicinal plants—one notable example being Neem (*Azadirachta indica*)—and sometimes wine. The use of sutures, medicinal ointments, and herbal applications such as aloe vera for wound healing was also practiced [5,7].

Bandaging was an art by 500 BC as by then surgeons knew that bandaging too tightly can cause gangrene. Around 300 BC, the Egyptian medicine transferred to the Greeks. During the visit of the Greek historian Herodotus to the Egypt (450 BC), he noticed different medicine practices; however, wound care had already existed. Around 800 BC, Greeks emerged [6]. It is also said that during the Trojan War, the Greek Army has its own surgeons for surgery and wound care. In Greece, Hippocrates (460–377 BC) made significant advancements in wound care by suggesting that wounds be kept dry and that wine or vinegar be used for washing. Hippocrates of Kos, who lived from around 460 to 377 BC, is often celebrated as the "Father of Medicine." He was a prominent Greek physician and thinker of the Classical period who played a pivotal role in shaping the foundations of modern medical practice. Hippocrates championed the use of careful observation and logical reasoning in diagnosing and treating illness, moving medicine away from superstition and toward a more scientific approach. He also helped to establish ethical standards for physicians, most famously through the Hippocratic Oath, which continues to influence medical ethics today. Boiled or soaked wool in wine was considered for wound bandages. For the purpose of wound ointment, oil, honey, and wine were recommended by him [8–10].

The medical knowledge and science were written in Greek from Hippocrates to the fall of the Roman Empire. Roman has a little understanding of medical science at that time; therefore, the Greeks were appointed as wound surgeons in Roman armies. During the peak time of the Roman Empire, there were thoughts developed to transfer the knowledge of science to a wider audience; however, there remained a restriction on how to do so until Latin encyclopedists appeared in Roman history. Marcus Varro, a well-known encyclopedist, described the theory of contagion for the first time around 50 BC. He suggested that certain illnesses might be caused by invisible "minute creatures" floating in the air that could enter the body through inhalation or ingestion. Although his idea lacked scientific validation at the time, it was a striking early insight that anticipated the germ theory of disease by many centuries [11]. After him, Aulus Cornelius Celsus, a great Roman encyclopedist, compiled the encyclopedia of eight book series named as *De Medicina* using perhaps his firsthand experience of surgery and wound care during his medical practices. For the first time, he differentiated between chronic sores and wounds and recommended different types of treatments. He described a number of different kinds of wounds and advocated their different treatments, including reversing post-surgery debridement wounds that are contused or contaminated before being sutured.

In his influential medical treatise *De Medicina*, Aulus Cornelius Celsus outlined a groundbreaking method for controlling bleeding through the ligation of blood vessels—a technique not commonly practiced before his time. By describing how to tie off vessels to manage hemorrhage, Celsus significantly advanced surgical practice. His clear understanding of anatomy and emphasis on careful, methodical intervention helped to lay the groundwork for modern hemostasis techniques [12].

Beyond bleeding control, Celsus also stressed the importance of wound care. He advocated for the use of dressings sometimes soaked in vinegar and recommended softening them with rose oil as wounds healed. These recommendations reflected a sophisticated understanding of infection prevention and pain management. His approach to wound treatment demonstrated a balance between cleanliness, comfort, and effectiveness, contributing greatly to the overall success of surgical outcomes [12].

Celsus's *De Medicina* served as a bridge between the empirical teachings of Hippocrates and the anatomical insights of Galen. It documented important advances from the Alexandrian medical school, including the first known descriptions of ligatures for hemostasis, wound healing by first intention (*per primam intentionem*), and even amputation procedures. His work represented a rational and systematic approach to medicine, one that prioritized both theoretical knowledge and practical application. In his work *De Medicina*, Celsus detailed a method for stopping bleeding. He explained that if there is a risk of severe hemorrhage due to the size of the wound and the amount of blood loss, the first step is to fill the wound with dry lint. A sponge soaked in cold water should then be placed on top and pressed firmly [12,13]. If bleeding continues, the lint should be reapplied this time soaked in vinegar. If these steps fail to control the bleeding, the veins responsible for the blood flow should be located, tied tightly in two places near the wound, and then cut between the ties. This allows each end of the vein to retract and close off naturally [6,11,13].

The third important documented record of scientific approaches was found in the encyclopedia "Historia Naturalis" by Caius Pliny [14]. He was a famous naturalist Roman author and philosopher. Contrary to the De Medicina, which is exclusively written from firsthand experience, the "Historia Naturalis," based on 37 books, was the compilation of others work and experience. After the destruction of Pompei, Claudius Galen came to Rome and appointed as emperor's Marcus Aureliu's physician and gladiatorial surgeon [14]. His main focus was physiology and anatomy in medicine based on condition visible to naked eye, rather than scientific experience. Roman work in medicinal science reached its peak with the first two centuries after Christ. He wrote the instructions for wound care. He stated that any hemorrhage wound can be treated through one of the four ways—applying direct pressure, twisting the wound end through anything like a hook, tying the cut while in a grasp, or applying styptics made up of aloe, frankincense, and egg white, the mixture is honey-like with a pinch of a fur. Later on, Galen used silk brought from China to tie off the cut wounds. It is also believed that he may have used vinegar as well inspired from the court physician of emperor Claudius named Scribonius Largus [6,8,15].

After Galen, nothing specific is available from European literature as most of the Europe cloaked in the Dark Ages; however, the knowledge is thrived somewhere else in the world including China, Constantinople, and India. In the 4th century, the knowledge center became the Byzantine empire centered at Constantinople. From Constantinople, the knowledge was shifted to the Arabs through exiled Nestorians who translated the Latin encyclopedia to Syrian languages of that time. Epitome, a masterpiece of summaries of medical knowledge, written by Paulus Aegineta's was a series of seven volumes. There was specific portion for surgery. Epitome and Nestorians work created the basis of medical knowledge of Islamic word, and during its expansion, the science of surgery and wound care reached its peak till the 9th century. However, due to certain cleanliness practices among Jews and Muslims, they mostly rely on physical treatment with little focus on surgical practices [6,8,15].

Medieval and Renaissance Practices

The wound care practices during the Medieval and Renaissance were a mix of practical and scientific knowledge and superstitions. With a little understanding of antiseptic practices emerged the usage of wine and honey. However, some of the societies had primarily relied on charm and prayers for the healing. Due to various restrictions such as limitations imposed during Roman rule and certain Muslim practices that regarded wounds as impure, surgical practices gradually shifted from trained surgeons to barber-surgeons and other lower-tier, yet professional, occupations. These practitioners handled wound treatment, chiropractic care, fractures, and other external injuries [16].

However, Islamic contributions to biological understanding and wound healing, based on knowledge inherited from ancient Greek and Roman practices, led to significant advancements and innovations. Several comprehensive medical texts and procedural manuals were compiled during this period. While barber-surgeons treated wounds, fractures, and injuries, apothecaries were responsible for preparing and dispensing medicines.

The Arabs were in contact with the Greek and Egyptian civilizations. Societal, administrative systems, and core knowledge such as medicine and medical practices were transferred from these two civilizations and later merged with medical practices of Indian and Chinese origin through trade routes. During the 5th century, Greek literature was translated into Arabic, forming the foundation for the advancement of medical practices in the Muslim world. Around the same time, there was a medical learning center in Persia known as Jundi-Shapur, which had been established in the 3rd century.

According to Islam, medicine practices focus on two dimensions of practices: preventive medicines and therapeutic medicine. Islam focuses on one's health and functions of the body and body parts. The Qur'an, the holy book of Islam, referred different body parts and declared them as the signs of God (23:14). Similarly, The Prophet advised the followers to seek treatment of sickness. As reported by Usāmah ibn Sharik, reported in *Sunan Ibn Mājah* 3436 "**Seek treatment, O servants of Allah! Verily Allah has not created any disease but He also created its cure—except old age.**" and by Abū Hurayrah in Ṣaḥīḥ *al-Bukhārī* "**There is no disease that Allah has created, except that He also created its treatment**." These directives created a positive drive considerably away from the superstitions and magic treatments of sickness and wounds. The belief that every disease has its cure compelled Muslims to explore the possible treatment from plants, minerals, and other natural ingredients or a mixture of all of them for every illness, and to record the findings in a scientific and practical manner.

The knowledge of medicine was found to be very attractive due to two basic reasons: Islam encouraged the pursuit of scientific knowledge and the profession has historically been respected. The fugitives Christian and Sabean practitioners who ran away from church persecution found themselves refuge in the buffer states of Byzantines and Persia. Numerous centers, such as Harran, Jundishapur, Ruha, and Al-Hira, were established to build practical traditions of medical knowledge. Different experts were appointed as royal physicians such as Jurji bin Bakhtishu, who was employed as Al-Mansur's court physician. Similarly, Al-Ma'mun appointed Hunayn Ibne Ishaq as the head of Dar Al Hikmah (the house of Wisdom). During that era, many literatures were translated to Arabic at different centers including knowledge of medicine, wound cleaning practices, and wound dressings.

The Islamic knowledge of medicine began to grow rapidly. The previously available literature was translated and practiced by Islamic Practitioners. The medical knowledge was proofed by practice, which was further researched and given new categories as per Islamic understanding and culture. For the first time, the art of diagnosis was developed, which consists of multiple observations including history of disease, investigation of urine, observation of body temperature, smell, and apparent condition including pulse.

The most prominent scholar of the 10th century is Abul-Qasim al-Zahrawi's (936–1013) whose western name is Albucasis. He was a teacher in medicine and surgeon by practice from Spain. He was believed to have strongly linked surgery with anatomy. His wound treatment practices were inspired by those of Galen's work. He used a variety of ointments depending upon the type of wound. Most Islamic contribution in medicine was the invention in medicinal chemistry and pharmacy. Islam produced many well-known scholars in the field of medicine. Ibn Sina (980–1037), also known in the West as Avicenna, was one of the most renowned Persian scholars who made profound contributions to philosophy, science, and particularly medicine. He meticulously compiled and organized existing medical knowledge into a comprehensive medical encyclopedia, *Al-Qanun fi al-Tibb* (The Canon of Medicine), enriched with detailed diagrams, illustrations, and systematic classifications. This work served as a foundational text not only in Islamic medical institutions but also in European medical schools, where it remained in use until the late 19th century. The *Canon* describes approximately 760 drugs and reflects Avicenna's lasting impact on medical science.

The story of wound care wouldn't be complete without mentioning the barbers and barber-surgeons. In the early Christian centuries, barbers were an integral part of monasteries, primarily tasked with maintaining the hair of the monks. But their familiarity with sharp tools soon led them to take on a more critical role—assisting monastery surgeons, especially when bloodletting or minor procedures were needed. Over time, their role grew more formal. In 1215, Pope Innocent III issued a significant decree at the Fourth Lateran Council that officially recognized barbers as barber-surgeons. This decision stemmed from various complexities within the Church, including evolving clerical laws and societal issues like marriage ceremonies. What began as informal help soon became standard practice, and the humble monastery barbers evolved into recognized practitioners in early surgical care [17]. After 1215, barber-surgeons became the primary practitioners for performing surgeries related to ergotism, particularly amputations. However, this status began to shift in 1268, when the profession was formally divided into two classes. From that point onward, barber-surgeons were categorized as "short-robed" surgeons, limited to procedures like amputations and bloodletting. In contrast, more complex cases—such as open wounds and bone fractures—were reserved for university-trained or "Master" surgeons. This marked a clear distinction in surgical responsibilities based on training and expertise [17].

Medical services are always in high demand during times of war and conflict. Throughout history, physicians and battlefield surgeons have been integral parts of military contingents. The role of warfare surgeons, however, saw particular growth during the Norman conquest of England under William the Conqueror 1066. As English and French cultures began to merge, many medical institutions adopted the French and Norman models. Notably, centers like the Abbey of Baldwin drew inspiration from establishments such as the Abbey of Saint-Ennemond, reflecting the broader influence of French-Norman medical practices during that period [17]. Some surgery practices were also exchanged during the first crusade (1096–1099). Although those were hostiles times, there were possible alliances with state to state such as a Christian state forming an alliance with a Muslim state against another Muslim state and vice versa. Arab medical practices significantly influenced European surgical methods, particularly in the care of battlefield injuries. However, as noted earlier, Europe was largely in its Dark Ages from the 9th to the 13th century—a time marked by stagnation in many fields. In contrast, that same era was a golden age for the Islamic world, flourishing in every aspect of life, from social and cultural advancements to medicine and wound care innovations [17].

The Era of Antiseptic Discovery (19th Century)

People once believed that most diseases were caused by filth or poor living conditions, a view known as the filth theory of disease. Following this idea, the U.S. Health Department took early steps to educate the public on the value of preventive medicine. Around the period before 1860, sanitarians strongly believed that by cleaning up the environment, improving drainage, providing clean drinking water, ensuring proper ventilation, and removing waste, people's health would naturally improve. While this approach did help in some ways, the theory eventually lost ground, mainly because it didn't truly address the real causes behind many diseases [18]. Louis Pasteur was the first to clearly propose that microorganisms are the underlying cause of many diseases. The emergence of germ theory in the 1860s significantly transformed the understanding of wound healing [19,20]. As the concept gained recognition, some medical practitioners began to adopt its principles. Among them was Joseph Lister, who pioneered antiseptic surgery. He introduced the use of carbolic acid to disinfect surgical instruments and reusable materials, aiming to prevent contamination by harmful microbes. This concept initialized the development of antiseptics [21].

For many centuries, surgeons and wound healers believed that suppuration and the presence of pus in the wound are signs of healing. With the discovery of "chloroform" in the mid-1800s, the surgeries increased significantly as a result of post-operative complications, which were also on the rise due to infections. Then, the wound healers have to believe that pus is a sign of infection not a sign of healing. This change in the thinking of the medical practitioners led to the groundbreaking work of Joseph Lister. In the 1960s, he started cleaning the wounds using carbolic acid as antiseptic and sterilizing gauze. His practices significantly reduced wound infections. The use of antiseptic wound dressings helped to suppress suppuration, pus formation, and the risk of infection. The introduction of antiseptics marked a pivotal turning point in both wound care and surgical practices [22].

With the discovery of creosote as a food preservative by Reichenbach, another significant use emerged when he observed its ability to remove dead skin tissue. He began testing its effectiveness against skin diseases in collaboration with a surgeon and a pharmacist. A series of remarkable results confirmed that it was effective in treating wounds, burns, gangrene, scabies, ulcers, and other conditions [22].

Marcellin Berthelot documented certain cases in which diluted solutions of creosote were used to treat skin diseases such as burns, cut wounds, ear infections, and other skin diseases. Pain relief was reported by ten patients and suppressed suppuration was reported by seven patients, whereas four people were healed without any suppuration (pus formation). Similarly, in 1836, a Scottish physician John Rose Cormack reported in his extensive literature review about creosote's medical uses for wound healing. He reported that creosote treatments effectively reduced pus formation in burns, promoted wound cicatrization, and provided pain relief. Such reports suggest an early approach to suppress suppuration and antiseptic methodology in wound care [22,23].

The original creation of Reichenbach's creosote, which was known as "German creosote," was a mixture containing mainly carbolic acid (phenol, along with other similar compounds such as cresols, guaiacol, and creosols). Each of the compounds is a derivative of phenol with slightly different chemical side groups; for example, cresols have a methyl group ($-CH_3$), guaiacol has an ester group ($-OCH_3$), and creosol has both of them *p* ($-CH_3$ and $-OCH_3$). On surface application to a wound on the skin, the German creosote slowly released these organic compounds that act as an antiseptic agent [22].

Soon after, a new debate started to differentiate between antiseptics mainly known as safe for the human body and disinfectants, which are toxic to living cells. Torald H. Sollmann, an American pharmacologist, reported based on laboratory trails that the germicidal power of cresols is three times higher than that of carbolic acid (phenol), while its toxicity to living tissues in comparatively less. Guaiacol (60%–90% creosote) has more germicidal power as compared to phenol. However, these findings may have not been much relevant to the actual clinical trials but still remains relevant to antiseptic practices [22,24,25].

In 1863, pharmacist Jules Lemaire published a book on *L'acide Phénique*, detailing his work with coal tar emulsified with saponin (coaltar saponiné); this preparation was originated by another pharmacist who discovered in 1950 that an alcoholic solution of coal tar mixed with saponin is surprisingly effective in gangrenous wounds. Soon after, other investigators supported the findings. His findings were supported by growing understanding that microbes in the air cause putrefaction and wound suppuration, aligning with earlier work by Pasteur. Lemaire's studies with phenol (carbolic acid) suggested to use it in disinfecting wounds, hospitals, and sewage, showing that it killed microbes and improved healing without pus formation.

Meanwhile, Joseph Lister, influenced by Pasteur's germ theory and possibly by reports of carbolic acid's success in sewage treatment in Carlisle, applied phenol to wounds in the 1860s. His antiseptic methods significantly reduced infections in compound fractures and revolutionized surgical practices. Although Lister's ideas faced resistance, especially in Britain and the U.S., his methods were quickly adopted in Germany and Scandinavia. Notably, U.S. surgeon David Yandell reported positive outcomes in 34 surgical cases using carbolic acid, while others like Samuel D. Gross remained skeptical of certain practices (e.g., the carbolic spray) but supported antiseptic surgery overall [26–28].

Similarly, during World War I, a significant care for wounds was emerged. Henry Drysdale Dakin tested some 200 compounds under the directions of a French-American surgeon, Alexis Carrel (1873–1944). He found that sodium hypochlorite was 30 times stronger than carbolic acid. He advised wound irrigation after every 2 hours with hypochlorite. During World War II, antibiotics were discovered in the form of penicillin. However, the irrigation with antiseptics such as carbolic acid or hypochlorite remains the main surface treatment [29,30].

Wound care has a history that predates even the Egyptian civilization. During the Egyptian era, grease-soaked gauze bandages were commonly used, though there was little understanding of proper wound management. As time progressed—especially by the late 19th century—wound care practices gradually became more sophisticated. Yet, the core objective remained the same to promote healing.

Traditional gauze dressings used in the 19th century had a significant drawback—they often adhered to the wound surface as it dried. When removed, this could cause trauma to the newly formed tissue, leading to pain and even fresh bleeding. These dressings, though simple, posed challenges that affected both the healing process and the comfort of the patient [31,32].

In the 20th century, however, there was a noticeable shift from basic wound care to a more comprehensive approach known as wound management. This modern perspective not only aimed to accelerate healing but also emphasized pain control, moisture balance, and protection of the wound bed. It marked a critical turning point in both clinical practice and patient well-being [33].

The 20th Century: Industrial and Scientific Advancements

World Wars and Rapid Medical Innovations

Caring for the wounded during wartime has always been a significant challenge, particularly the task of transporting injured soldiers to those who could provide proper medical care. From prehistoric methods to the development of modern field hospitals, and from transportation without wheels to the invention of air ambulances, all innovations have been driven by the need to care for military personnel who put their lives on the line in service of their nation.

World Wars I and II brought a lot of new wound types and new challenges for medical practitioners. World War I (1914–1919) brought about a scale of human suffering and injury that the world had never seen before. The war gift was gunfire and machine gun bursts, which caused multiple bullet wounds, often resulting in open injuries and fractured bones. The brutal combination of machine gun fire, artillery shell fragments, bayonets, barbed wire, and the first widespread use of poison gas left soldiers with devastating wounds, massive open lacerations, shattered bones, traumatic amputations, burns, and gas-induced lung injuries. These injuries created overwhelming pressure on British and French medical services, who were often unprepared for the sheer volume and complexity of cases arriving from the front.

With the introduction of motorized transport, British forces were able to set up Casualty Clearing Stations (CCS) around 6–9 miles behind the front lines. These makeshift surgical hospitals were staffed by teams of surgeons, anesthetists, and nurses—bringing women closer to the front lines than ever before in modern warfare. Originally designed to handle 150–400 patients at a time, CCS units were often swamped with over 1,000 wounded soldiers during heavy fighting [34,35].

However, there remained many challenges such as priority of wound treatment; faced with impossible choices, medical personnel had to shift their triage priorities. Rather than focusing solely on the most severe injuries, doctors began to treat those whose wounds were serious but more straightforward soldiers who had a higher chance of survival with timely care. A British field manual from the time starkly defined the purpose of triage: first, the conservation of manpower; and second, the interests of the wounded themselves. It was a grim but necessary strategy in the face of such immense human cost [36,37].

World War II encouraged significant improvements in wound care, primarily due to the extraordinary scale of casualties and the crucial need for effective treatments. The discovery of "the penicillin" was a historic milestone that saved uncountable lives with effective healing of wounds and surgical traumas. Other advancements, including the widespread use of penicillin and improved surgical techniques, significantly reduced mortality rates and had a lasting impact on civilian healthcare.

Introduction of Cotton, Gauze, and Adhesive Bandages

Gauze has been used for wound dressing since prehistoric times, and it was the most common option for covering open wounds. Although grease-soaked lint was also used in some practices, gauze remained the primary choice. Cotton in its raw form, gauze (a woven fabric specially designed for wound care), and adhesive bandages are common materials used in wound care and first aid. When there is a need to absorb blood or secreting fluid, cotton, in its raw form, can be used as padding or to absorb fluids in wound care.

Wound dressings refer to a wide range of materials (from lint to sophisticated bandages) used to cover and care for wounds of physical injuries or diseased tissues. The primary roles of these dressings include:

- **Maintaining a moist healing environment**: Prevents wound desiccation, which can slow healing. Moisture supports autolysis, cell migration, granulation, and re-epithelialization.
- **Preventing maceration**: Allows evaporation or absorbs excess wound exudate to protect healing tissue and reduce infection risk in highly secretory wounds.
- **Promoting hemostasis**: Helps to stop bleeding and supports early healing.
- **Protecting the wound**: Shields against mechanical damage, microbial invasion, dehydration, chemical injury, and pH alterations.
- **Reducing heat loss**: Maintains optimal temperature at the wound site for effective healing.

- **Controlling microbial growth**: Often includes antimicrobial agents to prevent infection.
- **Enhancing autolysis**: Supports the body's natural removal of dead tissue.
- **Supporting tissue repair**: Facilitates all stages of the healing process.
- **Providing compression**: Aids in stopping bleeding and reducing edema.
- **Offering structural support**: Stabilizes the wound area.
- **Improving patient comfort**: Minimizes pain and enhances mobility.
- **Reducing odor**: Improves hygiene and comfort for both patient and caregivers.
- **Enhancing appearance**: Promotes a cleaner, more manageable wound site.
- **Lowering treatment costs**: Efficient healing reduces the need for extended care.

Wounds may also have different characteristics depending upon the cause of the wound itself. The selection of the appropriate wound dressing largely depends on the type and physiological condition of the wound. An ideal wound dressing should have a combination of all or at least a few of the above-mentioned properties, such as maintaining a moist environment, which is essential for efficient wound healing. It must support epidermal cell migration, stimulate angiogenesis (the development of new blood vessels), and aid in the synthesis of connective tissues. Additionally, the dressing should allow for sufficient gas exchange between the wound and its environment, help maintain an optimal temperature to improve blood circulation, and protect the site from bacterial contamination. To ensure comfort and minimize trauma during dressing changes, the material should be non-adherent and easy to remove after healing. It should also assist in debridement by promoting the migration of white blood cells and the accumulation of enzymes necessary to remove dead tissue. Furthermore, all dressings must be sterile, non-toxic, and non-allergenic to prevent adverse reactions. The choice of dressing also relies on factors such as the degree of exudation, risk or presence of infection, necrotic tissue, anatomical location of the wound, and the stage of the healing process. Therefore, dressing selection should not be considered in isolation but rather as part of an integrated, patient-centered wound care strategy.

Another aspect of wound care was the use of precious metals in wound care historically even before the understanding of germs theory. Ancient civilizations like the Greeks, Egyptians, and Romans used metals like gold, silver, and copper to purify water and treat wounds, even before the emergence of the theory of microorganisms. A proper record of the use of silver nitrate to cure epilepsy in the 17th century. However, this practice ceased in the 20th century. During the 20th century, several antimicrobial applications of silver were observed through application of its salt as skin top ointments [38]. Several other different types of antimicrobial agents have been identified, which were previously in use on topical applications or in impregnated bandage forms, such as honey, silver compounds, chlorhexidine, hydrogen peroxide, iodine, proflavine, and some other uncommon compounds [39].

Emergence of Modern Wound Dressing Technologies

A major breakthrough in wound care came during the 19th century with the introduction of antiseptic theory and techniques. This development laid the foundation for modern wound dressing practices, which began to take shape in the 20th century. Traditional wound dressings of earlier times included gauze, lint, plasters, bandages (made from natural or synthetic materials), and cotton wool, which were mostly dry materials used as primary or secondary dressings. Wet-to-dry dressings were also widely used for cleaning wounds. Additionally, linen strips soaked in oil, natural ointments, plant extracts, or grease and then covered with plasters were commonly applied to support healing [40].

The 20th century marked a transformative period in wound care, shifting from basic and often unhygienic methods to scientifically driven, modern techniques. A major turning point was the move away from the outdated belief that wounds healed best when left dry and uncovered. Instead, research began to emphasize the advantages of maintaining a moist wound environment to accelerate healing and reduce complications [41–43].

Early 20th Century

Though cotton gauze had been introduced in the late 19th century, its use continued into the early 20th century alongside traditional dressings. However, growing awareness of hygiene and infection control began influencing wound care practices. In the early 20th century, particularly during World War I, wound care began evolving with the introduction of important medical innovations such as aseptic surgical techniques, X-ray imaging, and blood transfusions. Although traditional methods like wound cleansing and basic bandaging were still widely practiced, the adoption of more effective materials—such as absorbent dressings like "gamgee" and antiseptic agents like iodine –improved outcomes. A major breakthrough came in the 1940s with the introduction of antibiotics like penicillin, which significantly reduced infection rates and marked a transformative shift in modern wound management [5,43,44].

Mid-20th Century

The concept of "moist wound healing" (MWH) gained scientific backing, with studies showing that moisture significantly speeds up the healing process by supporting tissue regeneration and reducing scab formation.

In the 1960s, George Winter's research revolutionized wound care by proving that wounds heal faster in a moist environment than in a dry one. This was a major departure from the traditional belief that wounds should be exposed to air to dry out and form a scab. At the time, it was thought that scabbing protected the wound and promoted healing, but Winter's experiments, particularly on pig skin (which closely resembles human skin), showed otherwise. He found that wounds kept moist healed nearly twice as fast as those left to dry [45].

This discovery led to a fundamental shift in wound management, forming the basis of what is now known as **moist wound healing (MWH)**. Since then, multiple benefits of moist wound environments have been recognized:

- **Faster epithelialization**: Moisture accelerates the migration of skin cells, helping the wound close more quickly.
- **Lower risk of infection**: A sealed, moist environment acts as a barrier to external bacteria and supports natural immune defense mechanisms.
- **Reduced scarring**: Moist conditions minimize the need for scab formation, leading to smoother tissue regeneration and less visible scarring.
- **Less pain**: Keeping nerve endings moist reduces irritation and pain often caused by dry, exposed wounds.
- **Enhanced cellular activity**: Cells involved in repair—like fibroblasts and keratinocytes—function more effectively in a hydrated environment.
- **Stable wound temperature**: Moist dressings help maintain optimal warmth, which is essential for proper enzyme activity and tissue repair.

Following Winter's work, the development of **advanced wound dressings**—such as hydrocolloids, hydrogels, polyurethane foams, and transparent films—began. These products are designed to maintain an ideal moist environment while managing exudate (wound fluid), preventing infection, and ensuring patient comfort.

Today, MWH is considered a gold standard in modern wound care, widely supported by clinical evidence and used across hospitals and clinics around the world. Winter's research not only challenged outdated practices but also laid the foundation for innovations that have improved healing outcomes and patient experiences [3].

Late 20th Century

This period saw the development of advanced dressings like hydrocolloids, hydrogels, and alginates. These were tailored to address specific wound types and needs, from moisture management to infection control.

Key Developments

- **Occlusive dressings**: Introduced in the latter half of the century, these dressings create a sealed, moist environment that supports faster healing by promoting angiogenesis (formation of new blood vessels) and collagen synthesis while reducing infection risks.
- **Modern synthetic materials**: Materials like polyurethane foams and hydrogels became standard due to their effectiveness in absorbing exudate, retaining moisture, and enhancing patient comfort.
- **Scientific validation**: Pioneering research, notably by George Winter, provided clear evidence that wounds healed more efficiently in a moist environment, prompting a paradigm shift in clinical practice.

During the mid-20th century, modern wound dressings develop from the introduction of the "moist wound healing theory," which gained significant attraction in the 1960s when research confirmed that wounds heal more effectively in a moist environment. This paradigm shift moved clinical practice away from traditional dry dressings and laid the foundation for the development of advanced wound care materials. Early wound care practices had relied on dry, uncovered wounds or simple gauze, such as the woven absorbent cotton gauze introduced in 1891, offering limited protection and healing benefits. However, the introduction of the MWH concept revolutionized the approach. New types of moist bandages emerged soon after [45,34].

The first wave of modern dressings emerged mainly based on moist healing, including transparent films and hydrocolloids. These dressings not only retained moisture but also managed wound exudate and provided a barrier against contaminants. The next decades saw the expansion of dressing types, including foams and hydrogels, each designed to cater to specific wound conditions, such as varying levels of exudate or the need for cooling and pain relief [34].

By the mid-1990s, wound care advanced further with the development of specialized synthetic dressings such as alginates (derived from seaweed), silver-infused dressings for infection control, and growth factor-enriched formulations to promote tissue regeneration. The field also embraced bioengineered skin substitutes and cellular therapies, reflecting a growing emphasis on tailoring treatment to the wound's phase of healing and individual patient needs. These advancements continue to shape modern wound care by combining scientific innovation with patient-centered strategies [46–48].

Research on MWH demonstrates that maintaining a moist environment significantly enhances the healing process and reduces the risk of infection. Occlusive dressings, which retain moisture, have proven more effective than non-occlusive ones in preventing infections, reporting lower infection rates (3.3% vs. 5.4%, $p < 0.001$). This approach supports cellular activity, pain relief, and addresses psychological concerns such as stress and social isolation linked to chronic wounds [34,46].

The studies reviewed, including 50 controlled trials, highlight the importance of choosing dressings based on the wound's condition and healing stage. Moisture balance is essential; excessive exudate can cause leakage and discomfort, whereas insufficient moisture delays healing. Wound Bed Preparation (WBP), a structured approach to wound care, further enhances treatment outcomes by optimizing the wound environment. MWH is a clinically proven method that accelerates healing, improves patient comfort, and lowers complications, making it a cornerstone of modern wound management [49]. However, not all wounds are suitable for the moist dressings, some wounds are intentionally kept open to make them dry and to form natural protective layers such as burn wounds [50].

Advanced and Smart Wound Dressings (21st Century)

The 21st century's lead in wound dressing was the development and research based on wound healing support for different kinds of wounds through bioactive wound dressings. Bioactive wound dressings in the 21st century represent a transformative leap in wound care by combining advanced materials with therapeutic functionality to enhance healing outcomes. These dressings go beyond simply covering wounds—they actively interact with the wound environment to promote faster and more effective healing. Incorporating natural and synthetic polymers, antimicrobial agents, and even responsive smart technologies, bioactive dressings address critical wound care factors such as moisture regulation, infection control, and inflammation management [51–53].

Natural materials like collagen, chitosan, alginates, and hyaluronic acid are widely used in these dressings due to their biocompatibility and biological activity, while synthetic polymers such as polyurethane and polyethylene oxide offer added benefits like structural integrity and controlled drug release. Many bioactive dressings are infused with antimicrobial agents, including silver nanoparticles, honey, and antiseptics, to combat wound infection—an increasingly vital function in the face of growing antibiotic resistance [54–56].

In terms of delivery systems, these dressings often include anti-inflammatory agents, analgesics, or growth factors directly embedded in the matrix for localized treatment. Hydrogels and nanofibers are frequently employed due to their moisture-retaining properties and structural similarity to the extracellular matrix, which supports cellular migration and tissue regeneration. Some of the most innovative dressings now incorporate smart features, such as sensors that monitor wound pH, temperature, or bacterial activity and respond by releasing therapeutic agents accordingly [57–59].

Popular examples of bioactive dressings include those made from honey, hyaluronic acid, collagen, and bacterial cellulose. The benefits are substantial: improved healing rates through enhanced cellular activity, infection prevention, localized and sustained drug delivery, pain reduction, and fewer dressing changes—all of which contribute to better patient comfort and outcomes [60].

However, challenges remain. Many bioactive dressings require more rigorous clinical validation, and their high cost can limit accessibility in some healthcare settings. Ongoing material innovation is crucial, especially to improve biocompatibility, biodegradability, and the precision of drug delivery. Looking forward, personalized wound dressings tailored to specific wound types and patient needs are a promising direction in this evolving field, potentially revolutionizing how both acute and chronic wounds are treated [61,62].

Nanotechnology and drug delivery systems are reshaping the field of wound care by making dressings smarter, more efficient, and more responsive to the healing environment. These cutting-edge advancements allow for better infection control and faster healing, often at reduced overall treatment costs. At the core of this innovation are nanomaterials, which bring unique properties that enhance how drugs are delivered and how wounds are managed [63,64].

One of the main advantages of nanotechnology is targeted drug delivery. Nanoparticles can be engineered to carry therapeutic agents directly to the wound site, ensuring that treatment is concentrated where it's needed most while reducing unwanted side effects elsewhere in the body. In addition, many of these systems offer sustained drug release, maintaining consistent therapeutic levels over time and reducing the need for frequent dressing changes. Another key benefit is biocompatibility [65–66]. Many nanomaterials, especially those derived from natural polymers like chitosan or collagen, are not only well-tolerated by the body but also actively support tissue regeneration. Some nanoparticles, such as silver or zinc oxide, even possess inherent antimicrobial properties, helping prevent or control infections. Nanotechnology has also enabled the development of "smart" wound dressings. These advanced dressings can monitor conditions such as pH, moisture, and temperature and respond automatically by releasing appropriate therapeutic agents essentially acting as both a sensor and a treatment system in one [63,66].

Specific applications include:

- Hydrogels infused with nanoparticles to keep the wound moist and deliver drugs.
- Nanofibers, which form scaffolds that promote cell growth and tissue repair.
- Metallic or oxide nanoparticles for antimicrobial and anti-inflammatory effects.
- Nanoemulsions, which improve drug penetration deep into the wound bed.

Looking ahead, the field is moving toward personalized wound care—customizing dressings based on individual patient and wound characteristics. The development of smart bandages with built-in sensors and controlled drug release is already underway. Additionally, combining nanotechnology with stem cell therapy and regenerative factors could significantly improve recovery in chronic or complex wounds. However, some challenges remain. Producing these nanomaterials on a large scale while keeping costs reasonable is still a hurdle. Regulatory approval processes can also be lengthy and complicated. Most importantly, while early results are promising, long-term safety and biocompatibility of nanomaterials still require more research. Nanotechnology is opening exciting new possibilities in wound care, with the potential to significantly improve healing outcomes, especially in complex or chronic cases [67–69].

Current times and future prospectives are focused on smart wound dressings of the 21st century, which integrate **biosensors, colorimetric sensors**, and **wireless monitoring systems** to track wound conditions such as pH, temperature, and moisture in real time. These advanced bandages support early detection of infection and enable personalized care interventions [70,71].

- A sensor-equipped bandage for **real-time pH monitoring** has been shown to correlate wound pH levels with healing stages, using flexible electronics to help clinicians make timely decisions [70]. Other devices combine **pH-sensitive dyes (like bromothymol blue)** that change color from yellow to blue when the wound pH rises above 7, indicating infection. These have been successfully applied to commercial dressings like Aquacel and Promogran.

pH monitoring wound dressings represent a modern advancement in wound care by offering a non-invasive and continuous method for assessing healing progress. These dressings are designed to detect changes in the pH level of wound exudate, which is a critical marker of infection, inflammation, or delayed healing. By incorporating pH-sensitive materials, such as dyes that change color in response to acidic or alkaline environments, these dressings allow clinicians and caregivers to visually assess the wound without needing to remove the dressing, thereby minimizing discomfort and reducing the risk of further contamination. Common types of these dressings include hydrogels, electrospun fibers, and polymer films embedded with natural or synthetic pH indicators. Some innovative examples involve the use of natural compounds like *Curcuma longa* extract or anthocyanins derived from red cabbage, which are integrated into hydrogels or nanocellulose matrices to provide clear and visible color changes. Optical fiber-based systems are also being explored for more precise, sensor-driven monitoring. The benefits of such dressings include early detection of complications, improved clinical decision-making, fewer dressing changes, and potentially lower healthcare costs. Their ability to continuously monitor wound conditions makes them a promising tool for enhancing patient outcomes in both acute and chronic wound management [70].

- Several waterproof **"smart" dressings** detect infection parameters (pH, temperature, moisture) via microelectronic, colorimetric, or electrochemical sensors and transmit this data wirelessly for remote monitoring [72,73].
- Novel designs feature **liquid pathways** that drain excess wound fluid while simultaneously sensing pH changes, all in one wearable device ideal for chronic wounds management [74,75].
- Flexible and electronically printed wound dressings represent a new generation of advanced medical technology that combines flexible electronics with conventional dressing materials. These smart dressings are capable of continuously monitoring critical wound parameters such as temperature, pH, and moisture levels in real time. Some versions are equipped with embedded sensors that can detect early signs of infection and even trigger targeted therapeutic responses when needed. By enabling timely intervention and personalized treatment, these dressings aim to enhance the overall wound healing process, minimize complications, and reduce the need for frequent manual inspections or dressing changes. Flexible electronics printed on biocompatible materials enable **wearable "lab-on-a-bandage" systems**, collecting wound biomarkers and transmitting alerts remotely—potentially revolutionizing outpatient care [76,77].

These **smart dressings** bring multiple benefits:

- **Timely infection detection** without disturbing the wound.
- **Dynamic wound monitoring** to support clinical decisions.

- **Remote healthcare integration**, enabling doctors to track healing via smartphone or cloud platforms.
- **Reduced infection risk, better healing outcomes**, and improved patient comfort.

Challenges and Future Prospects

Current wound dressing technologies face several challenges in effectively managing complex wounds and adapting to dynamic healing environments. Many traditional dressings are passive, lacking the ability to respond to changes in wound conditions or provide real-time feedback. This often leads to delayed treatment decisions, especially in cases of infection or inflammation. Moreover, existing dressings are not always ideal for wounds located on high-stress or mobile areas such as joints and the neck, where flexibility and adherence are crucial. Pain and discomfort during dressing changes are also common issues, particularly with dressings that adhere tightly to the wound bed [41,78].

Another significant limitation is the risk of infection, especially with gauze-based dressings that are prone to bacterial contamination. Additionally, frequent dressing changes and clinical assessments not only increase the overall treatment cost but also place a considerable burden on healthcare systems. Material limitations—such as poor biodegradability, limited biocompatibility, or inadequate mechanical strength—further restrict the performance and effectiveness of current dressings [79].

Specific examples illustrate these limitations. Hydrocolloid dressings, while effective for some wound types, are not ideal for infected wounds and may cause maceration if exudate levels are high. Hydrogels support MWH but can easily detach and may not protect against infection. Foam dressings offer cushioning but can restrict mobility and are less suitable for infected wounds. Traditional gauzes can cool the wound through evaporation and are easily contaminated, potentially hindering the healing process. To overcome these issues, research is increasingly focused on developing smart wound dressings equipped with integrated sensors and drug delivery systems. These next-generation dressings aim to actively monitor wound conditions, provide real-time diagnostic information, and respond therapeutically to promote faster and more effective healing [80–82].

Future advancements in wound dressing technologies aim to address critical challenges such as managing chronic wounds, integrating intelligent monitoring systems, enhancing infection control, and improving patient comfort. Chronic wounds, such as diabetic foot ulcers and venous leg ulcers, remain difficult to treat due to their complex pathophysiology and the presence of comorbidities. Next-generation dressings are expected to include bioactive agents, growth factors, and anti-inflammatory compounds to specifically target these complications and support tissue regeneration. One of the most promising developments lies in the field of smart wound dressings. These intelligent systems are designed to monitor wound parameters like pH, temperature, and moisture levels in real time and deliver drugs on demand based on the wound's condition. Smart dressings have the potential to enable early detection of infections, personalize treatments, and significantly reduce the frequency of dressing changes and hospital visits—ultimately lowering healthcare costs and improving patient outcomes [83–85].

Infection control, particularly the management of biofilms bacterial colonies highly resistant to antibiotics, is another pressing concern. Future dressings are likely to include anti-biofilm technologies and advanced antimicrobial agents capable of disrupting these resilient structures. Material innovation also plays a crucial role in next-generation dressings. There is a growing interest in developing biocompatible, biodegradable, and mechanically robust materials, including natural polymers and engineered nanomaterials. These materials can be tailored to support different wound types and healing stages, offering more targeted and effective care [83,86].

Smart dressings are emerging as a powerful tool in the move toward personalized wound care. By integrating tiny sensors and drug delivery systems, these advanced dressings can track key indicators like temperature, pH, and bacterial presence directly at the wound site. Based on this real-time information, they can respond by releasing targeted treatments such as antibiotics or growth factors to support and accelerate healing. Despite their potential, there are still hurdles to overcome. Making these dressings both affordable and reliable, especially in a wide range of wound conditions, and ensuring they can be smoothly adopted in everyday clinical settings, remains a significant challenge [51,58,87].

One of the most promising directions for the future of wound care is the development of personalized wound dressings, designed to meet the unique needs of each patient and the specific nature of their wound. Achieving this will require a more in-depth understanding of the intricate biological processes that influence healing. By aligning dressing design with these individual factors, care can become far more precise and effective. Smart dressings, which are capable of real-time monitoring and delivering medication directly where it's needed, represent a major step forward in this direction, making personalized wound care not just a concept, but a practical and achievable goal [58,87,88].

Comfort and usability remain essential considerations. Dressings that are soft, non-adherent, easy to apply and remove, and potentially self-healing can enhance patient comfort and compliance. Emerging research explores self-removable and self-repairing materials that minimize trauma and disturbance to the wound bed during dressing changes. Personalized wound care is expected to become a future norm. Customized dressings, adaptable in composition, structure, and therapeutic delivery based on individual wound characteristics and real-time sensor data, will offer tailored solutions for more effective wound management [89–92].

Summary

The evolution of wound dressings represents a remarkable transformation from ancient, rudimentary practices to the modern-day application of advanced biomedical science and technology. Historically, wound care was largely empirical, guided by trial, tradition, and basic observation. Materials such as honey, animal fats, plant extracts, and grease-soaked cloths were used to cover wounds, not necessarily to heal them but to shield them from further harm. These early methods, though primitive, laid the foundation for centuries of empirical healing, long before germ theory or cellular biology could explain the mechanisms at play.

A major shift occurred in the 19th century with the rise of antiseptic techniques, particularly through the work of Joseph Lister, who introduced carbolic acid to reduce surgical infections. This was coupled with the broader acceptance of Louis Pasteur's germ theory, revolutionizing both surgical and wound care practices by identifying microorganisms as the root cause of infection. The antiseptic era significantly lowered mortality rates and marked a new understanding that wound environments must be protected not just physically, but biologically. This era also saw the rise of sterilized cotton gauze and lint, which remained dominant throughout the early 20th century.

The next revolutionary moment came in the 1960s, when George Winter demonstrated that wounds healed faster in moist conditions than in dry ones. This discovery contradicted centuries of medical doctrine and led to the concept of MWH. The realization that maintaining a moist environment could enhance epithelialization, reduce pain, and minimize scarring shifted the paradigm of wound care entirely. It catalyzed the development of modern dressings—hydrogels, hydrocolloids, foams, alginates, and films—that could maintain moisture, absorb exudate, protect against infection, and support cellular activity.

In recent decades, wound dressings have evolved beyond passive coverings into active therapeutic agents. Bioactive dressings incorporating growth factors, enzymes, antimicrobial agents, and tissue-regenerating compounds now form an integral part of modern wound management. These dressings not only address the wound environment but also interact with biological processes at the molecular level to accelerate healing, manage pain, and reduce infection risk. The introduction of nanotechnology and smart materials has enabled the creation of dressings that can monitor wound parameters like pH, temperature, and moisture in real time, and respond dynamically to changes by releasing appropriate therapeutic agents.

Despite these advancements, significant challenges remain. Chronic wounds such as diabetic foot ulcers, pressure ulcers, and venous leg ulcers continue to place a heavy burden on patients and healthcare systems. Infection control, particularly biofilm-associated infections, remains a critical area requiring innovative antimicrobial strategies. Additionally, issues of cost-effectiveness, accessibility, patient compliance, and dressing-related pain during removal continue to influence treatment outcomes. Material science must continue to evolve to produce dressings that are not only effective but also biocompatible, biodegradable, and tailored to specific wound types and healing stages.

Looking ahead, the future of wound care lies in the integration of personalized medicine, real-time diagnostics, and responsive therapies. Smart dressings embedded with flexible electronics and sensors are being developed to offer clinicians real-time data, potentially transforming wound care into a proactive, rather than reactive, discipline. Personalized wound care solutions—where dressing composition and therapeutic payloads are customized based on the patient's physiology and wound status—are likely to become standard. Research into self-healing materials,

AI-driven monitoring systems, and regenerative therapies using stem cells and tissue scaffolds holds tremendous promise.

In conclusion, the journey of wound dressing evolution is a testament to humanity's enduring quest to heal and protect. What began as simple coverings has now become a sophisticated blend of science, engineering, and medicine, an essential component of modern healthcare that not only saves limbs but lives. With continued interdisciplinary collaboration, wound care will continue to improve, ensuring faster healing, better patient outcomes, and a higher quality of life for millions around the world.

REFERENCES

1. M. A. Gilmore, 'Phases of wound healing', *Dimens. Oncol. Nurs.*, vol. 5, no. 3, pp. 32–34, 1991.
2. S. Maxson, E. A. Lopez, D. Yoo, A. Danilkovitch-Miagkova, and M. A. LeRoux, 'Concise review: role of mesenchymal stem cells in wound repair', *Stem Cells Transl. Med.*, vol. 1, no. 2, pp. 142–149, 2012, doi:10.5966/sctm.2011-0018.
3. J. B. Shah, 'The history of wound care', *J. Am. Coll. Certif. Wound Spec.*, vol. 3, no. 3, pp. 65–66, 2012, doi:10.1016/j.jcws.2012.04.002.
4. W. Ahmad, Z. Aquil, and S. S. Alam, 'Historical background of wound care', *Hamdan Med. J.*, vol. 13, no. 4, pp. 189–195, 2020. doi:10.4103/HMJ.HMJ_37_20.
5. S. Bhattacharya, 'Wound healing through the ages', *Indian J. Plast. Surg. Off. Publ. Assoc. Plast. Surg. India*, vol. 45, no. 2, pp. 177–179, 2012, doi:10.4103/0970-0358.101255.
6. G. Majno, *The Healing Hand: Man and Wound in the Ancient World.* Harvard University Press, 1975.
7. V. S. Kumar and V. Navaratnam, 'Neem (Azadirachta indica): prehistory to contemporary medicinal uses to humankind', *Asian Pac. J. Trop. Biomed.*, vol. 3, no. 7, pp. 505–514, 2013, doi:10.1016/S2221-1691(13)60105-7.
8. R. D. Forrest, 'Early history of wound treatment', *J. R. Soc. Med.*, vol. 75, 1982, doi:10.1177/014107688207500310.
9. C. Yapijakis, 'Hippocrates of Kos, the father of clinical medicine, and *Asclepiades of Bithynia*, the father of molecular medicine: review', *In Vivo*, vol. 23, no. 4, pp. 507–514, 2009.
10. Encyclopædia Britannica, Inc., *Hippocrates|Biography, Works, & Facts|Britannica.* https://www.britannica.com/biography/Hippocrates (accessed August 5, 2025).
11. RCPE, *The History of Germ Theory in the College Collections.* Royal College of Physicians of Edinburgh. https://www.rcpe.ac.uk/heritage/heritage-blog/history-germ-theory-college-collections (accessed August 5, 2025).
12. N. Papavramidou, V. Thomaidis, and A. Fiska, 'The ancient surgical bloodletting method of arteriotomy', *J. Vasc. Surg.*, vol. 54, no. 6, pp. 1842–1844, 2011, doi:10.1016/j.jvs.2011.05.100.
13. J. W. Blatchford, 'The surgery of Celsus' De Medicina', *Ann. Surg. Open*, vol. 5, no. 3, p. e482, 2024, doi:10.1097/AS9.0000000000000482.
14. S. Tan, 'Medicine in stamps Galen (130–201A.D.): history's most enduring medic', *Sing. Med. J.*, vol. 36, no. 6, pp. 641–642, 2002.
15. G. I. Broughton, J. E. Janis, and C. E. Attinger, 'A brief history of wound care', *Plast. Reconstr. Surg.*, vol. 117, no. 7S, p. 6S, 2006, doi:10.1097/01.prs.0000225429.76355.dd.
16. Longwood University, *Medieval Surgeons Surprisingly Skilled in Healing.* https://www.longwood.edu/news/2015/medieval-surgeons-surprisingly-skilled-in-healing/ (accessed August 5, 2025).

17. P. Hernigou, J. Hernigou, and M. Scarlat, 'Medieval surgery (eleventh–thirteenth century): barber surgeons and warfare surgeons in France', *Int. Orthop.*, vol. 45, no. 7, pp. 1891–1898, 2021, doi:10.1007/s00264-021-05043-z.
18. H. D. Kramer, 'The germ theory and the early public health program in the United States', *Bull. Hist. Med.*, vol. 22, no. 3, pp. 233–247, 1948.
19. R. Vallery-Radot, *The Life of Pasteur.* National Library of Medicine Institution. https://catalog.nlm.nih.gov/discovery/fulldisplay/alma9918881184306676/01NLM_INST:01NLM_INST (accessed July 23, 2025).
20. P. Debré and E. Forster, *Louis Pasteur.* Johns Hopkins University Press, 1998. doi:10.56021/9780801858086.
21. W. W. Sager, E. B. Vedder, and C. Rosenberg, 'Antiseptics and wound healing', *Am. J. Surg.*, vol. 38, no. 2, pp. 348–350, 1937, doi:10.1016/S0002-9610(37)90445-8.
22. C. T. Ambrose, 'The conquest of pus—a history of bitumen, creosote and carbolic acid', *J. Anc. Dis. Prev. Remedies*, vol. 6, no. 2, 2018, doi:10.4172/2329-8731.1000179.
23. J. R. Cormack, 'A treatise on the chemical, medicinal, and physiological properties of creosote, illustrated by experiments, &c.', *Medico-Chir. Rev.*, vol. 25, no. 49, pp. 69–71, 1836.
24. F. W. Tilley, 'Phenol coefficients', *Am. J. Public Health*, vol. 11, no. 6, pp. 513–519, 1921, doi:10.2105/ajph.11.6.513.
25. G. F. Reddish, 'Limitations of the phenol coefficient', *Industrial & Engineering Chemistry*, vol. 29, no. 9, pp. 1044–1047, 1937. doi:10.1021/ie50333a017 (accessed July 30, 2025).
26. M. Worboys, 'Joseph Lister and the performance of antiseptic surgery', *Notes Rec. R. Soc.*, vol. 67, no. 3, pp. 199–209, 2013, doi:10.1098/rsnr.2013.0028.
27. J. Y. Simpson, 'Carbolic acid and its compounds in surgery', *The Lancet*, vol. 90, no. 2305, pp. 546–549, 1867, doi:10.1016/S0140-6736(02)56223-1.
28. S. N. Michaleas, K. Laios, A. Charalabopoulos, G. Samonis, and M. Karamanou, 'Joseph Lister (1827–1912): a pioneer of antiseptic surgery', *Cureus*, vol. 14, no. 12, p. e32777, 2022, doi:10.7759/cureus.32777.
29. P. Dutkowski, O. De Rougemont, and P.-A. Clavien, 'Alexis carrel: genius, innovator and ideologist', *Am. J. Transplant.*, vol. 8, no. 10, pp. 1998–2003, 2008, doi:10.1111/j.1600-6143.2008.02364.x.
30. G. Vernon, 'Alexis Carrel: "father of transplant surgery" and supporter of eugenics', *Br. J. Gen. Pract.*, vol. 69, no. 684, p. 352, 2019, doi:10.3399/bjgp19X704441.
31. P. Sipos, H. Gyõry, K. Hagymási, P. Ondrejka, and A. Blázovics, 'Special wound healing methods used in ancient Egypt and the mythological background', *World J. Surg.*, vol. 28, no. 2, pp. 211–216, 2004, doi:10.1007/s00268-003-7073-x.
32. A. A. Rogers, R. S. Walmsley, M. G. Rippon, and P. G. Bowler, 'Adsorption of serum-derived proteins by primary dressings: implications for dressing adhesion to wounds', *J. Wound Care,* vol. 8, no. 8, pp. 403–406, 1999. https://www.magonlinelibrary.com/doi/abs/10.12968/jowc.1999.8.8.25910 (accessed July 31, 2025).
33. D. Queen, H. Orsted, H. Sanada, and G. Sussman, 'A dressing history', *Int. Wound J.*, vol. 1, no. 1, pp. 59–77, 2004, doi:10.1111/j.1742-4801.2004.0009.x.
34. H. Ellis, *The Cambridge Illustrated History of Surgery*, 2nd edn. Cambridge University Press, 2009. https://cir.nii.ac.jp/crid/1970586434841502729 (accessed July 31, 2025).
35. H. Ellis and S. Abdalla, *A History of Surgery*, 3rd edn. CRC Press, 2018. doi:10.1201/9780429461743.
36. R. A. Pollock, 'Triage and management of the injured in World War I: the diuturnity of Antoine De Page and a Belgian Colleague', *Craniomaxillofacial Trauma Reconstr.*, vol. 1, no. 1, pp. 63–70, 2008, doi:10.1055/s-0028-1098965.
37. K. V. Iserson and J. C. Moskop, 'Triage in medicine, Part I: concept, history, and types', *Ann. Emerg. Med.*, vol. 49, no. 3, pp. 275–281, 2007, doi:10.1016/j.annemergmed.2006.05.019.

38. R. J. White, 'An historical overview of the use of silver in wound management', *Br. J. Community Nurs.*, vol. 6, no. Supl, pp. 3–8, 2001, doi:10.12968/bjcn.2001.6.Supl.12619.
39. https://www.worldwidewounds.com/2004/february/Cooper/Topical-Ant.
40. A. N. M. Alamgir, 'Fibers, surgical dressings, and bandages of natural origin', in *Therapeutic Use of Medicinal Plants and Their Extracts: Pharmacognosy*, A. N. M. Alamgir (Ed.), Springer, 2017, vol. 1, pp. 355–378. doi:10.1007/978-3-319-63862-1_8.
41. E. Rezvani Ghomi, S. Khalili, S. Nouri Khorasani, R. Esmaeely Neisiany, and S. Ramakrishna, 'Wound dressings: current advances and future directions', *J. Appl. Polym. Sci.*, vol. 136, no. 27, p. 47738, 2019. doi:10.1002/app.47738.
42. S. D. Bhoyar, K. Malhotra, and B. Madke, 'Dressing materials: a comprehensive review', *J. Cutan. Aesthetic Surg.*, vol. 16, no. 2, pp. 81–89, 2023, doi:10.4103/JCAS.JCAS_163_22.
43. Flushing Hospital Medical Center, *Wound Healing through the Ages.* Health Beat Health Beat. https://flushinghospital.org/newsletter/wound-healing-through-the-ages-2/ (accessed August 5, 2025).
44. BBC Bitesize, *Developments in Medicine in the Early 20th Century—Medicine on the British Sector of the Western Front, 1914–1918- GCSE History Revision—Edexcel.* BBC Bitesize. https://www.bbc.co.uk/bitesize/guides/z8p4cmn/revision/5 (accessed August 5, 2025).
45. G. D. Winter, 'Formation of the scab and the rate of epithelization of superficial wounds in the skin of the young domestic pig', *Nature*, vol. 193, pp. 293–294, 1962, doi:10.1038/193293a0.
46. Z. Liang, P. Lai, J. Zhang, Q. Lai, and L. He, 'Impact of moist wound dressing on wound healing time: a meta-analysis', *Int. Wound J.*, vol. 20, no. 10, pp. 4410–4421, 2023, doi:10.1111/iwj.14319.
47. S. A. Alobaid, S. Shrestha, M. Tasseff, B. Wang, M. L. van Hoek, and P. K. Dutta, 'Activity of silver-zinc nanozeolite-based antibiofilm wound dressings in an in vitro biofilm model and comparison with commercial dressings', *Discov. Nano*, vol. 20, no. 1, p. 26, 2025, doi:10.1186/s11671-025-04208-8.
48. K. Ousey, C. Roberts, and D. Leaper, 'Silver-containing dressings', in *Wound Healing Biomaterials*, M. S. Ågren (Ed.), Woodhead Publishing, 2016, pp. 403–437. doi:10.1016/B978-1-78242-456-7.00020-9.
49. M. Varga, *Moist Wound Healing : Past and Present a Historical Perspective on the Importance of Moist Wound Healing.* Academia.edu, 2021. https://www.academia.edu/64053324/Moist_Wound_Healing_Past_and_Present_A_historical_perspective_on_the_importance_of_moist_wound_healing (accessed August 3, 2025).
50. G. D. Winter and J. T. Scales, 'Effect of air drying and dressings on the surface of a wound', *Nature*, vol. 197, no. 4862, pp. 91–92, 1963, doi:10.1038/197091b0.
51. A. Alberts, D.-I. Tudorache, A.-G. Niculescu, and A. M. Grumezescu, 'Advancements in wound dressing materials: highlighting recent progress in hydrogels, foams, and antimicrobial dressings', *Gels*, vol. 11, no. 2, Art. no. 2, 2025, doi:10.3390/gels11020123.
52. F. Moradifar, N. Sepahdoost, P. Tavakoli, and A. Mirzapoor, 'Multi-functional dressings for recovery and screenable treatment of wounds: a review', *Heliyon*, vol. 11, no. 1, p. e41465, 2025, doi:10.1016/j.heliyon.2024.e41465.
53. Byram Healthcare, *Wound-Care Type-of-Wound-Dressing.* Byram Healthcare, 2025. https://www.byramhealthcare.com/wound-care/type-of-wound-dressing (accessed August 5, 2025).
54. G. Yaşayan, E. Alarçin, A. Bal-Öztürk, and M. Avci-Adali, 'Natural polymers for wound dressing applications', in *Studies in Natural Products Chemistry*, vol. 74, Atta-ur-Rahman (Ed.), in Bioactive Natural Products, vol. 74., Elsevier, 2022, pp. 367–441. doi:10.1016/B978-0-323-91099-6.00004-9.

55. T. T.-P. Ho et al., 'Natural polymer-based materials for wound healing applications', *Adv. NanoBiomed. Res.*, vol. 4, no. 5, Article e202300131, 2024. doi:10.1002/anbr.202300131.
56. B. Sheokand, M. Vats, A. Kumar, C. M. Srivastava, I. Bahadur, and S. R. Pathak, 'Natural polymers used in the dressing materials for wound healing: past, present and future', *J. Polym. Sci.*, vol. 61, no. 14, pp. 1389–1414, 2023, doi:10.1002/pol.20220734.
57. P. Price, K. Fogh, C. Glynn, D. L. Krasner, J. Osterbrink, and R. G. Sibbald, 'Why combine a foam dressing with ibuprofen for wound pain and moist wound healing?' *Int. Wound J.*, vol. 4, pp. 1–3, 2007. doi:10.1111/j.1742-481X.2007.00310.x.
58. L. Su, Y. Jia, L. Fu, K. Guo, and S. Xie, 'The emerging progress on wound dressings and their application in clinic wound management', *Heliyon*, vol. 9, no. 12, p. e22520, 2023, doi:10.1016/j.heliyon.2023.e22520.
59. Y. Liu, W. Chen, Y. Gao, and K. Wei, 'Anti-inflammatory dressing based on hyaluronic acid and hydroxyethyl starch for wound healing', *Int. J. Biol. Macromol.*, vol. 282, p. 137078, 2024, doi:10.1016/j.ijbiomac.2024.137078.
60. M. G. Nur et al., 'Recent advances in bioactive wound dressings', *Wound Repair Regen. Off. Publ. Wound Heal. Soc. Eur. Tissue Repair Soc.*, vol. 33, no. 1, p. e13233, 2025, doi:10.1111/wrr.13233.
61. G. Polverino, F. Russo, and F. D'Andrea, 'Bioactive dressing: a new algorithm in wound healing', *J. Clin. Med.*, vol. 13, no. 9, p. 2488, 2024, doi:10.3390/jcm13092488.
62. R. Yu, H. Zhang, and B. Guo, 'Conductive biomaterials as bioactive wound dressing for wound healing and skin tissue engineering', *Nano-Micro Lett.*, vol. 14, p. 1. doi:10.1007/s40820-021-00751-y.
63. A. T. T. Prabhu, V. Baliga, S. Bhat, S. T. Thenkondar, Y. Nayak, and U. Y. Nayak, 'Transforming wound management: nanomaterials and their clinical impact', *Pharmaceutics*, vol. 15, no. 5, p. 1560, 2023. doi:10.3390/pharmaceutics15051560.
64. W. Wang, K.-j. Lu, C.-h. Yu, Q.-l. Huang, and Y.-Z. Du, 'Nano-drug delivery systems in wound treatment and skin regeneration', *J. Nanobiotechnol.,* vol. 17, p. 82. doi:10.1186/s12951-019-0514-y.
65. A. Khan, H. M. Mostafa, K. H. Almohammed, N. Singla, Z. Bhatti, and M. I. Siddique, 'Advances in nanotechnology in drug delivery systems for burn wound healing: a review', *Biomed. Pharmacol. J.*, vol. 18, pp. 373–386. https://biomedpharmajournal.org/vol18no1/advances-in-nanotechnology-in-drug-delivery-systems-for-burn-wound-healing-a-review/ (accessed August 5, 2025).
66. N. K. Rajendran, S. S. D. Kumar, N. N. Houreld, and H. Abrahamse, 'A review on nanoparticle based treatment for wound healing', *J. Drug Deliv. Sci. Technol.*, vol. 44, pp. 421–430, 2018, doi:10.1016/j.jddst.2018.01.009.
67. M. R. Dhondale, A. Jha, M. Kumar, G. Ajmal, G. V. Bonde, and B. Mishra, 'Electrospun nanofiber-based drug delivery platform: advances in diabetic foot ulcer management', *Expert Opin. Drug Deliv.,* vol. 18, no. 1, pp. 25–42, 2020. 10.1080/17425247.2021.1823966
68. P. Jiang et al., 'Current status and progress in research on dressing management for diabetic foot ulcer', *Front. Endocrinol.*, vol. 14, p. 1221705, 2023, doi:10.3389/fendo.2023.1221705.
69. M. Parani, G. Lokhande, A. Singh, and A. K. Gaharwar, 'Engineered nanomaterials for infection control and healing acute and chronic wounds', *ACS Appl. Mater. Interf.*, vol. 8, no. 16, pp. 10049–10069, 2016.doi:10.1021/acsami.6b00291
70. F. Mariani et al., 'Advanced wound dressing for real-time pH monitoring', *ACS Sens.*, vol. 6, no. 6, pp. 2366–2377, 2021, doi:10.1021/acssensors.1c00552.
71. Q. Pang, F. Yang, Z. Jiang, K. Wu, R. Hou, and Y. Zhu, 'Smart wound dressing for advanced wound management: real-time monitoring and on-demand treatment', *Mater. Des.*, vol. 229, p. 111917, 2023, doi:10.1016/j.matdes.2023.111917.

72. J. Wu, X. Fan, J. Ma, W. Wang, and H. Chen, 'Asymmetric wettable, waterproof, and breathable nanofibrous membranes for wound dressings', *ACS Appl. Bio Mater.,* vol. 4, no. 9, pp. 6756–6766, 2021. doi:10.1021/acsabm.0c01624
73. Y. Zheng, X. Chen, L. Li, and M. Chen. 'Waterproof and breathable wound dressing composited by expanded polytetrafluoroethylene backing and hydrogel', *Macromol. Biosci.*, vol. 22, no. 11, p. e2200131, 2022. doi:10.1002/mabi.202200131.
74. E. Szunerits, M. Boukherroub, and R. Gref. 'State-of-the-art and future challenges of smart wound dressings for diabetic foot ulcer treatment', *Adv. NanoBiomed Res.*, 2024. doi:10.1002/anbr.202400040
75. E. Gianino, C. Miller, and J. Gilmore, 'Smart wound dressings for diabetic chronic wounds', *Bioengineering*, vol. 5, no. 3, p. 51, 2018, doi:10.3390/bioengineering5030051.
76. Q. Pang, D. Lou, S. J. Li, G. Wang, B. B. Qiao, S. R. Dong, L. Ma, C. Y. Gao, and Z. H. Wu, 'Smart flexible electronics-integrated wound dressing for real-time monitoring and on-demand treatment of infected wounds', *Adv. Sci.,* vol. 7, no. 6, p. 1902673. doi:10.1002/advs.201902673.
77. H. Ehtesabi, S.-O. Kalji, and L. Movsesian, 'Smartphone-based wound dressings: a mini-review', *Heliyon*, vol. 8, no. 7, p. e09876, 2022, doi:10.1016/j.heliyon.2022.e09876.
78. K. M. Pasaribu et al., 'A review: current trends and future perspectives of bacterial nanocellulose-based wound dressings', *Int. J. Biol. Macromol.*, vol. 279, p. 135602, 2024, doi:10.1016/j.ijbiomac.2024.135602.
79. T. D. Moreira, V. B. Martins, A. H. da Silva Júnior, C. Sayer, P. H. H. de Araújo, and A. P. S. Immich, 'New insights into biomaterials for wound dressings and care: challenges and trends', *Prog. Org. Coat.*, vol. 187, p. 108118, 2024, https://doi.org/10.1016/j.porgcoat.2023.108118.
80. Oncology Nursing Society, *Hydrocolloid and Hydrogel Dressings.* Oncology Nursing Society. https://www.ons.org/clinical-tools/pep/intervention/hydrocolloid-and-hydrogel-dressings (accessed August 5, 2025).
81. ScienceDirect Topics, *Hydrocolloid Dressing: An Overview.* https://www.sciencedirect.com/topics/medicine-and-dentistry/hydrocolloid-dressing (accessed August 5, 2025).
82. P. R. Hartmeier, N. B. Pham, K. Y. Velankar, F. Issa, N. Giannoukakis, and W. S. Meng, 'Hydrogel dressings for chronic wound healing in diabetes: beyond hydration', *J. Pharm. Drug Deliv. Res.*, vol. 10, no. 1, p. 1000197, 2021.
83. V. Gounden and M. Singh, 'Hydrogels and wound healing: current and future prospects', *Gels*, vol. 10, no. 1, p. 43, 2024, doi:10.3390/gels10010043.
84. S. Matoori, A. Veves, and D. J. Mooney, 'Advanced bandages for diabetic wound healing', *Sci. Transl. Med.*, vol. 13, no. 585, p. eabe4839, 2021, doi:10.1126/scitranslmed.abe4839.
85. M. Abrigo, S. L. McArthur, and P. Kingshott, 'Electrospun nanofibers as dressings for chronic wound care: advances, challenges, and future prospects', *Macromol. Biosci.*, vol. 14, no. 6, pp. 772–792, 2014, doi:10.1002/mabi.201300561.
86. A. Bal-Öztürk, B. Özkahraman, Z. Özbaş, G. Yaşayan, E. Tamahkar, and E. Alarçin, 'Advancements and future directions in the antibacterial wound dressings: a review', *J. Biomed. Mater. Res. B Appl. Biomater.* doi:10.1002/jbm.b.34736.
87. H. Derakhshandeh, S. S. Kashaf, F. Aghabaglou, I. Ghanavati, and A. Tamayol, 'Smart bandages: the future of wound care', *Trends Biotechnol.*, vol. 36, no. 12, pp. 1259–1274, 2018, doi:10.1016/j.tibtech.2018.07.007.
88. Linknovate Stories, *Game-Changing Innovations in Wound Healing.* Linknovate Stories. https://blog.linknovate.com/5-game-changing-innovations-in-wound-healing/ (accessed August 5, 2025).
89. S. W. Care, 'Multidisciplinary approach to wound care', *Skilled Wound Care.* https://www.skilledwoundcare.com/post/multidisciplinary-approach-to-wound-care (accessed August 5, 2025).

90. K. Bechert and S. E. Abraham, 'Pain management and wound care', *J. Am. Coll. Certif. Wound Spec.*, vol. 1, no. 2, pp. 65–71, 2009, doi:10.1016/j.jcws.2008.12.001.
91. E. H. Beers, 'Palliative wound care: less is more', *Surg. Clin. North Am.*, vol. 99, no. 5, pp. 899–919, 2019, doi:10.1016/j.suc.2019.06.008.
92. A. W. Care, 'Comfort-focused pain management solutions in wound care', *Adv. Wound Care.* https://advanced-wounds.com/pain-management-solutions/ (accessed August 5, 2025).

3 Nanomaterials for Wound Regeneration

Shagufta Riaz, Sehrish Iftikhar, Maleeha Akram, Hina Shafique, and Aleeza Fatima

INTRODUCTION

Importance of Wound Healing in Medical Science

Wound healing is a critical biological process essential for restoring tissue integrity and preventing complications such as infections and delayed recovery. This intricate mechanism involves the body's response to injury, where damaged tissues are repaired to restore both structural and functional integrity, reducing healthcare costs and advancing treatment modalities. The process of wound healing not only protects against pathogens but also facilitates recovery, thereby enhancing the quality of life for patients [1]. Proper wound healing is critical in maintaining skin integrity, which serves as the body's first line of defense against infections. Disruption can lead to severe complications, including sepsis. The immune response plays a vital role in this process, with phases of inflammation and proliferation crucial for preventing chronic wounds [2,3]. Successful healing restores tissue function, allowing individuals to return to normal activities. This is particularly important in post-amputation care, where effective healing can significantly impact recovery and rehabilitation [3]. Rapid healing minimizes hospital stays and long-term interventions, thus lowering healthcare costs. Efficient wound management can prevent complications that require extensive medical resources [4]. Innovations in wound care, such as advanced dressings and stem cell therapies, are driven by the need for effective healing solutions. These advancements not only improve patient outcomes but also push the boundaries of medical science [5]. For patients with chronic conditions like diabetes, effective wound healing is vital to prevent severe complications, including ulcers and potential amputations [6].

Challenges in Traditional Wound Healing Methods

Traditional wound healing methods have been foundational in medical care, but they face several challenges that limit their effectiveness, especially in addressing complex or chronic wounds. They fail to adequately protect against infections, accelerate healing, and manage moisture, leading to prolonged recovery times and complications. Traditional dressings often lack antimicrobial properties, making wounds vulnerable to microbial contamination. This can lead to chronic infections, which

DOI: 10.1201/9781003616726-4

complicate healing and may require advanced interventions. Conventional treatments do not effectively promote healing, especially for chronic wounds. The absence of advanced therapeutic features, such as growth factors, can result in extended recovery periods [7,8]. Chronic conditions like diabetes and venous insufficiency require targeted therapies that traditional methods do not provide. These methods often overlook the underlying causes of chronic wounds [7,9]. Many traditional dressings fail to maintain the necessary moist environment for optimal healing, which is crucial for cell activity and tissue repair [10]. Simple bandages may not offer sufficient structural support, risking further tissue damage, particularly in complex wounds [7,8]. Traditional wound care often leads to visible scarring (Figure 3.1) due to inadequate modulation of the healing phases. Unlike modern treatments, traditional methods do not incorporate advanced features such as antimicrobial agents or bioactive materials, which are essential for enhancing wound healing. In contrast, emerging therapies, including cellular and immunotherapies, show promise in addressing these limitations by targeting the underlying causes of chronic wounds and enhancing healing processes [7,9].

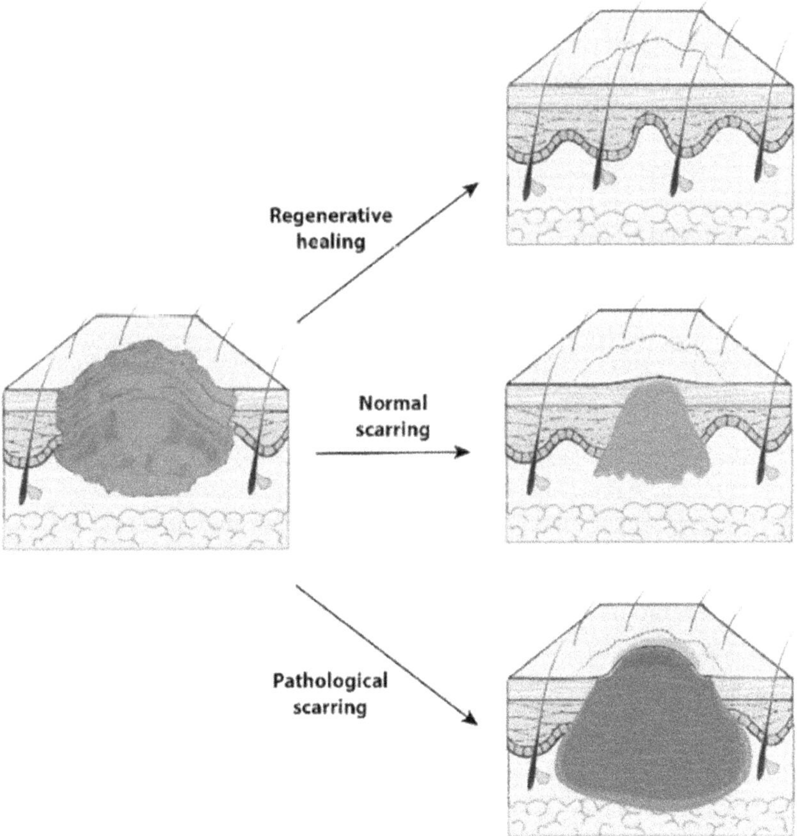

FIGURE 3.1 The spectrum of scarring [11].

Role of Nanotechnology in Wound Care

Nanotechnology is revolutionizing wound care by significantly enhancing healing processes, minimizing infection risks, and fostering tissue regeneration. The incorporation of nanomaterials into wound management strategies has led to remarkable advancements, especially in the creation of smart dressings and nanoparticles (NPs) tailored to meet specific healing requirements. Nanotechnology involves the utilization of materials at the nanoscale, which exhibit unique properties such as high surface-to-volume ratios, increased reactivity, and improved bioavailability. These characteristics enable nanotechnology to effectively address critical challenges in wound management, including infection control, tissue regeneration, and sustained drug delivery.

Antimicrobial Properties

One of the key advantages of using NPs in wound care is their ability to deliver antimicrobial agents in a controlled manner. This controlled release ensures sustained therapeutic effects, allowing for prolonged protection against infections while minimizing the frequency of treatment applications. The integration of these NPs into wound dressing enhances their effectiveness and contributes to improved healing outcomes [12]. NPs such as silver (AgNPs), zinc oxide (ZnO NPs), and titanium dioxide (TiO_2 NPs) possess strong antimicrobial properties, making them effective in preventing infections in both chronic and acute wounds. These NPs work by disrupting bacterial membranes and interfering with microbial DNA, which is crucial for combating infections. Notably, they have demonstrated efficacy against antibiotic-resistant bacteria, including MRSA, significantly reducing infection rates in various wound types [12,13].

Smart Dressings

Smart dressings equipped with sensors have the capability to monitor wound conditions, identifying signs of infection and inflammation, which facilitates timely medical interventions [12]. The incorporation of hydrogels and electroactive polymers into these dressings enhances their mechanical properties and supports tissue regeneration. Recent advancements in nanotechnology have led to the creation of intelligent wound dressings that can autonomously respond to changes in the wound environment. These innovative dressings not only detect infections but also automatically release suitable treatments, thereby optimizing healing outcomes [14].

Tissue Regeneration

These materials replicate the extracellular matrix (ECM), promoting cell growth and accelerating the wound healing process. They can be tailored to incorporate bioactive agents, which enhance healing outcomes [15]. Polymer- and lipid-based nanostructures facilitate the precise delivery of therapeutic agents, improving the treatment of challenging wounds. Nanotechnology plays a crucial role in enhancing cellular activities vital for wound healing. Specifically, nanomaterials can stimulate processes such as cell proliferation, migration, and angiogenesis (the formation of new blood vessels), thereby expediting tissue repair [13,16].

Tissue Engineering

Nanocomposites and nanoscaffolds play a vital role in the creation of bioengineered skin substitutes, which are essential for treating large wounds and burns. These innovative substitutes support cellular activities, fostering new tissue growth and improving wound closure. By facilitating the development of such advanced materials, nanocomposites and nanoscaffolds significantly enhance the healing process for extensive injuries [17,18].

Moisture Management

Nanotechnology-based wound dressings effectively regulate the wound environment by maintaining a moist atmosphere, which is essential for epithelialization and minimizing scarring. These advanced dressings also incorporate nanomaterials that enhance oxygen permeability and absorb excess exudate, thereby improving healing conditions. By ensuring a moist wound environment, these dressings significantly contribute to faster healing and better overall outcomes [19,20].

Controlled Drug Delivery

Nanocarriers, such as liposomes and dendrimers, enable sustained and targeted delivery of bioactive compounds, including growth factors and antibiotics. This targeted approach reduces side effects and enhances treatment efficacy, addressing chronic wound challenges [17,21].

Overview of the Wound Healing Process

The wound healing process is a complex and dynamic series of events that can be categorized into four main phases: hemostasis, inflammation, proliferation, and remodeling. Each phase plays a crucial role in restoring skin integrity and function, and any disruption can lead to chronic wounds or complications. Four overlapping phases: hemostasis, where bleeding stops; inflammation, which removes infection; proliferation, where new tissue forms; and remodeling, where the wound matures and strengthens, ultimately reforming the skin barrier to prevent infection and fluid loss (Figure 3.2).

Hemostasis

Hemostasis is the critical initial phase of wound healing, focusing on stopping bleeding and forming a stable clot. This phase begins immediately after an injury, during which blood vessels constrict to minimize blood loss. Platelets aggregate at the wound site, releasing growth factors that initiate the healing process. Recent advancements in hemostatic materials have enhanced the effectiveness of this phase, employing various biopolymers and innovative technologies. The following sections will explore key aspects of hemostasis in wound healing [22].

Physiological Hemostatic Mechanisms

Hemostasis is a complex physiological process that involves three main steps.

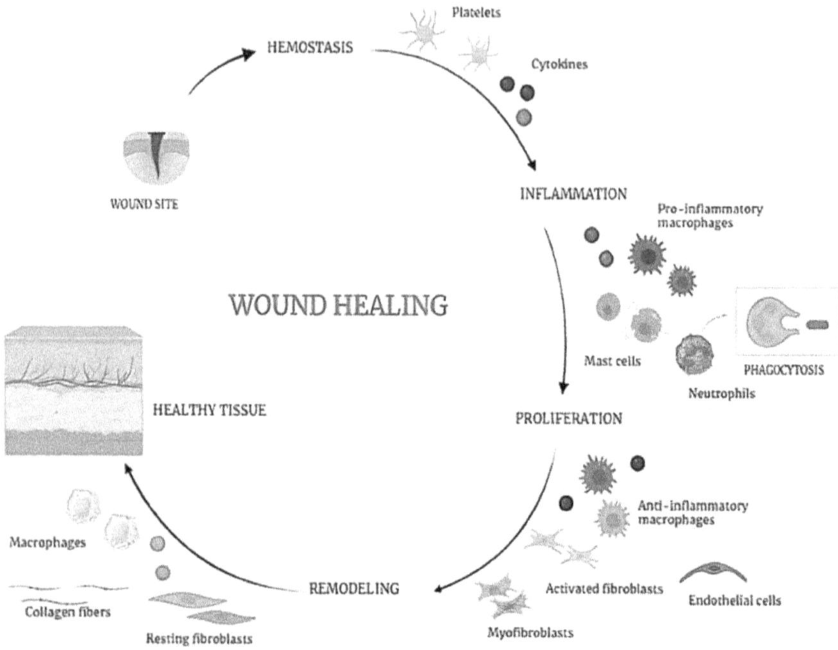

FIGURE 3.2 Schematic diagram depicting different stages of wound healing.

Vasoconstriction

Immediately after an injury, blood vessels constrict to reduce blood loss. This occurs when the integrity of the vascular walls and endothelial cells is compromised, exposing the subendothelial matrix to blood. The exposed matrix triggers platelet capture, adhesion, and activation, leading to the formation of a platelet plug. Smooth muscle contraction in the blood vessel further helps to prevent blood loss at the site of injury [23]. The whole process of blood hemostasis has been shown in Figure 3.3.

Primary Hemostasis

This phase involves several key actions by platelets:

- **Activation**: Platelets become activated upon encountering the exposed subendothelial matrix.
- **Adhesion**: Platelets adhere to collagen and other components exposed at the injury site, facilitated by von Willebrand factor (vWF).
- **Aggregation**: Activated platelets change shape and release mediators that attract additional platelets, forming a temporary platelet plug.

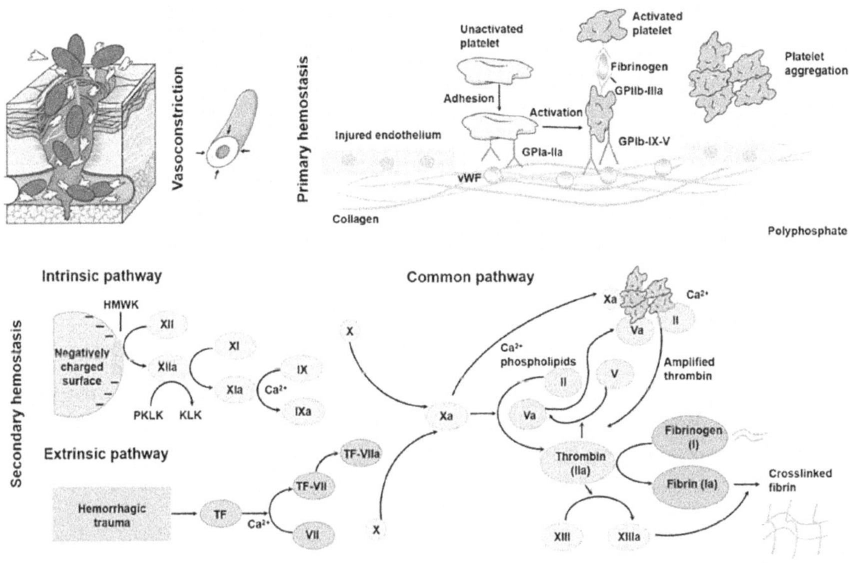

FIGURE 3.3 Schematic of the complex mechanism of blood vessel hemostasis [23].

- **Secretion**: Platelets release substances such as adenosine diphosphate (ADP) and serotonin, which enhance vasoconstriction and promote further platelet aggregation [23].

Secondary Hemostasis

This phase reinforces the platelet plug through the coagulation cascade:

- The coagulation cascade is activated by tissue factor (TF) and other procoagulant proteins in response to vessel injury.
- Factor VIIa forms a complex with TF, activating factors IX and X.
- The activation of factor X leads to the production of thrombin from prothrombin.
- Thrombin converts fibrinogen into fibrin strands, which polymerize to form a stable fibrin mesh that solidifies the clot.
- Factor XIII is also activated by thrombin, cross-linking fibrin strands to enhance clot stability.

Coagulation Pathways

Two primary pathways promote blood coagulation:

- **Tissue factor pathway**: This pathway is initiated by the exposure of TF from damaged tissues, activating factors IX and X.

- **Contact pathway**: This pathway involves factor XII and leads to the activation of factor XI, which subsequently activates factor IX [23].

Both pathways converge on the common pathway, culminating in thrombin production, which is essential for platelet activation and fibrin formation.

Physical Hemostatic Methods

Various methods can be employed to achieve effective hemostasis, tailored to the type of vascular bleeding. Here are some detailed methods.

Finger Pressure Hemostasis

This method involves applying direct pressure to the artery against the underlying bone near the injury site. It is particularly effective for controlling arterial bleeding in superficial areas. By pressing on the artery with a finger or palm, blood circulation is temporarily halted, allowing time for further treatment [24].

Tourniquet Application

A tourniquet is used to compress a limb and stop arterial bleeding quickly. While this method is reliable, it is essential to apply it correctly to avoid excessive wrapping, which can lead to skin damage and tissue ischemia if left on for too long. Tourniquets are most effective for limb injuries where rapid control of bleeding is necessary [25].

Pneumatic Hemostasis

This technique utilizes a gas-filled tourniquet that compresses the limb to block blood flow. Commonly used in orthopedic surgery, pneumatic hemostasis helps to maintain a clear surgical field and minimizes bleeding. However, it can cause complications such as paralysis, shock, and skin damage if not monitored closely [25].

Electrocoagulation Hemostasis

Electrocoagulation involves using a probe that generates heat through electrical current to promote coagulation at the wound site. Heat causes edema in the surrounding tissue, reducing blood vessel diameter and forming a thrombus to stop bleeding. This method is simple and economical but requires careful timing; prolonged application can lead to deeper tissue damage [26].

Ultrasonic Cutting and Blood-Stopping Knife

This advanced technique employs ultrasonic energy to cut tissue while simultaneously promoting coagulation. The ultrasonic knife amplifies kinetic energy to break protein bonds in tissues, leading to coagulation and minimal damage to the surrounding areas. Although effective, its operation can be slow and costly [27].

Laser Hemostasis

Laser hemostasis uses focused heat energy to evaporate water in cells and promote vascular wall collagen degeneration, leading to thrombosis formation. This method is particularly effective for capillary and arteriolar bleeding while causing minimal damage to the surrounding tissues. However, it can produce toxic smoke and may lead to adhesion post-operation.

Microwave Knife Hemostasis

Microwave knives generate heat through radiation, causing tissue solidification and achieving hemostatic effects. This method offers rapid healing with less postoperative bleeding but primarily affects blood vessels within a limited range (approximately 3 mm) [28].

Radiofrequency Knife Hemostasis

This technique uses radiofrequency energy to create a plasma electric field that destroys protein bonds in tissues, promoting coagulation with minimal thermal damage. It is effective for small blood vessels but requires significant saline in the liquid environment for optimal operation [29]. These methods highlight various approaches to managing bleeding effectively during trauma care, each with specific applications and considerations based on the type of injury and severity of bleeding.

Inflammation

The inflammation phase of wound healing is a critical and complex process that initiates the body's response to injury. This phase is characterized by the recruitment of inflammatory cells, the release of cytokines, and the activation of various signaling pathways that facilitate tissue repair. Understanding the dynamics of this phase is essential for improving wound healing outcomes and addressing chronic wounds. Following hemostasis, the inflammatory phase begins, which is characterized by the recruitment of immune cells to the wound site. This phase is essential for preventing infection and clearing debris, involving cytokines and chemokines that facilitate communication between cells [30,31].

Key Characteristics of the Inflammation Phase

- **Cellular response**: Inflammatory cells, such as neutrophils and macrophages, are among the first responders to the injury site, playing a vital role in clearing debris and pathogens [30,31].

Neutrophils produce extracellular trapping nets of neutrophils, trigger phagocytosis, and produce oxidative bursts and degranulation to remove bacteria and necrotic tissue (Figure 3.4). It's cleared by burial, reverse metastasis of neutrophils, and secondary necrosis of neutrophils, while macrophages remove cell fragments, pathogens, and apoptotic cells and produce a large number of proinflammatory cytokines to recruit immune cells. Polarization to M2 type is influenced by TH2 cytokines, apoptotic cells, nucleotides, and temporary extracellular bases [31].

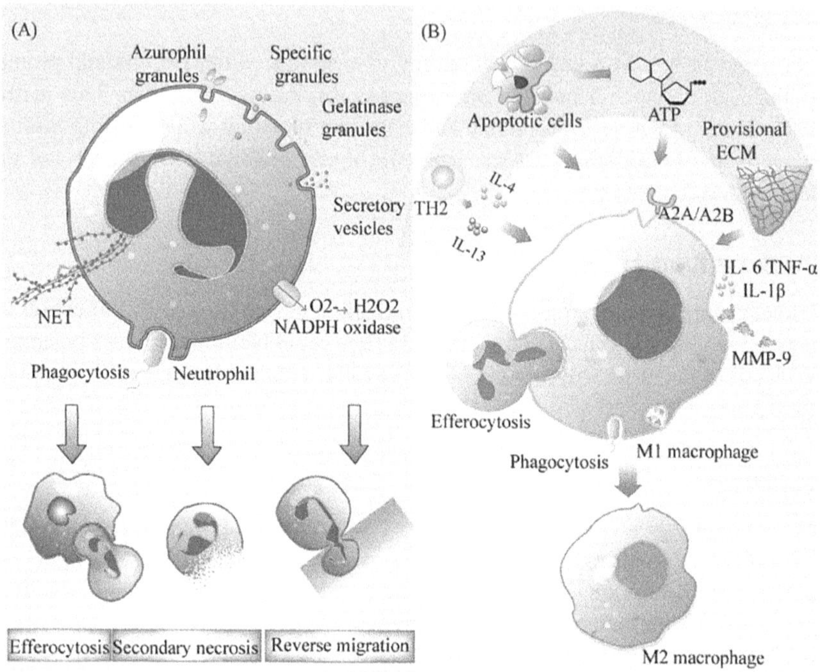

FIGURE 3.4 Role of the neutrophils and macrophages in wound inflammation [31].

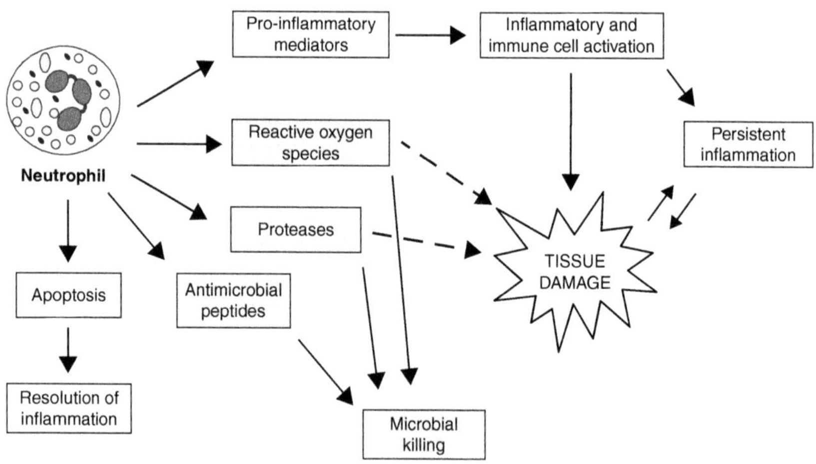

FIGURE 3.5 Overview of neutrophil activity [32].

Neutrophils are recruited to the wound site quickly after injury, where they carry out a variety of functions (Figure 3.5). They produce an array of proinflammatory mediators that recruit and activate other inflammatory cells, enhancing inflammation. In normal wounds, recruited neutrophils will eventually undergo apoptosis and be engulfed by macrophages, initiating a resolution program that terminates the

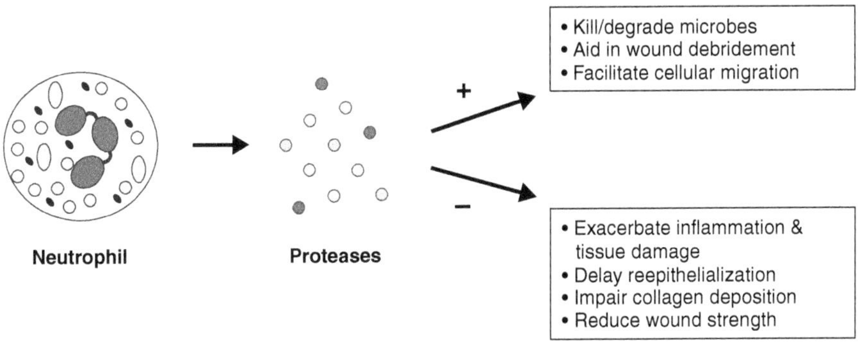

FIGURE 3.6 Neutrophil activity during wound healing [32].

inflammatory response. However, in non-healing wounds, inflammatory cells often continue to be recruited and activated, leading to persistent inflammation. Activated neutrophils help prevent wound infection by generating reactive oxygen species (ROS) and producing proteases and antimicrobial peptides. These substances kill and degrade potentially pathogenic microbes, but ROS and proteases, in particular, can cause tissue damage when released extracellularly. Excessive proteases can be especially harmful, causing unwanted degradation of the ECM and additional tissue damage. This can lead to a harmful cycle, whereby the damage caused by neutrophil-derived proteases causes even more inflammation (Figure 3.6). This leads to more tissue damage, eventually stalling the wound healing process and preventing complete closure of the wound [32].

Neutrophil-derived proteases have both beneficial and detrimental effects on wound healing. Activated neutrophils produce a number of proteases that can have positive (+) or negative (–) effects on the cutaneous repair process. Neutrophil-derived proteases help kill and degrade microbes and break down components of the ECM, which can debride the wound and facilitate cellular migration when present at appropriate levels. Conversely, excessive levels of proteases in the tissue resulting from overly active neutrophils or prolonged neutrophil recruitment can be detrimental by causing additional tissue damage and further inflammation. Consequently, defective collagen deposition, reduced wound strength, and delayed re-epithelialization can occur.

Cytokine and mediator release: The phase involves the release of cytokines and growth factors, which regulate the inflammatory response and promote healing [30,33]. During inflammation, the formation of a blood clot re-establishes hemostasis and provides a provisional matrix for cell migration. Cytokines play an important role in the evolution of granulation tissue through recruitment of inflammatory leukocytes and stimulation of fibroblasts and epithelial cells.

- **MicroRNA involvement**: Recent studies highlight the role of microRNAs in modulating the inflammatory response, suggesting potential therapeutic targets for enhancing wound healing (Figure 3.7).

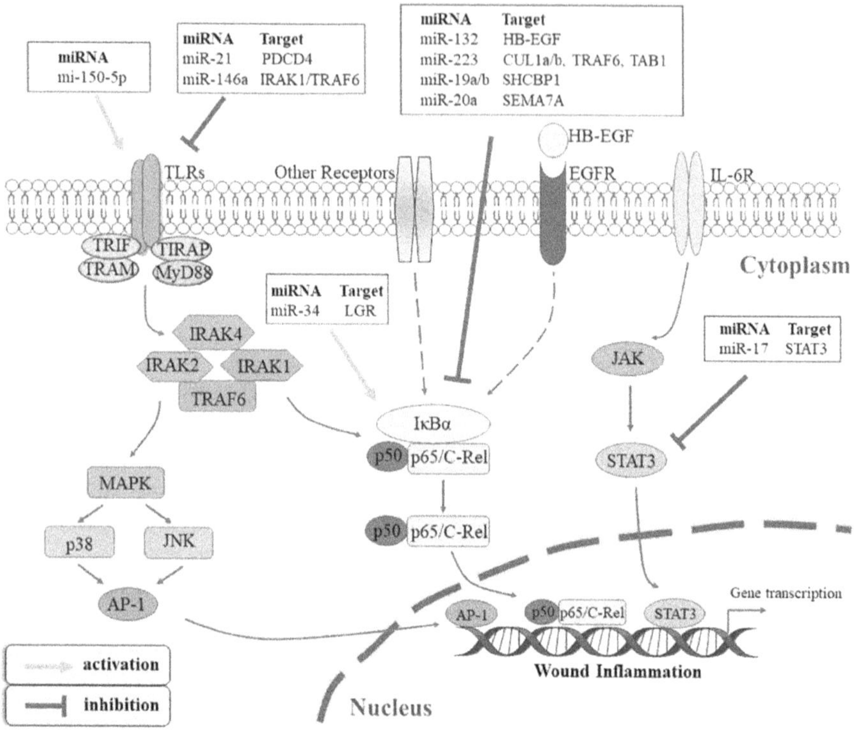

FIGURE 3.7 The schematic overview of miRNA-regulated inflammatory signaling pathways that occur during wound healing [34].

Proliferation

During proliferation, new tissue forms as fibroblasts produce collagen and ECM, promoting tissue granulation. Angiogenesis occurs, supplying nutrients and oxygen to the healing tissue, while epithelial cells migrate to cover the wound [22,35]. Approximately 3 days after injury, monocytes are recruited to the injury site, where they differentiate into macrophages and support healing. Macrophages are important players facilitating the inflammatory–proliferative phase transition during wound healing (Figure 3.8).

As inflammation subsides, proliferation becomes a major theme with a focus on covering the wound surface (i.e., re-epithelialization), restoring the vascular network, and forming granulation tissue. Re-epithelialization requires migration and proliferation of keratinocytes. In a few hours to 1 day after injury, the existing wound-edge keratinocytes start to migrate. To generate more cells to cover the wound, keratinocytes at the basal layer of the wound edge and epithelia stem cells from nearby hair follicles or sweat glands start proliferating approximately 2–3 days after injury.

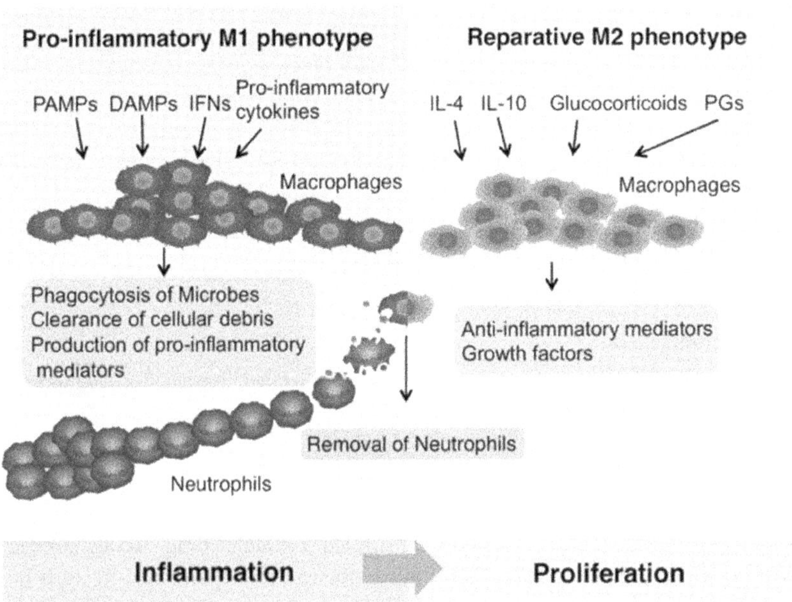

FIGURE 3.8 Schematic showing proliferation.

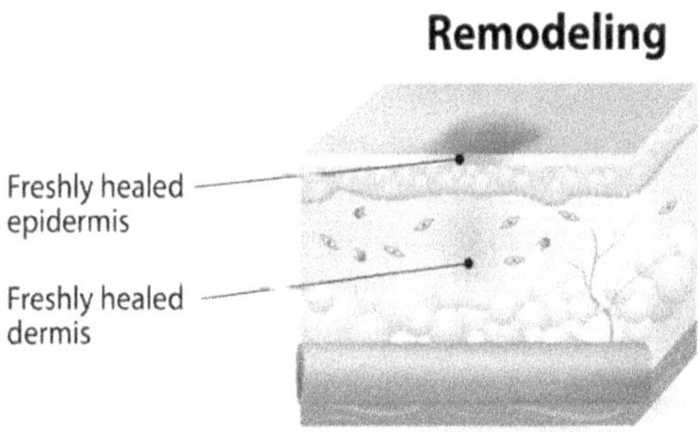

FIGURE 3.9 Remodeling process in wound healing [38].

Remodeling

The final phase involves the maturation of the newly formed tissue, where collagen is reorganized to increase tensile strength. This phase can last for months to years, resulting in scar formation, which may have reduced functionality compared to the original tissue [36,37]. The remodeling process in wound healing is a critical phase that follows inflammation and proliferation, characterized by the reorganization and maturation of newly formed tissue. This phase can last for months or even years, depending on the wound's severity and the individual's health. The remodeling phase is essential for restoring tissue integrity and function, and it involves several key processes (Figure 3.9).

Key Processes in Remodeling

- **Matrix reorganization**: The ECM undergoes significant changes, where collagen fibers are realigned and cross-linked to enhance tensile strength.
- **Cellular activity**: Fibroblasts play a crucial role by synthesizing collagen and other ECM components, while myofibroblasts contribute to wound contraction [38].
- **Hormonal and immune factors**: Hormones like insulin and cortisol, along with cytokines such as TGF-β1, influence the remodeling process, affecting cellular behavior and tissue repair.

Overall Mechanism

(i) Hemostasis: Immediately after the onset of an injury, exposed collagen binds to inactive platelets and activates them, causing vasoconstriction and reducing blood flow. Activated platelets release clotting factors, which promote platelet aggregation. These clotting factors also activate thrombin present in the blood plasma, initiating the coagulation cascade. Activated thrombin activates fibrin strands and adheres together on the wound site to form a platelet plug. (ii) Inflammation: Following Hemostasis, acute inflammation occurs. Cytokines and growth factors are released, attracting leukocytes to the wound area. Neutrophils arrive first, followed by monocytes, which differentiate into macrophages, and lymphocytes. (iii) Proliferation: During this phase, keratinocytes, endothelial cells, and activated fibroblasts migrate to and proliferate in the wound area, promoting tissue repair and closure. Fibroblasts transform into myofibroblasts, aiding in wound contraction and further accelerating closure. Angiogenesis, which is the process by which new blood vessels form from existing ones, also starts to occur. (iv) Remodeling: The final phase involves the maturation and reorganization of wound tissue. This can result in either partial healing with scarring or complete regeneration of the tissue (Figure 3.10). Stretching and pulling forces help collagen fibers align properly, restoring tissue strength and function [14].

NANOMATERIALS IN WOUND REGENERATION

Nanomaterials are materials that have at least one dimension in the nanoscale range, typically 1–100 nm. Materials at this scale exhibit unique physical, chemical, and biological properties that vary from their bulk. Nanomaterials can be classified into various kinds consisting of NPs, nanofibers, nanotubes, nanosheets, and nanocomposites depending on their shape and structure. They may be synthesized by the usage of a number of methods, which include top-down (breaking down bulk substances) and bottom-up (building from atomic or molecular tiers) processes.

Properties of Nanomaterials

Nanomaterials possess a range of different properties that make them suitable for several applications including wound healing. Key points are as follows.

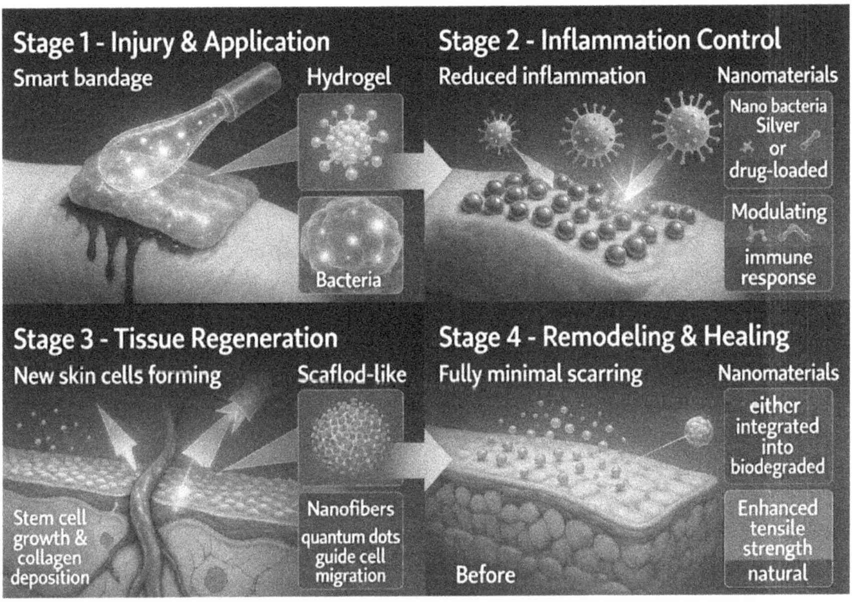

FIGURE 3.10 The schematic showing healing process consisting of different healing stages.

Size-Dependent Properties

The small size and large surface area of nanomaterials enhance their reactivity and interaction with biological systems. At the nanoscale, quantum effects produce unique optical, electronic, and magnetic properties.

Mechanical Properties

Generally, the nanomaterials possess better strength, elasticity, and toughness than the same sort of bulk materials. Due to their mechanical versatility, they can be integrated into almost any substrate including wound healing dressings.

Chemical Reactivity

This increases the chemical reactivity in the sense that catalytic activities as well as efficient drug delivery are facilitated. The surface functionalization is easily programmable to enhance the biocompatibility and targeting qualities.

Antimicrobial Properties

Nanomaterials such as silver nanoparticles (AgNPs) and zinc oxide exhibit intrinsic antimicrobial properties, which can prevent infections in wounds.

Optical Properties

Nanomaterials like quantum dots and gold nanoparticles (AuNPs) possess unique optical characteristics, such as fluorescence or plasmonic resonance, which are useful for imaging and diagnostics.

Thermal Properties

Certain nanomaterials, such as graphene and carbon nanotubes (CNTs), display exceptional thermal conductivity, which can aid in controlling wound environments.

Biocompatibility

Many nanomaterials, especially those derived from natural sources like nanocellulose or chitosan, are biocompatible, making them ideal for biomedical applications.

Controlled Release

Nanomaterials can act as carriers for drugs, growth factors, or other therapeutic agents enabling controlled and sustained release to promote wound healing.

Electrical Properties

Conductive nanomaterials, such as graphene or conductive polymers, can be used to stimulate wound healing through electrical signals.

Degradability

Biodegradable nanomaterials ensure minimal toxicity and safe clearance from the body after serving their function.

Types of Nanomaterials Used in Wound Care

Nanomaterials are essential in wound healing because of the high surface area, compatibility, and configurable properties, as depicted in Figure 3.11. Some of the well-used nanomaterials in wound regenerative therapy are metal NPs (including

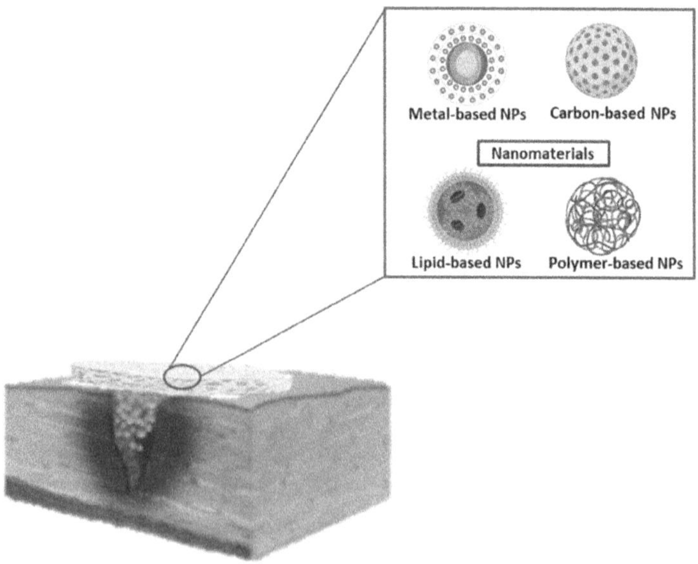

FIGURE 3.11 Types of nanomaterials for wound care.

silver, gold, and zinc oxide), polymeric NPs like chitosan and polylactic acid, and carbon-based nanomaterials including graphene oxide and CNTs. Nanofibers and hydrogels functionalized with NPs form the structural framework for tissue repair, while bioactive nanocomposites possess multiphenolic properties to enhance tissue repair. These materials provide an opportunity for improving the quality and speed of wound healing as well as reducing the infection rate.

Metal and Metal Oxide Nanoparticles

It has been developed earlier that using metal and metal oxide NPs with applications in wound care is a suitable solution because of their antibacterial, non-cytotoxic, and tissue regenerating properties evidenced in recent literature. AgNPs have attracted a lot of attention because of their potent antimicrobial effects by states such as ROS production and bacterial cell membrane destruction; they have been used in infection prevention and enhanced wound healing in dressings (Kawata et al., 2023). ZnO NPs provide antibacterial and anti-inflammatory activities, enhancing fibroblast viability and collagen deposition in vitro and in vivo (Singh et al., 2022). The titanium dioxide (TiO_2) NPs are known for disinfection and skin healing, and CuO NPs display high antibacterial effects against MDR strains (Khan et al., 2023). However, problems such as cytotoxicity and environmental concern remain unexplored, and still underlying studies are emphasizing a green approach and the development of more potential nanoparticle agents for safe and enhanced wound healing.

Polymer-Based Nanomaterials

NPs such as nanofibers and hydrogels have attracted important interest in wound healing applications due to their biocompatibility and multifunctionality of delivering various agents. Examples of nanofibers include the electrospun, which use a chitosan PCL polymer because their similarity with the ECM enhances cell adherence and tissue reconstruction (Wang et al., 2022). Promising wound dressings include hydrogels that provide a moist healing environment and deliver drugs in a controlled manner using polymers like gelatin, alginate, or PEG, minimizing infection and wound healing time (Ahmed et al., 2023). Polymer matrices with antimicrobial active antimicrobial agents like AgNPs or antibiotics in composite systems have improved chronic wound healing properties (Kumar et al., 2022). Additional and more advanced polymeric systems, namely smart hydrogels exhibiting pH, temperature, or enzymatic sensitivity, enhance the therapy's efficacy by incorporating factors that mimic the wound milieu. Nevertheless, the issue of moving from radical to traditional treatments and practical difficulties associated with scaling present certain concerns for extended clinical applications.

Carbon-Based Nanomaterials

Carbon-based NPs, such as graphene and CNTs, are relatively novel inserts in wound care owing to their excellent mechanical properties, antibacterial characteristics, and biocompatibility factors. Graphene oxide and its antibacterial properties through oxidative stress and membrane damage enhance fibroblast conductions with angiogenesis (Zhang et al. 2022). CNTs have favorable characteristics including a large surface area and electrical conductivity, which allow better drug release and biosensing of wound healing (Lee et al., 2023). Alkali-treated graphene oxide (GO) has been used in conjunction with polymers such as chitosan or PVA and exhibits enhanced on-site antibacterial properties and improved rates of wound healing in vivo (Kumar et al., 2023). However, there exists a major drawback where the issues of cytotoxicity and biodegradability arise again, meaning that further work to develop more enhanced safety characteristics has to be carried out. New trends in functionalization and sustainable synthesis methods give new opportunities to carbon-based nanomaterials in further development of wound healing technologies.

Lipid-Based Nanomaterials

Lipid-based NPs like liposome and micelles are widely used in wound care because of their biocompatibility, the ability to encapsulate both hydrophilic and hydrophobic drugs, and controlled release. Liposomes, constituted with phospholipid bilayers, have been applied for the controlled administered release of growth factors, antibiotics, and anti-inflammatory agents to the site of injury in improving healing rates and diminishing the incidence of infection, as cited by Ahmed et al. (2023). Using self-assembled micelles from amphiphilic molecules, hydrophobic drugs are delivered consequent of micelle formation to desired sites with minimal systemic side effects, as shown by the studies by Sharma et al. (2022). These lipid-based systems can also be incorporated into hydrogels or wound dressings for better therapeutic effects, as mentioned in Figure 3.11. New generations of liposomes using stimuli responsiveness such as pH or enzymes have also improved their performance in chronic wound situations. However, challenges like stability and large-scale production are still a hindrance for clinical translation, which propels further research to perfect their performance.

Mechanisms of Action of Nanomaterials in Wound Healing

Wound healing mechanism of action of nanomaterials is shown in Figure 3.12.

Antimicrobial Properties

Nanomaterial can kill bacteria through several processes in the case of wound healing and clears the environment for fresh healing to occur. Some of the key actions include production of ROS that interfere with microbial membrane, proteins, and DNA resulting in cell death. Further, metal NPs such as silver and zinc help to produce ions that inactivate bacterial enzymes and disable metabolic activities. Nanomaterials also inhibit biofilm formation through failure in bacterial attachment and through the ability to enter fully developed biofilms. A surface charge and high surface-to-volume ratio of NPs facilitate adhesion and interaction with bacterial cell membranes, inducing structural damaging. Chitosan and carbon-based NPs can be incorporated into nanomaterial system without adding extra antimicrobial agents to combat microbial biofilms because of their ability to bind with negative charges on the microbial membrane, thereby causing membrane rupture and leakage of contents. They not only act against infections and eruptions, but also help decrease inflammation processes, which contribute to the quick formation of a coagulum and, ultimately, tissue repair [39]. This paper has also outlined that CDs elicit

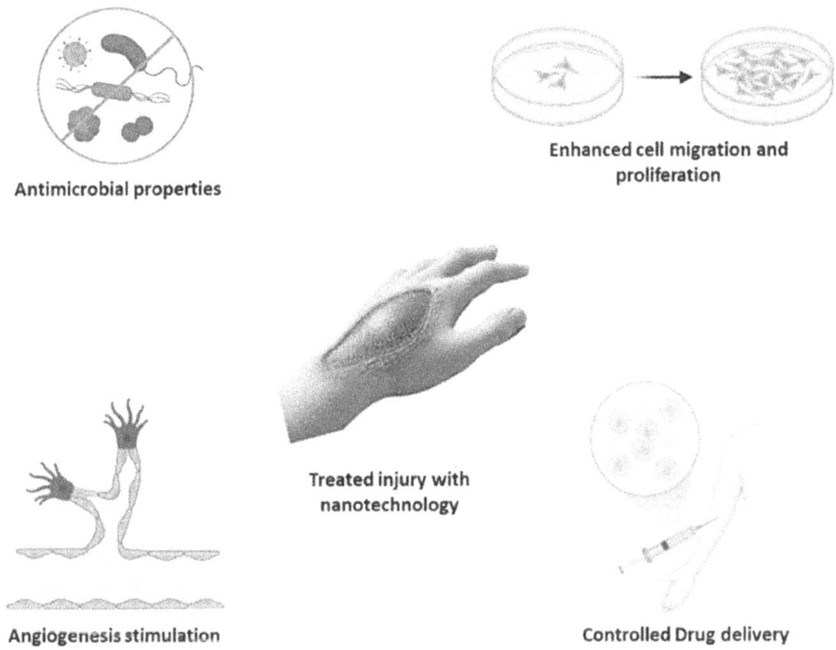

FIGURE 3.12 Treatment of wound via nanotechnology.

promising antimicrobial activities through mechanisms such as physical disruption of the microbial cells, induction of oxidative stress, and lipid remodeling. All these multifaceted mechanisms act harmoniously in the fight against pathogenic microorganisms and create realistic new potential therapeutic wound healing.

Angiogenesis Stimulation

Nanomaterials affect angiogenesis in wound healing by increasing the proliferation, migration, and tubulogenesis of endothelial cells, all of which are critical events in blood vessel formation. Gold and zinc oxide NPs act as angiogenic factors by upregulating vascular endothelial growth factor (VEGF) [40]. For example, AuNPs stimulate the PI3K/Akt and MAPK signaling, which are relevant for endothelial cells as well as angiogenesis. Also, other nanomaterials can directly release growth factors or nitric oxide (NO) to the wound area and improve angiogenic outcomes. Graphene oxide (GO) and other carbon-based materials help regulate VEGF and integrin, thereby helping in vascularization. By combining the mechanism, we can enhance the delivery of oxygen and nutrients in the wound area while also enhancing tissue repair and wound healing [41].

Enhanced Cell Proliferation and Migration

Nanomaterials promote cell proliferation and migration in wound healing, but there is no study on the photodegradation of nanomaterials. Due to their large surface area and the ability for its modification, they enhance the delivery of growth factors and other bioactive molecules in tissue regeneration. NPs or nanofibers and nanocomposites are used as scaffold materials because they replicate the ECM for the cells to adhere and migrate. This structure also helps the important cells like fibroblast, keratinocyte, and endothelial cells to migrate toward the repaired site [42]. Nanomaterials have also been found to modulate the production of signaling molecules like integrins and focal adhesion proteins, which amplify cell motility. Besides, their antimicrobial features exclude high chances of getting infections, thus providing a better healing environment. Together, all these mechanisms help achieve faster wound closure and better tissue healing, as suggested by current advancements in nanomedicine.

Controlled Drug Delivery

The role of nanomaterials in wound healing particularly associated with controlled drug delivery is evident, as presented in literature. The large surface area and good biocompatibility of nanofibers and its capability for loading and controlled release of bioactive molecules allow local and efficacious delivery of therapeutic agents like antibiotics, growth factors, and anti-inflammatory drugs at the wound site. These nanocarrier systems like NPs, nanofibers, and nanogels participate in the management of drug release through stimuli like pH, temperature, or enzyme activity for a controlled and site-specific drug delivery [43,44]. This reduces side effects on other parts of the body, increases drug stability, and optimizes the healing process by encouraging faster tissue development, minimizing inflammation, and preventing infections, thereby shortening the healing period, as pointed out by research done recently.

Applications of Nanomaterials in Wound Care

Nanomaterials found various applications in almost every field of life. They have a significant role in the medical field. Some of these are given below.

Nanoparticles-Based Dressings

Nanomaterials are innovative components in wound healing, especially NP dressings that capture major features of wound healing. These are special dressings that have incorporated antimicrobial/anti-inflammatory regenerative agents using NPs like silver, zinc oxide, and copper oxide for microbial inhibition and wound healing. Aside from hydrogels, other nanoparticle-based dressing materials are films, foams, and electrospun nanofibers. Nanoparticle-incorporated films give improved barrier protection as well as the ability to tailor drug delivery and nanoparticle-incorporated foams have high absorbency of wound exudates and promote moist wound healing [45]. Here, electrospun nanofibers with NPs provide a three-dimensional structure of interconnected pores that mimic the ECM to support cell growth and tissue repair. Polymeric and lipid-based nanoparticle delivery allows the controlled release of quantities of drugs such as antibiotics and growth factors. Cerium oxide NPs attenuate oxidative stress; gold and silica NPs stimulate angiogenesis and tissue remodeling. Stimuli-responsive NPs incorporated in smart dressings provide targeted drug delivery in response to specific stimuli, and oxygen-releasing NPs contribute to hypoxic wound healing. Materials like nanocellulose and chitosan are biocompatible, which improves mechanical characteristic and biodegradability, envisaging a green and patient-centric approach.

Nanofiber Scaffolds for Skin Regeneration

Nanofiber scaffolds containing nanomaterials have demonstrated high potential for skin-tissue engineering because they facilitate cell attachment, spreading, migration, and proliferation in a highly porous network that resembles the ECM. These scaffolds, created often through electrospinning toward creating nanoweb-like structures, can be incorporated with functional NPs like silver, zinc oxide, or gold for imparting antimicrobial characteristics, encouraging angiogenesis, and minimizing oxidative stress [46]. At the same time, nanofiber scaffolds enable the engineering of drug delivery to promote cell growth factors, cytokines, and/or antibiotics in tissue regeneration and elimination of infection. Nanocellulose and chitosan enhance integration of scaffold with skin, whereas stimuli-sensitive nanomaterials allow for controlled release of therapy relative to wound conditions [47]. Given the structural, biological, and functional advantages epitomized in nanofiber scaffold, this work confirms nanofibers as novel nanomaterials with prospects for skin wound healing and regeneration.

Hydrogels and Nanocomposites

The utilization of nanomaterials within hydrogels and nanocomposites makes a revolutionary new approach in wound healing by utilizing structural reinforcement in addition to therapeutic capacities. NPs including silver or zinc oxide incorporated hydrogels exhibit long-term antimicrobial activity, improvement in oxidative stress, and maintenance of moist wound healing environment. The incorporation of NPs with biopolymers such as chitosan or nanocellulose results in improved properties that include mechanical strength, biocompatibility, and drug releasing mechanisms in nanocomposite dressings. These systems allow the selective and localized delivery of therapeutic substances such as antibiotics, growth factors, anti-inflammatory drugs, and stimulants of angiogenesis and tissue regeneration. Advanced hydrogels and nanocomposites are termed stimuli-responsive, which means that they change their properties in response to local pH, temperature, or the presence of infection agents within the wound site. Nanohydrogels and nanocomposite-based dressings are able to overcome these limitations through the incorporation of nanomaterials, which provide hydrogel with the desirable structural and functional characteristics of a multicomponent nanocomposite, which enhances wound healing care in acute and chronic wounds [48].

Role in Chronic Wound Management

Multiple NPs, such as bioactive glasses, carbon dots (CDs), zinc oxide, europium oxide, and molybdenum disulfide nanosheets, have been utilized mainly as reinforcement in adhesive self-healing hydrogels. A prime example would be nano-bioactive glasses (NBGs), which typically consist of silica and other elements such as calcium (Ca) and phosphorus (P). NBGs have offered numerous unique biological properties, such as osteogenic differentiation, bone/soft tissue bonding activity, and angiogenesis, and have shown a vital role in activating coagulation factors that improve chronic wound healing. Most recently, nanoenzymes, a category of synthetic nanomaterials capable of emulating the catalytic functions of natural enzymes, including peroxidase (POD) and glucose oxidase (GOx) activities, have introduced fresh possibilities for advancing the therapeutic of chronic wounds. Such nanoenzymes hold the potential to address hyperglycemia and bacterial infections, thereby promoting the repair of such wounds. Nanosheets of molybdenum disulfide combined with bovine serum albumin (BSA)-functionalized Au nanoparticles (AuNPs) were integrated into an ODex/glycol CS (GC) hydrogel [49].

Recent advances in Nanomaterials for Wound Regeneration

Wound healing is a multi-step process that fully depends on biochemical and physiological responses, which occur in four phases; the first is hemostasis. Nanomaterials have offered a promising platform in the treatment of wounds since the traditional methods have been shown to pose some challenges. The characteristics of nanomaterials include a large surface-area-to-volume ratio, the possibility of controlling their properties, and the bioavailability of therapeutic substances. Recent advances have focused on three main areas: the intelligent nanomaterials in specific therapy, the three-in-one nanomaterials, and the combinational use of nanomaterials with wearable electronics. They are revolutionizing the wound care field in a faster, more customized, and more productive way.

Smart Nanomaterials for Targeted Therapy

Targeted therapy is meant to bring therapeutic agents to a specific area in the body such as the wound site without affecting the rest of the body. Zwitterionic NPs, nanogels, and nanosheets are stimuli-responsive nanomaterials including pH, temperature, and ROS, which may be abnormally changed in wound surroundings.

pH-Responsive Nanomaterials

The surgical site has marked inflammation because of bacterial invasion and tissue turnover, and this results in low pH in the wound site: pH-sensitive NPs take advantage of this to release their loads of medicine or chime in cases of low pH (Figure 3.13). For instance, NPs fabricated from a biodegradable polymer with a suitable antibiotic or growth factor can be incorporated and subsequently serve its purpose by breaking down when in contact with the acidic environment [50].

Temperature-Sensitive Nanogels

Smart nanogels that are sensitive to temperature can be employed for stimuli-triggered drug delivery by using temperature (Figure 3.14). These materials are stable at physiological temperature and release their contents at slightly elevated temperatures, which may result from inflammation at the site of the wound [51].

ROS-Responsive Nanoparticles

When ROS accumulates, oxidative stress is experienced leading to impaired wound healing. ROS-responsive NPs are constructed to target ROSs, as well as carrying antioxidants or anti-inflammatory agents (Figure 3.15). These nanomaterials possess the dual functionality of combating oxidative stress and enhancing tissue healing [52].

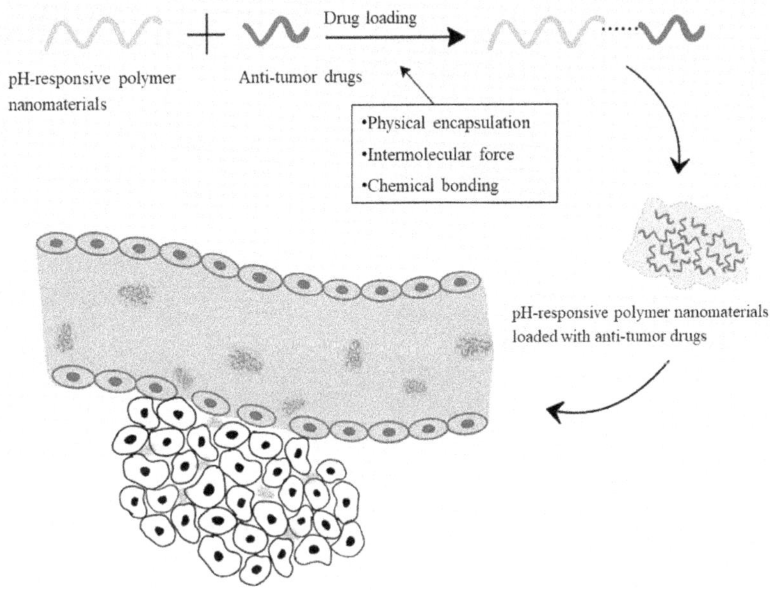

FIGURE 3.13 pH-responsive nanomaterials.

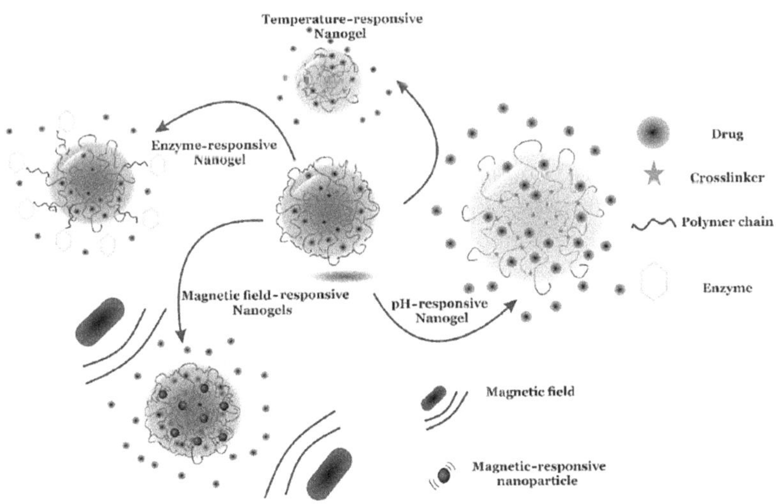

FIGURE 3.14 Temperature-responsive nanogels.

Biodegradable Nanosystems

Smart nanomaterials are gradually being designed to be biodegradable after their therapeutic use so that they do not remain in the human body's lumen (Figure 3.16). This boosts their security and usefulness in clinical practices [53].

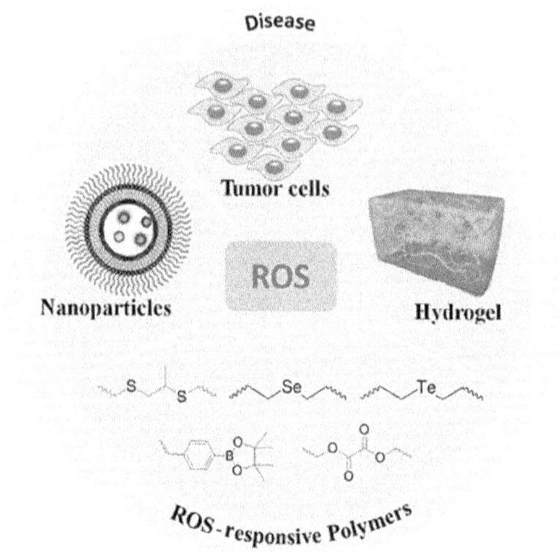

FIGURE 3.15 ROS-responsive nanogels.

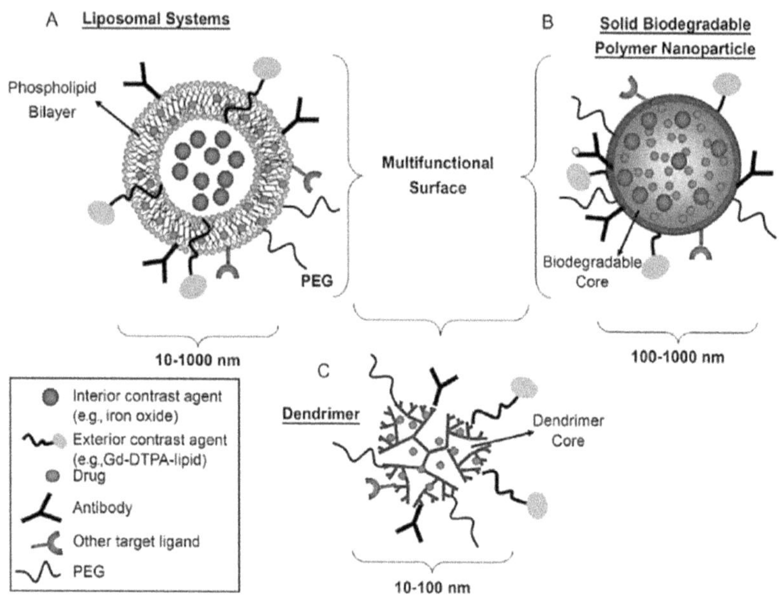

FIGURE 3.16 Biodegradable nanosystems.

Multifunctional Nanomaterials for Combined Effects

Multifunctional nanomaterials are intended and developed to Howell various aspects of the wound healing process, including preventing bacterial infection, promoting tissue regeneration, and fighting inflammation. Such materials adapt numerous therapeutic aspects at once and can therefore provide a balanced solution for wound treatment.

Antimicrobial Properties

Infected wounds are one of the largest critical issues in clinical practice. Current research reveals that NPs containing silver, zinc oxide, and chitosan are active against a range of microbes. Therefore, incorporating these agents into wound dressings makes it possible to prevent as well as treat infecting agents (Figure 3.17).

Promotion of Angiogenesis

Particulate matrices that incorporate angiogenic factors such as VEGF or platelet-derived growth factor (PDGF) can stimulate the formation of new blood vessels to meet oxygen and other nutrient needs of the healing tissue (Figure 3.18). Angiogenesis is achieved from this as it speeds up the healing process and prevents the development of chronic ulcers.

Anti-Inflammatory Effects

Inflammation, particularly when it persists, often can slow down the process of healing. Nanomaterials that can work in multiple ways and include anti-inflammatory medicines like corticosteroids or ingredients from natural foods like curcumin can rewrite the body's inflammation level to make it ideal for tissue healing [54] (Figure 3.19).

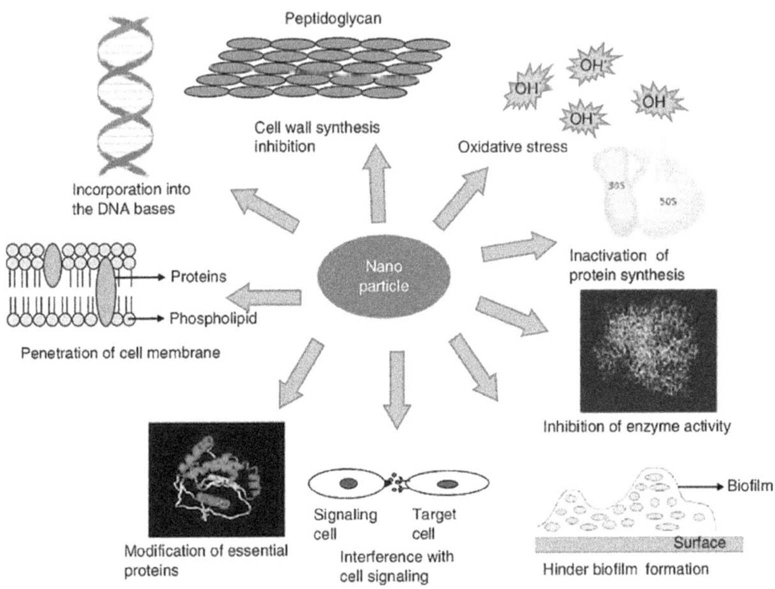

FIGURE 3.17 Antimicrobial properties

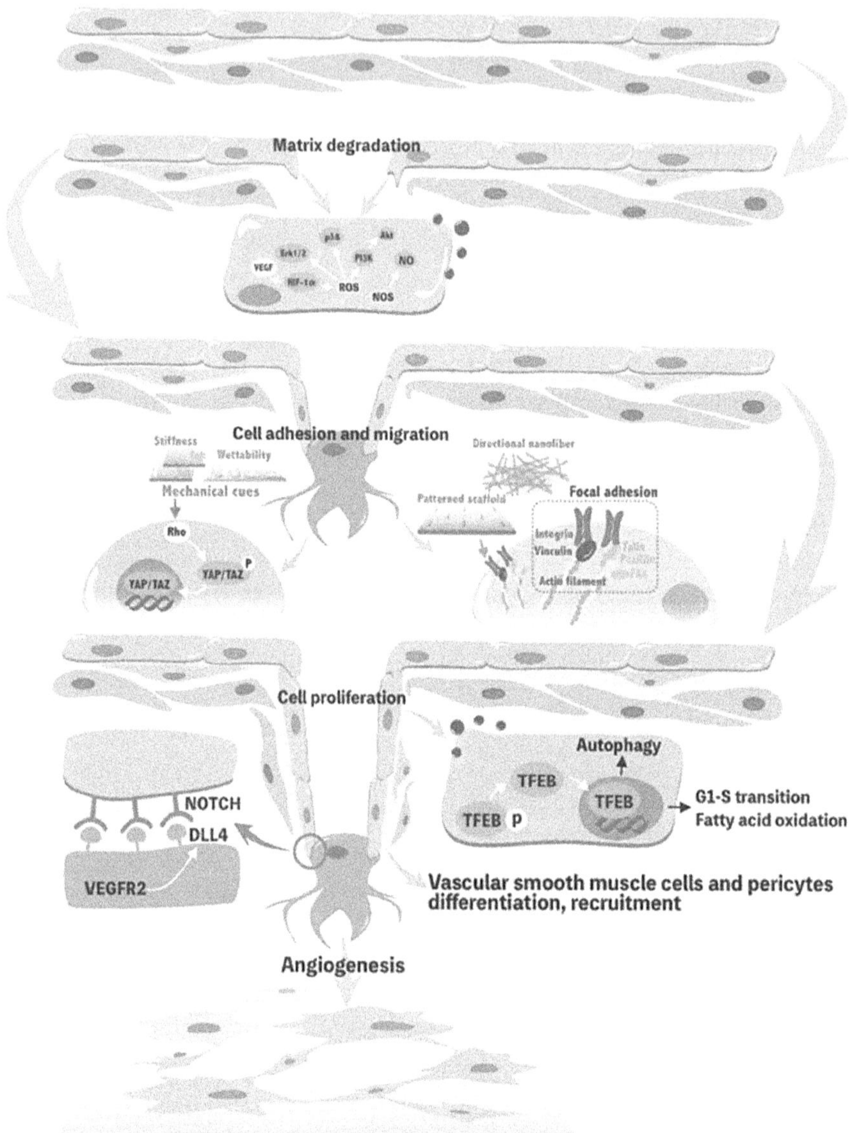

FIGURE 3.18 Angiogenic effect of nanoparticles.

Enhanced Cell Proliferation

Composite nanomaterials that offer structural support are nanofibers and hydrogels, which replicate the function of ECM as well as being conducive to cell accumulation. These scaffolds can be additionally decorated with bioactive molecules to augment the modality of tissue regeneration (Figure 3.20).

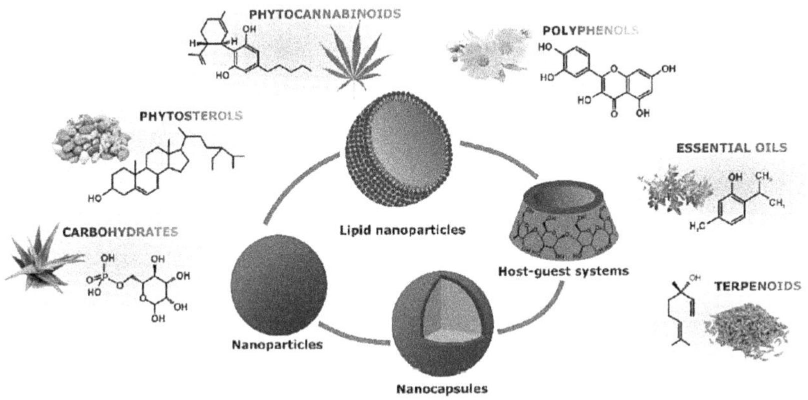

FIGURE 3.19 Anti-inflammatory effect of nanoparticles.

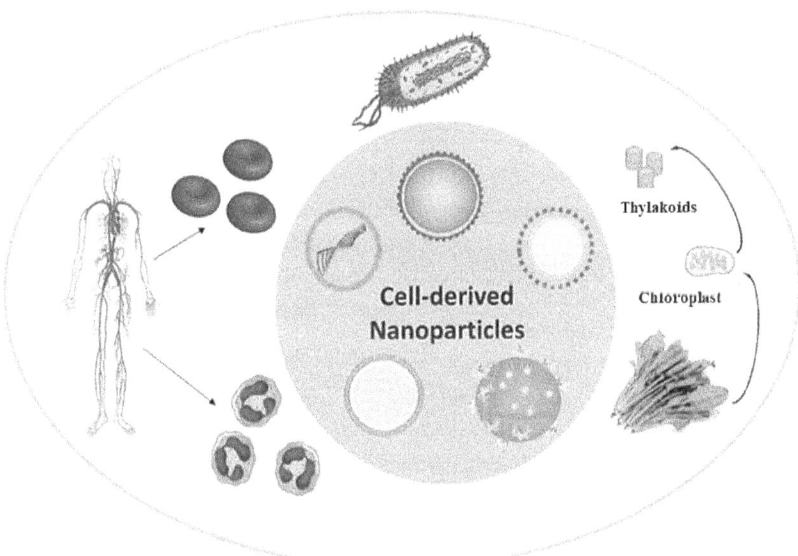

FIGURE 3.20 Cell proliferation.

Controlled Drug Release

Multifunctional nanomaterials can encapsulate multiple therapeutic agents, which have different release profiles, by using nanocarriers like liposomes or dendrimers. It also enables one drug to be given successively by the other with an agenda of enhancing the therapeutic value of the substances during different phases of healing.

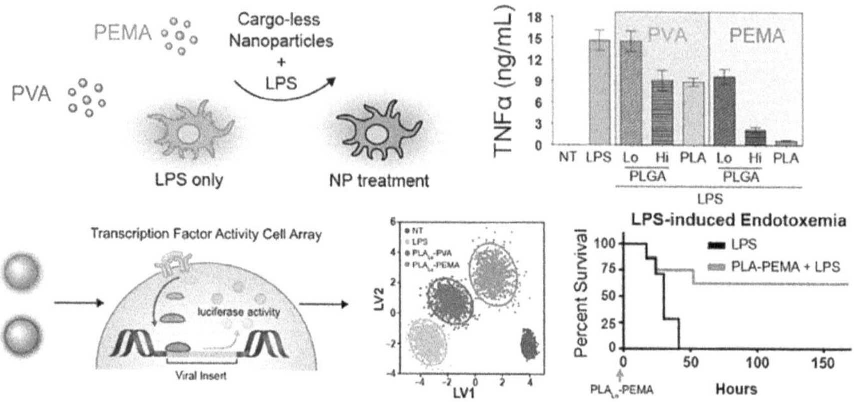

FIGURE 3.21 Immunomodulatory effects.

Immunomodulatory Effects

Some of the nanomaterials can help adjust the immune response and activities of proinflammatory and anti-inflammatory cytokines (Figure 3.21). These aid in migrating the wound from the inflammation phase to the proliferation phase more easily [14].

Integration with Wearable Devices for Real-Time Monitoring

The integration of nanomaterials with wearables pushes wound care to a whole new micro level of personalization. These smart systems can precisely observe the conditions of the wound in parallel and offer important information to clinicians and patients regarding any necessary interventions at the appropriate time.

Biosensors for Wound Monitoring

Nanomaterial-based biosensors embedded into wearable health monitoring terminals can detect and monitor vital life metrics including pH, glucose, lactate, and oxygenation. For instance, flexible sensors created from graphene or AuNPs integrate into tissue perfectly and are sensitive to the slightest variations in wound characteristics (Figure 3.22).

Therapeutic Delivery Systems

One useful application of nanomaterials is based on the use of wearable devices containing drug reservoirs. These systems can be designed to deliver the therapeutics in line with some features, which include changes in pH or temperature hence being effective.

Wireless Connectivity

Sophisticated wearable gadgets use wireless technologies to allow data to be transferred to doctors among others. This facilitates monitoring from a distance and infrequent clinic visits, which may be essential in patients with chronic wounds (Figure 3.23).

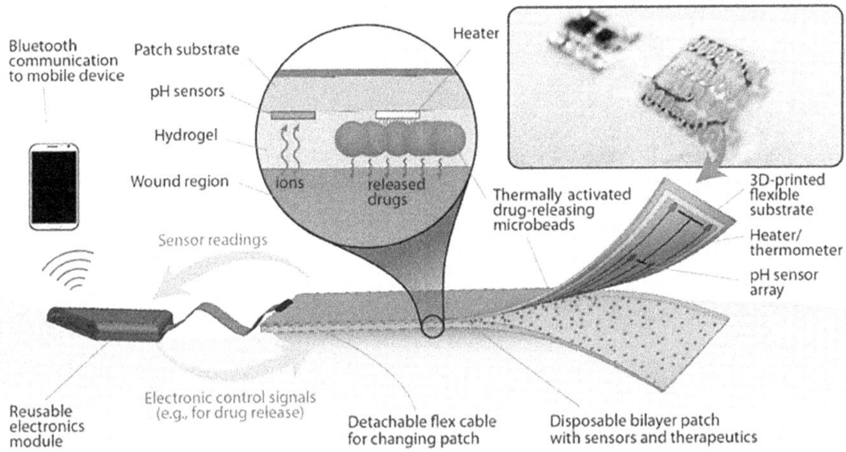

FIGURE 3.22 Biosensors for wound monitoring.

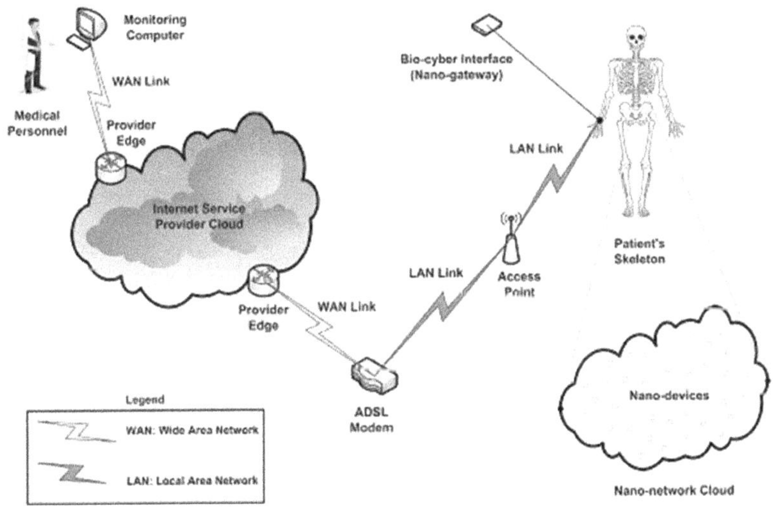

FIGURE 3.23 Wireless connectivity in nanoparticles.

Self-Healing Materials

The use of self-healing nanomaterials in wearable devices allows for the device to remain long-lasting and functional (Figure 3.24). These materials cannot be easily breached and can self-heal if ever damaged, which prolongs the functioning of the specific device in question [55].

Energy Harvesting

Ultra-thin devices like piezoelectric or triboelectric nanogenerators exist to convert the motions of the human body or its surroundings into energy. This energy can be used to fuel the wearable device so that the device can become independent of the power supply from other parts.

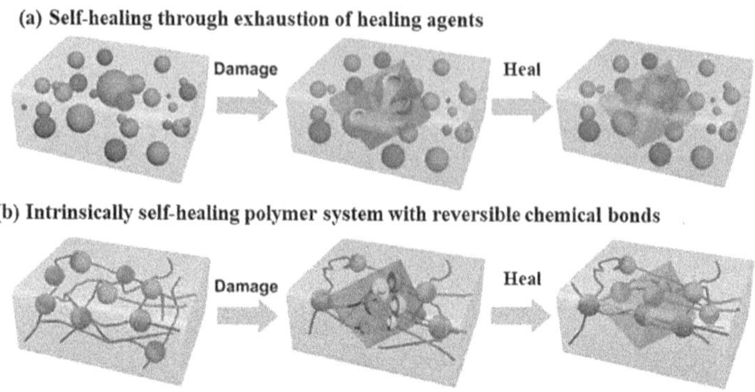

FIGURE 3.24 Self-healing methods.

Advantages and Limitations of Nanomaterials in Wound Healing

Nanomaterials are novel in wound healing applications since they hold great promise as these materials have presented the healing matrix. This includes a high SA:V ratio, controllable physicochemical properties, and molecular-level compatibility with biosystems. Despite the numerous advantages they offer, challenges like biocompatibility, toxicity, and regulatory issues must be dealt with for the use of these nanomaterials to be expanded. In the next section of the paper, the benefits as well as drawbacks of nanomaterial application in wound care will be described in detail [56].

Benefit

Enhanced Efficacy

The therapeutic agents can be introduced at the site of the wound with a high degree of accuracy using nanomaterials. For instance, NPs can be used to encapsulate drugs that will only be released continuously to the targeted area. This focused exposure reduces system acute exposure and therefore enhances the cure rates of chronic wounds, such as diabetic ulcers. In addition, the use of narrow material such as AgNPs is also an effective antibacterial and has to reduce the infection rate, which hinders the process of healing.

Reduced Side Effects

Many of the clinical practices involving wound care can cause systemic therapy with risks such as organ toxicity or drug resistance. In contrast to nanomaterials, which provide site-specific targeting, they cause much less systemic effects. For example, lipid-based NPs can be employed to deliver anti-inflammatory agents to the cellular level and reduce inflammation but with minimal damage to the rest of the surrounding tissue.

Cost-Effectiveness in Long-Term Care

Even though the cost of nanomaterials might be relatively high at the onset, they are economically feasible for commercial use. Wound healing is an important concern because it reduces avoidable time, hospitalization, or repeated procedures. Also, the use of nanomaterials in dressings, including nanofibrous scaffolds, enhances the rate of tissue replacement, which may reduce the days taken for healing and the costs that accompany it.

Challenges

Biocompatibility and Toxicity Concerns

However, there is a major issue with the biocompatibility of nanomaterials in these applications exposed. Some may bring about oxidative stress or inflammation in the biological systems when they are introduced into systems. For example, staying concentrations of metal-based NPs including minute silver or zinc oxide can lead to cytotoxicity impacting the health of tissues. These materials must be subjected to rigorous tests to vastly minimize the long-term side effects once applied in clinical usage.

Regulatory and Scalability Issues

As mentioned above, nanomaterials go through numerous regulatory barriers before they can be allowed for their use. Regulatory bodies including the U.S. Food and Drug Administration and the European Medicines Agency want full preclinical and clinical information on all these materials before certifying them. Nonetheless, nanomaterials again come with a rather complicated structure, which makes it very difficult to standardize testing protocols. Further, the similarly related constraint is the issue of up-scaling nanomaterials for commercial purposes. Most manufacturing operations are precise and are conducted under strict conditions, making them more time-consuming.

Future Direction and Technology

Nanomaterials have become promising tools for wound healing applications due to their distinctive properties and therapeutic potential, particularly in the form of biopolymer nanoformulations. These formulations, made from biocompatible and biodegradable polymers, enable controlled drug delivery, promote faster wound closure, and minimize scarring. However, to fully realize their potential and facilitate clinical translation, several challenges must be addressed. A key challenge lies in optimizing drug release kinetics [57]. Biopolymeric nanoformulations can encapsulate diverse therapeutic agents, such as growth factors, antimicrobials, and anti-inflammatory drugs, highlighting the need for precise control over their release profiles [58].

Future research should prioritize developing innovative strategies to regulate drug release in biopolymer nanoformulations. Stimuli-responsive systems, capable of reacting to changes in the wound microenvironment or external triggers, present a promising approach. Additionally, a thorough understanding of the in vivo pharmacokinetics and pharmacodynamics of these formulations is critical for optimizing dosage and administration frequency [59]. Another challenge is enhancing the stability and shelf-life of biopolymer nanoformulations. Biopolymers are often prone to degradation, which can alter their properties over time, reducing drug encapsulation efficiency and therapeutic effectiveness. Addressing this requires robust formulation techniques and optimized storage conditions to maintain structural integrity and ensure consistent drug release.

Potential solutions include advanced cross-linking methods, lyophilization processes, and protective coatings to improve stability and longevity [60].

Emerging Technologies in Nanomedicine for Wound Care

Nanotechnology has revolutionized wound care, transforming biomedical dressings with advanced functionalities. Its integration into wound care solutions has significantly improved the efficiency of healing processes and the management of bacterial infections, marking a notable advancement in medical practices. Nanotechnology-enhanced dressings exhibit superior mechanical strength and controlled drug release, enabling more precise and effective therapeutic applications [61]. This review highlights recent advancements in wound healing technologies, emphasizing innovative medical dressings such as nanoenzymes. Additionally, smart materials like hydrogels and electroactive polymers bring dynamic features to dressings, fostering tissue regeneration. Emerging approaches, including biofabrication, microfluidic systems, bio-responsive scaffolds, and personalized therapies, hold great potential to accelerate wound healing and reduce scarring. Utilizing nanoscale materials and methods to promote healing, lower infection rates, and improve patient outcomes is the main goal of emerging nanomedicine technologies for wound care [62]. Here is a summary of significant advancements:

NANOPARTICLE FOR ANTIMICROBIAL ACTION

Silver Nanoparticle

AgNPs play a crucial antimicrobial role in wound healing through multiple mechanisms that target bacterial cells and inhibit biofilm formation. Their nanoscale dimensions and high surface area enable them to disrupt bacterial membranes, penetrate cells, and cause intracellular damage. AgNPs generate oxidative stress, release metal ions, and interact with biological molecules such as DNA and enzymes. By aggregating on bacterial membranes, they interfere with essential biological functions and disrupt enzyme activity critical for energy metabolism and oxidative stress defense [56]. Furthermore, AgNPs inhibit the production of exopolysaccharides required for biofilm formation and disrupt quorum sensing, the bacterial communication system responsible for biofilm development and virulence regulation. Wound dressings incorporating flexible fabrics coated with AgNPs have been developed to leverage these properties. Research also suggests that AgNPs may contribute to reduced inflammation during wound healing. This effect is attributed to mechanisms such as silver-induced neutrophil apoptosis and the suppression of matrix metalloproteinase (MMP) activity, which may help mitigate the inflammatory response [63].

Gold Nanoparticle

AuNPs play significant anti-inflammatory and antioxidative roles in the wound healing process while also exhibiting notable antibacterial activity against both

Gram-negative and Gram-positive bacteria. Additionally, AuNPs have demonstrated antifungal properties, being effective against both unicellular and multicellular fungi, either as standalone agents or when combined with biopolymers such as chitosan [64]. Gold nanocomposites, such as chitosan-AuNPs (Chi/AuNPs), have been shown to be safe, as they do not adversely affect normal human skin cell lines. AuNPs have also been incorporated into chitosan hydrogels, enhancing antimicrobial resistance, reducing bacterial infections, and promoting wound healing. However, compared to AgNPs, AuNPs are less frequently utilized in wound care. This is due to challenges such as higher costs, lower antibacterial potency, concerns regarding biocompatibility and regulatory approval, and variations in their mechanisms of action [65].

Zinc Oxide Nanoparticle

Zinc oxide NPs have demonstrated significant potential in wound healing, primarily through the generation of electron–hole pairs that produce ROS, contributing to their antimicrobial properties. Additionally, these NPs play a role in promoting the re-epithelialization process, which is a critical step in wound healing [66].

POTENTIAL FOR PERSONALIZED WOUND HEALING SOLUTIONS

Personalized wound care is an emerging field that focuses on customizing treatments to match the unique biological characteristics of individual patients. The approach integrates factors such as genetic makeup, age, gender, comorbidities, and specific wound types (chronic, diabetic, or burn wounds). Personalization involves tailoring treatment plans that optimize healing based on these variables [67].

- **Genetic and phenotypic factors**: Studies have shown that genetic differences affect wound healing responses. Variations in genes related to inflammation, collagen synthesis, and cellular regeneration (e.g., VEGF, TGF-β) influence healing rates and scar formation [68]. Personalized treatments can target these pathways to optimize recovery.
- **Comorbidities and risk factors**: Conditions like diabetes, obesity, and vascular diseases can hinder the healing process. Personalized solutions assess these risk factors, enabling the use of more effective treatments, such as advanced wound dressings and targeted therapies, that are suited to individual patients' needs [69].

NANOTECHNOLOGY AND SMART MATERIALS FOR PERSONALIZED TREATMENT

Nanotechnology has been instrumental in the development of personalized wound care by enhancing drug delivery systems and designing responsive dressings. Nanomaterials like NPs and nanofibers offer controlled and targeted release of therapeutics, which can be adjusted based on the wound's specific requirements [70].

- **Nanoparticles for targeted drug delivery**: NPs, including silver, gold, and zinc oxide, can be engineered to release antimicrobial agents or growth factors at controlled rates, ensuring that the healing process is optimized for the patient's wound condition.
- **Smart wound dressings**: Smart materials, such as hydrogels and electroactive polymers, can respond to changes in the wound environment, such as pH or temperature, offering a personalized therapeutic approach. These materials can adjust drug release or even monitor wound conditions in real time, enhancing healing efficiency.

BIOMARKERS AND DIAGNOSTICS FOR PERSONALIZED CARE

The integration of advanced diagnostics and biomarker identification can further refine personalized wound healing strategies. For instance, monitoring biomarkers related to inflammation, infection, and tissue regeneration can guide treatment decisions, allowing healthcare providers to adjust therapies based on the wound's progress [71].

- **Biomarkers for infection detection**: New diagnostic tools that detect infection markers, such as MMPs and C-reactive protein (CRP), enable timely intervention, ensuring that antimicrobial treatments are used when needed, without overuse.
- **Regenerative medicine and stem cells**: Personalized wound healing is increasingly incorporating regenerative medicine approaches, such as stem cell therapies, to promote tissue regeneration. Stem cells can be isolated and cultured from the patient's own tissues to reduce rejection and optimize healing.

REGULATORY AND ETHICAL CONSIDERATIONS

Regulatory and ethical considerations play a crucial role in the development and implementation of personalized wound healing solutions, particularly those involving emerging technologies such as nanomaterials, stem cells, and bioengineered dressings. Regulatory bodies, such as the Food and Drug Administration and the European Medicines Agency, are responsible for ensuring the safety and efficacy of these novel therapies. One of the primary challenges in this area is the rigorous safety and efficacy testing required before approval. For example, wound healing technologies that incorporate NPs or stem cells must undergo comprehensive in vitro and in vivo studies to assess their potential risks, including cytotoxicity, biocompatibility, and long-term effects [72]. The approval process for personalized therapies, such as those involving patient-specific materials or genetic-based interventions, is complex and often requires tailored pathways that account for individual patient variations, further complicating timelines for approval. Additionally, with the integration of smart wound dressings and personalized health monitoring, there are significant concerns about patient data privacy, with regulations like the General Data Protection Regulation (GDPR) and the Health Insurance Portability and Accountability Act

(HIPAA) ensuring secure collection and use of health data [73]. Ethically, personalized wound care raises several important issues. First, ensuring informed consent is vital, especially when patients are receiving novel treatments that are not widely available. Clear communication about the potential risks and benefits of such treatments is necessary to allow patients to make fully informed decisions about their care. Another ethical challenge involves equity and accessibility, as the cost of advanced personalized therapies could limit their availability to certain populations, potentially exacerbating healthcare disparities [73].

Personalized treatments, particularly those involving regenerative medicine and genetic modifications, also raise ethical questions surrounding the manipulation of human cells and tissues. Concerns about the long-term effects of stem cell-based therapies, including the possibility of tumor formation or genetic alterations, must be carefully considered. Additionally, there are ethical concerns about animal testing used in the development of these treatments. While animal models provide valuable insights, efforts should be made to minimize harm through alternative methods, such as in vitro models or computer-based simulations [74].

Finally, regulatory and ethical oversight must address the long-term monitoring of personalized therapies. Since the effects of these advanced treatments may not be fully evident in the short term, it is essential to establish frameworks for ongoing monitoring to identify and manage any complications that may arise. Public perception and trust in new technologies also play a key role in their acceptance. Ethical considerations should include efforts to educate both the public and healthcare providers about the potential benefits and risks associated with personalized wound healing therapies to foster informed decision-making. Balancing innovation with safety, equity, and patient-centered care is essential to ensure the successful clinical translation of these advanced technologies [75].

REFERENCES

1. S. Kumar et al., "Current understanding to accelerate wound healing: mechanism and clinical importance," *Recent Adv. Wound Heal.*, Nov. 2021, doi:10.5772/INTECHOPEN.101429.
2. J. Blackburn, Z. Kopecki, and K. J. Ousey, "Skin integrity, antimicrobial stewardship and infection control: a critical review of current best practice," *Wound Pract. Res.*, vol. 32, no. 1, pp. 34–43, Mar. 2024, doi:10.33235/WPR.32.1.34-43.
3. D. S. Kirwin, H. E. Diaz, T. C. Frantz, C. F. Janney, C. L. Hardy, and W. H. Lyford, "Wound healing: cellular review with specific attention to postamputation care," *Cutis*, vol. 113, no. 3, pp. 125–131, Mar. 2024, doi:10.12788/CUTIS.0970.
4. Y. H. Almadani, J. Vorstenbosch, P. G. Davison, and A. M. Murphy, "Wound healing: a comprehensive review," *Semin. Plast. Surg.*, vol. 35, no. 3, pp. 141–144, Aug. 2021, doi:10.1055/S-0041-1731791.
5. G. Albahri et al., "The therapeutic wound healing bioactivities of various medicinal plants," *Life (Basel, Switzerland)*, vol. 13, no. 2, Feb. 2023, doi:10.3390/LIFE13020317.
6. P. Rybkowska, "Optimizing skin wound healing: the crucial role of the innate immune system and inflammatory microenvironment," *Forum Leczenia Ran*, vol. 5, no. 2, pp. 77–86, Jun. 2024, doi:10.15374/FLR2024008.
7. L. Huelsboemer et al., "Cellular therapeutics and immunotherapies in wound healing - on the pulse of time?," *Mil. Med. Res.*, vol. 11, no. 1, Dec. 2024, doi:10.1186/S40779-024-00528-5.

8. J. D. Chin, L. Zhao, T. G. Mayberry, B. C. Cowan, M. R. Wakefield, and Y. Fang, "Photodynamic therapy, probiotics, acetic acid, and essential oil in the treatment of chronic wounds infected with *Pseudomonas aeruginosa*," *Pharm.,* vol. 15, no. 6, p. 1721, Jun. 2023, doi:10.3390/PHARMACEUTICS15061721.
9. A. Miron et al., "Antimicrobial biomaterials for chronic wound care," *Pharm.,* vol. 15, no. 6, p. 1606, May 2023, doi:10.3390/PHARMACEUTICS15061606.
10. R. Szabó and I. Barcs, "The importance of infection prevention and control in chronic wound care," *Bőrgyógyászati és Venerológiai Szle.*, vol. 98, no. 6, pp. 316–320, Dec. 2022, doi:10.7188/BVSZ.2022.98.6.4.
11. H. E. DesJardins-Park, S. Mascharak, M. S. Chinta, D. C. Wan, and M. T. Longaker, "The spectrum of scarring in craniofacial wound repair," *Front. Physiol.*, vol. 10, no. MAR, p. 445822, Mar. 2019, https://doi.org/10.3389/fphys.2019.00322.
12. M. S. F. Alencar et al., "Evidence-based practices on nanotechnology in wound treatment," *Cad. Pedagógico.*, vol. 21, no. 12, pp. e10234–e10234, Nov. 2024, doi:10.54033/CADPEDV21N12-037.
13. F. N. Cetin, A. Mignon, S. Van Vlierberghe, and K. Kolouchova, "Polymer- and lipid-based nanostructures serving wound healing applications: a review," *Adv. Healthc. Mater.*, vol. 14, no. 1, p. 2402699, Jan. 2025, doi:10.1002/ADHM.202402699.
14. S. Nasra, S. Pramanik, V. Oza, K. Kansara, and A. Kumar, "Advancements in wound management: integrating nanotechnology and smart materials for enhanced therapeutic interventions," *Discov. Nano.,* vol. 19, no. 1, pp. 1–31, Oct. 2024, doi:10.1186/S11671-024-04116-3.
15. V. Kotteeswaran, M. Saravanakumar, R. M. Alexander, R. S. Nair, and K. M. Ramnath, "Advancement of nanofibers in wound healing: a review," *Biomed. Pharmacol.* J., vol. 17, no. 3, pp. 1407–1431, Sep. 2024, doi:10.13005/BPJ/2953.
16. V. Sanapalli et al., "Nanoparticles for delivering micro and macromolecules for the management of diabetic wounds," *Cell Biochem. Funct.*, vol. 42, no. 8, Dec. 2024, doi:10.1002/CBF.70006.
17. W. Fu et al., "Opportunities and challenges of nanomaterials in wound healing: advances, mechanisms, and perspectives," *Chem. Eng. J.*, vol. 495, p. 153640, Sep. 2024, doi:10.1016/J.CEJ.2024.153640.
18. M. Singh, H. Dabas, A. Rehman, and P. R. Solanki, "Skin tissue engineering based on nanotechnology for wound management," In: P. R. Solanki, A. Kumar, R. P. Singh, J. Singh, & K. R. B. Singh (Eds.), *Nanotechnological Asp. Next-Generation Wound Manag*, Academic Press, pp. 233–244, Jan. 2024, doi:10.1016/B978-0-323-99165-0.00010-1.
19. D. Bhattacharya, B. Ghosh, and M. Mukhopadhyay, "Development of nanotechnology for advancement and application in wound healing: a review," *IET Nanobiotechnol.*, vol. 13, no. 8, p. 778, Oct. 2019, doi:10.1049/IET-NBT.2018.5312.
20. T. Ashwini et al., "Transforming wound management: nanomaterials and their clinical impact," *Pharmaceutics*, vol. 15, no. 5, May 2023, doi:10.3390/PHARMACEUTICS15051560.
21. H. Chopra et al., "Recent updates in nanotechnological advances for wound healing: a narrative review," *Nanotechnol. Rev.*, vol. 12, no. 1. doi:10.1515/ntrev-2023–0129.
22. J. Du, J. Wang, T. Xu, H. Yao, L. Yu, and D. Huang, "Hemostasis strategies and recent advances in nanomaterials for hemostasis," *Molecules*, vol. 28, no. 13, p. 5264, Jul. 2023, doi:10.3390/MOLECULES28135264.
23. J. Li, J. Chen, and R. Kirsner, "Pathophysiology of acute wound healing," *Clin. Dermatol.*, vol. 25, no. 1, pp. 9–18, Jan. 2007, doi:10.1016/J.CLINDERMATOL.2006.09.007.
24. R. Derner and J. Buckholz, "Surgical hemostasis by pneumatic ankle tourniquet during 3027 podiatric operations," *J. Foot Ankle Surg.*, vol. 34, no. 3, pp. 236–246, May 1995, doi:10.1016/S1067-2516(09)80054-9.

25. A. Z. Pathan, S. Aijaz, S. Sheikh, and S. Sattar, "Randomized trial comparing radial hemostasis techniques; catechol conjugated chitosan pad (InnoSEAL) versus pneumatic compression band," *Catheter. Cardiovasc. Interv.*, vol. 98, no. 2, pp. E181–E187, Aug. 2021, doi:10.1002/CCD.29578.
26. S. Seki et al., "Laparoscopic hemostasis for abdominal brunt massive hemorrhage due to endometriosis," *Asian J. Endosc. Surg.*, vol. 15, no. 2, pp. 376–379, Apr. 2022, doi:10.1111/ASES.13008.
27. S. Takao, H. Shinchi, K. Maemura, and T. Aikou, "Ultrasonically activated scalpel is an effective tool for cutting the pancreas in biliary-pancreatic surgery: experimental and clinical studies," *J. Hepatobiliary. Pancreat. Surg.*, vol. 7, no. 1, pp. 58–62, Mar. 2000, doi:10.1007/S005340050155.
28. A. Al-Aown et al., "Laparoscopic radical and partial nephrectomy: the clinical efficacy and acceptance of the techniques," *Urol.* Ann., vol. 6, no. 2, p. 101, 2014, doi:10.4103/0974-7796.130521.
29. A. P. Sah, "Clinical outcomes and experience of a multiyear consecutive case series of total knee arthroplasty procedures conducted with a bipolar sealer system for hemostasis," *J. Knee Surg.*, vol. 35, no. 12, pp. 1378–1384, Oct. 2022, doi:10.1055/S-0041-1723972.
30. F. Pereira Beserra, L. Fernando Sérgio Gushiken, M. Fernanda Hussni, and C. Helena Pellizzon, "Regulatory mechanisms and chemical signaling of mediators involved in the inflammatory phase of cutaneous wound healing," In: K. H. Doğan (Ed.), *Wound Healing—Current Perspectives*, IntechOpen, 2019. doi:10.5772/intechopen.81731.
31. Z. Wang, F. Qi, H. Luo, G. Xu, and D. Wang, "Inflammatory microenvironment of skin wounds," *Front. Immunol.*, vol. 13, p. 789274, Mar. 2022, doi:10.3389/FIMMU.2022.789274.
32. T. A. Wilgus, S. Roy, and J. C. McDaniel, "Neutrophils and wound repair: positive actions and negative reactions," *Adv. Wound Care*, vol. 2, no. 7, pp. 379–388, Sep. 2013, doi:10.1089/WOUND.2012.0383.
33. S. K. Shukla, A. K. Sharma, V. Gupta, and M. H. Yashavarddhan, "Pharmacological control of inflammation in wound healing," *J. Tissue Viability*, vol 28, no. 4, pp. 218–222, Nov. 2019, doi:10.1016/J.JTV.2019.09.002.
34. Y. Jiang, X. Xu, L. Xiao, L. Wang, and S. Qiang, "The role of microRNA in the inflammatory response of wound healing," *Front. Immunol.*, vol. 13, p. 852419, Mar. 2022, https://doi.org/10.3389/fimmu.2022.852419.
35. M. Abazari, A. Ghaffari, H. Rashidzadeh, S. M. Badeleh, and Y. Maleki, "A systematic review on classification, identification, and healing process of burn wound healing," *Int. J. Low. Extrem. Wounds*, vol. 21, no. 1, pp. 18–30, Mar. 2022, doi:10.1177/1534734620924857.
36. O. Krizanova, A. Penesova, J. Sokol, A. Hokynkova, A. Samadian, and P. Babula, "Signaling pathways in cutaneous wound healing," *Front. Physiol.*, vol. 13, p. 1030851, Nov. 2022, doi:10.3389/FPHYS.2022.1030851.
37. M. Fernández-Guarino, M. L. Hernández-Bule, and S. Bacci, "Cells and processes in wound healing: more recent advances," *Biomedicines*, vol. 11, no. 9, p. 2526, May 2023, doi:10.20944/PREPRINTS202305.0643.V1.
38. T. Lestari, S. Syukur, G. Revilla, R. S. Rita, and R. Rustini, "The burn wound healing process : a review," *Int. J. Progress. Sci. Technol.*, vol. 40, no. 1, pp. 77–88, Aug. 2023, doi:10.52155/ijpsat.v40.1.5565.
39. R. Dhar, M. Chakraborty, and T. K. Dutta, "A comprehensive assessment of the antimicrobial and immunomodulatory effects of frequently consumed fermented foods: insights in the management of COVID-19," *J. Appl. M*icrobiol., vol. 134, no. 1, pp. 1–18, Jan. 2023, doi:10.1093/JAMBIO/LXAC034.

40. F. Wang et al., "Graphene oxide framework structures and coatings: impact on cell adhesion and pre-vascularization processes for bone grafts," *Int. J. Mol. Sci.*, vol. 23, no. 6, p. 3379, Mar. 2022, https://doi.org/10.3390/ijms23063379.
41. S. Mukherjee et al., "Graphene oxides show angiogenic properties," *Adv. Healthc. M*ater., vol. 4, no. 11, pp. 1722–1732, Aug. 2015, doi:10.1002/ADHM.201500155.
42. A. Bal-Öztürk et al., "Innovative approaches in skin therapy: bionanocomposites for skin tissue repair and regeneration," *Mater. Adv.*, vol. 5, no. 12, pp. 4996–5024, Jun. 2024, doi:10.1039/D4MA00384E.
43. S. Riaz, A. Riaz, A. Younus, M. Mubin, and M. Ashraf, "Application of bionanomaterials for cancer therapy," In: J. A. Malik, M. R. Goyal, & M. J. M.Sadiq (Eds.), *Sustainable Nanomaterials for Biomedical Engineering: Impacts, Challenges, and Future Prospects,* Apple Academic Press/Taylor & Francis, pp. 307–341, May 2023, https://doi.org/10.1201/9781003333456-14.
44. J. Li et al., "Chitosan-based nanomaterials for drug delivery," *Molecules,* vol. 23, no. 10, p. 2661, Oct. 2018, doi:10.3390/MOLECULES23102661.
45. F. Jonidi Shariatzadeh, S. Currie, S. Logsetty, R. Spiwak, and S. Liu, "Enhancing wound healing and minimizing scarring: a comprehensive review of nanofiber technology in wound dressings," *Prog. Mater. Sci.*, vol. 147, p. 101350, Jan. 2025, doi:10.1016/J.PMATSCI.2024.101350.
46. S. Saurav et al., "Harnessing natural polymers for nano-scaffolds in bone tissue engineering: a comprehensive overview of bone disease treatment," *Curr. Issues Mol. Biol.,* vol. 46, no. 1, pp. 585–611, Jan. 2024, doi:10.3390/CIMB46010038.
47. N. S. Sumitha, N. G. Krishna, and G. S. Sailaja, "Chitosan-TEMPO-oxidized nanocellulose magnetic responsive patches with hyperthermia potential for smart melanoma therapy," *ACS Appl. Polym. Mater.*, vol. 5, no. 11, pp. 9170–9179, Nov. 2023, https://doi.org/10.1021/acsapm.3c01654.
48. Y. Li, L. Yang, Y. Zeng, Y. Wu, Y. Wei, and L. Tao, "Self-healing hydrogel with a double dynamic network comprising imine and borate ester linkages," *Chem. Mater.*, vol. 31, no. 15, pp. 5576–5583, Aug. 2019, https://doi.org/10.1021/acs.chemmater.9b01301.
49. P. Nezhad-Mokhtari, M. Hasany, M. Kohestanian, A. Dolatshahi-Pirouz, M. Milani, and M. Mehrali, "Recent advancements in bioadhesive self-healing hydrogels for effective chronic wound care," *Adv. Colloid Interface Sci.*, vol. 334, p. 103306, Dec. 2024, doi:10.1016/J.CIS.2024.103306.
50. S. Chen et al., "Cerium oxide nanoparticles in wound care: a review of mechanisms and therapeutic applications," *Front. Bioeng. Biotechnol.*, vol. 12, p. 1404651, May 2024, https://doi.org/10.3389/fbioe.2024.1404651.
51. T. Sangnim, V. Puri, D. Dheer, D. N. Venkatesh, K. Huanbutta, and A. Sharma, "Nanomaterials in the wound healing process: new insights and advancements," *Pharmaceutics*, vol. 16, no. 3, Mar. 2024, doi:10.3390/PHARMACEUTICS16030300.
52. A. Barroso, H. Mestre, A. Ascenso, S. Simões, and C. Reis, "Nanomaterials in wound healing: from material sciences to wound healing applications," *Nano Sel.*, vol. 1, no. 5, pp. 443–460, Nov. 2020, doi:10.1002/NANO.202000055.
53. A. Kushwaha, L. Goswami, and B. S. Kim, "Nanomaterial-based therapy for wound healing," *Nanomater.* vol. 12, no. 4, p. 618, Feb. 2022, doi:10.3390/NANO12040618.
54. S. Hamdan et al., "Nanotechnology-driven therapeutic interventions in wound healing: potential uses and applications," *ACS Cent. Sci.*, vol. 3, no. 3, pp. 163–175, Mar. 2017, https://doi.org/10.1021/acscentsci.6b00371.
55. S. Patel et al., "Wearable electronics for skin wound monitoring and healing," *Soft Sci.*, vol. 2, no. 2, p. N/A-N/A, Jun. 2022, doi:10.20517/SS.2022.13.
56. M. A. Shalaby, M. M. Anwar, and H. Saeed, "Nanomaterials for application in wound healing: current state-of-the-art and future perspectives," *J. Polym. Res.,* vol. 29, no. 3, pp. 1–37, Feb. 2022, doi:10.1007/S10965-021-02870-X.

57. R. Abbasi, G. Shineh, M. Mobaraki, S. Doughty, and L. Tayebi, "Structural parameters of nanoparticles affecting their toxicity for biomedical applications: a review," *J. Nanoparticle Res.*, vol. 25, no. 3, pp. 1–35, Feb. 2023, doi:10.1007/S11051-023-05690-W.
58. P. U. Muñoz-González, J. M. Flores-Moreno, I. A. Quintero-Ortega, D. Mantovani, B. Mendoza-Novelo, and G. González-García, "Water-dispersible fluorescent silicon nanoparticles that modulate inflammatory response in macrophages," *ACS Appl. Nano Mater.*, vol. 6, no. 13, pp. 11187–11197, Jul. 2023, https://doi.org/10.1021/acsanm.3c01210.
59. Y. Zhou et al., "Microstructure-united heterogeneous sodium alginate doped injectable hydrogel for stable hemostasis in dynamic mechanical environments," *Int. J. Biol. M*acromol., vol. 248, p. 125877, Sep. 2023, doi:10.1016/J.IJBIOMAC.2023.125877.
60. A. Abdel-Halim, "Strategies for cancer therapy," *Egypt. Pharm. J.*, vol. 22, no. 2, pp. 165–176, Apr. 2023, doi:10.4103/EPJ.EPJ_188_22.
61. M. Zarei, G. Lee, S. G. Lee, and K. Cho, "Advances in biodegradable electronic skin: material progress and recent applications in sensing, robotics, and human–machine interfaces," *Adv. Mater.*, vol. 35, no. 4, p. 2203193, Jan. 2023, doi:10.1002/ADMA.202203193.
62. R. Bhattacharjee et al., "Nanotheranostics to target antibiotic-resistant bacteria: strategies and applications," *OpenNano*, vol. 11, p. 100138, May 2023, doi:10.1016/J.ONANO.2023.100138.
63. S. S. Mathew-Steiner, S. Roy, and C. K. Sen, "Collagen in wound healing," *Bioeng.*, vol. 8, no. 5, p. 63, May 2021, doi:10.3390/BIOENGINEERING8050063.
64. A. Etxabide, P. A. Kilmartin, and J. I. Maté, "Color stability and pH-indicator ability of curcumin, anthocyanin and betanin containing colorants under different storage conditions for intelligent packaging development," *Food Control*, vol. 121, p. 107645, Mar. 2021, doi:10.1016/J.FOODCONT.2020.107645.
65. Y. Yang, Y. Du, J. Zhang, H. Zhang, and B. Guo, "Structural and functional design of electrospun nanofibers for hemostasis and wound healing," *Adv. Fiber Mater.*, vol. 4, no. 5, pp. 1027–1057, Jun. 2022, doi:10.1007/S42765-022-00178-7.
66. L. Sethuram and J. Thomas, "Therapeutic applications of electrospun nanofibers impregnated with various biological macromolecules for effective wound healing strategy: a review," *Biomed. Pharmacother.*, vol. 157, Jan. 2023, doi:10.1016/J.BIOPHA.2022.113996.
67. S. A. El-Sherbeni and W. A. Negm, "The wound healing effect of botanicals and pure natural substances used in in vivo models," *Inflammopharmacology*, vol. 31, no. 2, pp. 755–772, Apr. 2023, doi:10.1007/S10787-023-01157-5.
68. Á. Serrano-Aroca et al., "Scaffolds in the microbial resistant era: fabrication, materials, properties and tissue engineering applications," *Mater. Today Bio.*, vol. 16, p. 100412, Dec. 2022, doi:10.1016/J.MTBIO.2022.100412.
69. C. Mukherjee et al., "Recent advances in biodegradable polymers: properties, applications and future prospects," *Eur. Polym. J.*, vol. 192, p. 112068, 2023, doi:10.1016/j.eurpolymj.2023.112068.
70. M. S. B. Reddy, D. Ponnamma, R. Choudhary, and K. K. Sadasivuni, "A comparative review of natural and synthetic biopolymer composite scaffolds," *Polym.*, vol. 13, no. 7, p. 1105, Mar. 2021, doi:10.3390/POLYM13071105.
71. Z. Jiang et al., "Nanofiber scaffolds as drug delivery systems promoting wound healing," *Pharm.*, vol. 15, no. 7, p. 1829, Jun. 2023, doi:10.3390/PHARMACEUTICS15071829.
72. P. Li et al., "Design of 3D polycaprolactone/ε-polylysine-modified chitosan fibrous scaffolds with incorporation of bioactive factors for accelerating wound healing," *Acta Biomater.*, vol. 152, pp. 197–209, Oct. 2022, doi:10.1016/J.ACTBIO.2022.08.075.

73. G. Amokrane et al., "Electrospun poly(ϵ-caprolactone) fiber scaffolds functionalized by the covalent grafting of a bioactive polymer: surface characterization and influence on in vitro biological response," *ACS Omega*, vol. 4, no. 17, pp. 17194–17208, Oct. 2019, https://doi.org/10.1021/acsomega.9b01647.
74. Y. L. Chung, P. Y. Chou, and M. J. Sheu, "The wound-healing activity of PEDOT-PSS in animals," *Int. J. Mol. Sci.,* vol. 24, no. 16, p. 12539, Aug. 2023, doi:10.3390/IJMS 241612539.
75. Q. Tang et al., "Flexible, breathable, and self-powered patch assembled of electrospun polymer triboelectric layers and polypyrrole-coated electrode for infected chronic wound healing," *ACS Appl. Mater. Interfaces*, vol. 15, no. 14, pp. 17641–17652, Apr. 2023, https://doi.org/10.1021/acsami.3c00500.

4 Core–Shell Technology for Wound Dressings

Muhammad Qamar Khan
and Muhammad Abbas Haider Alvi

INTRODUCTION TO CORE–SHELL TECHNOLOGY

Core–shell technology represents a sophisticated materials engineering approach in which two distinct components, an inner **core** and an outer **shell**, are combined into a single-structured system. This architecture enables the optimized use of materials by assigning specific functions to each layer, making the technology highly suitable for biomedical applications, especially **advanced wound dressings** [1].

Concept of Core–Shell Structures

In a core–shell system, the *core* typically contains the primary functional agents, such as a drug, growth factor, or bioactive compound, while the *shell* serves as a protective barrier, controlling the release of the core material and enhancing stability. The two layers are engineered to work synergistically:

Core: It includes active agent reservoir, moisture retention, or structural support. **Shell**: It includes protection from degradation, mechanical strength, and interaction with the biological environment. This dual-layered configuration mimics natural systems such as cells or biomineral shells, enabling more precise control over material behavior compared to single-component dressings (Figure 4.1).

Relevance to Wound Management

Wound healing is a complex, staged process involving hemostasis, inflammation, proliferation, and remodeling. Each phase has unique requirements, such as:

- moisture regulation,
- infection control,
- controlled drug delivery, and
- structural support for tissue regeneration.

Traditional wound dressings often fail to meet these multiple requirements simultaneously. Core–shell technologies offer an integrated solution by allowing multifunctionality within one material system.

DOI: 10.1201/9781003616726-5

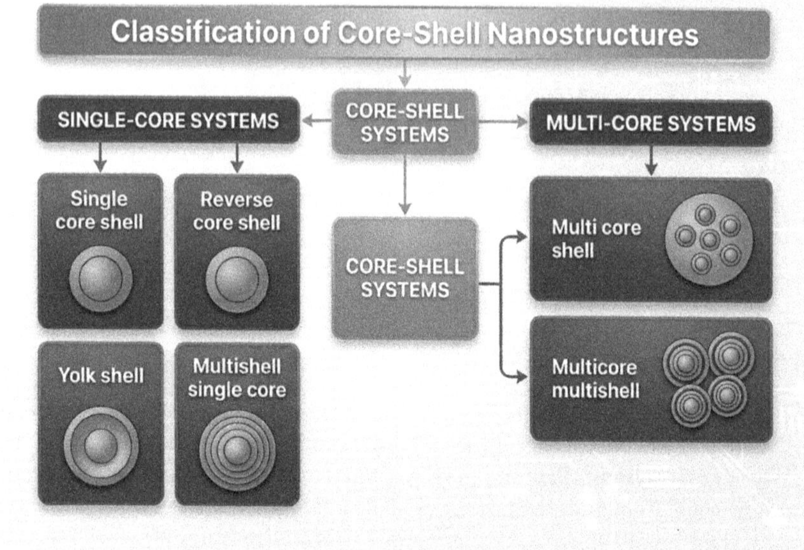

FIGURE 4.1 Core–shell nanostructures.

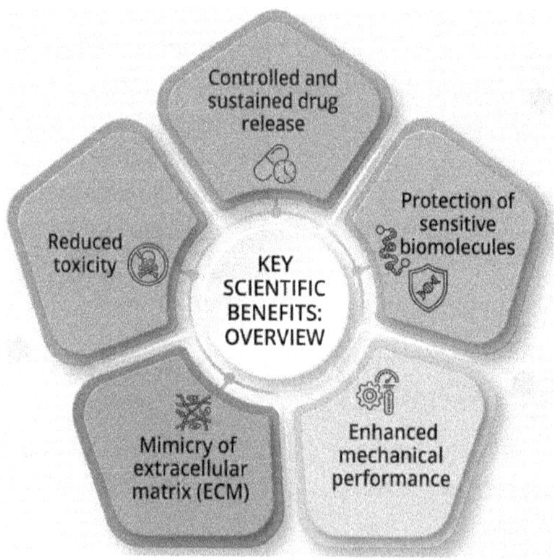

FIGURE 4.2 Advantages over conventional dressings.

Advantages Over Conventional Dressings

Core–shell wound dressings provide several superior features [2] (see Figure 4.2), including:

- **Controlled and sustained drug release**: The shell moderates the diffusion of therapeutic agents from the core, preventing rapid depletion and reducing dosing frequency.

- **Protection of sensitive biomolecules**: Growth factors, peptides, and antibiotics can be shielded from degradation by environmental factors such as oxygen or enzymes.
- **Enhanced mechanical performance**: The shell can be engineered for strength, while the core may remain soft or absorbent.
- **Mimicry of extracellular matrix (ECM)**: Core–shell nanofibers closely resemble ECM architecture, promoting cell attachment and migration.
- **Reduced toxicity**: By isolating reactive agents in the core, contact with surrounding tissue is minimized.

These capabilities make core–shell structures ideally suited for chronic wounds, burns, diabetic ulcers, and surgical sites.

Evolution of Core–Shell Technology in Biomedicine

Initially developed for fields like catalysis and electronics, core–shell systems were later adapted to biomedical engineering with advancements in nanotechnology and polymer sciences. Key developments include:

- coaxial electrospinning for nanofiber fabrication,
- hydrogel-based core–shell beads for drug encapsulation, and
- bioresorbable polymer shells that degrade at controlled rates.

As research advanced, core–shell wound dressings evolved from simple drug-loaded fibers to sophisticated, responsive systems capable of reacting to pH, temperature, or bacterial enzymes [3].

Importance in Modern Healthcare

The rise in chronic diseases (e.g., diabetes), aging populations, and antibiotic-resistant infections has intensified the need for smarter wound care solutions. Core–shell technology offers:

- personalized treatment strategies,
- enhanced therapeutic efficiency,
- minimized infection risks, and
- improved patient comfort and outcomes.

Thus, core–shell systems are becoming a central component of next-generation wound dressings.

PRINCIPLES OF CORE–SHELL FIBER ARCHITECTURE

Building upon the foundational concepts presented in Section 4.1, core–shell fiber architecture represents the structural backbone of many advanced wound dressings. This architecture translates the general idea of core–shell systems into **fiber-based**

materials, enabling high surface area, tunable porosity, and biomimicry of natural tissue structures.

Structural Configuration of Core–Shell Fibers

Core–shell fibers consist of two concentric layers:

- **Core**: It contains active therapeutic agents (e.g., antimicrobials, growth factors), hydrogels for moisture balance, or supportive polymers.
- **Shell**: It functions as a protective layer controlling the release of core materials, providing mechanical strength, and forming the primary interface with the wound.

The dual layer design allows for spatial separation of functionalities—an essential advantage over single layer fibers where all components are directly exposed to the environment.

Mechanisms Governing Functionality

The behavior and performance of core–shell fibers in wound dressings stem from several key mechanisms:

Diffusion controlled release: The shell regulates the diffusion of encapsulated agents in the core, ensuring:

- sustained drug delivery,
- avoidance of initial burst release, and
- optimized therapeutic window across wound healing phases.

Barrier protection: The shell shields core materials from:

- enzymatic degradation,
- environmental oxygen,
- light-induced degradation, and
- premature interaction with microbes.

This mechanism directly supports the advantages discussed earlier.

Mechanical reinforcement: The shell layer contributes stiffness and tensile strength, while the softer or functional core provides elasticity and bioactivity. This synergy is critical for dressings that must flex with the skin yet maintain structural integrity.

Micro- to Nanoscale Fiber Architecture

Core–shell wound dressings are typically fabricated at micro- or nanoscale dimensions, which enhances their performance:

- **High surface-area-to-volume ratio**: It improves oxygen exchange and fluid absorption.
- **ECM-like structure**: It supports fibroblast adhesion and keratinocyte migration, aiding faster re-epithelialization.
- **Porosity control**: It enables exudate management and reduces maceration.

These characteristics reinforce the points in Section 4.1 relating to ECM mimicry and improved healing environments [4].

Selection of Materials for Core and Shell

The functional requirements of each layer dictate material choice, ensuring compatibility with wound healing needs.

Core materials: These are often selected for:

- drug loading capacity,
- moisture retention, and
- biodegradability.
- **Examples**: hydrogels (alginate, PVA), therapeutic polymers (chitosan), proteins, and nanoparticles.

Shell materials: These are chosen for:

- mechanical protection,
- barrier function, and
- controlled degradation.
- **Examples**: PLA, PCL, gelatin, and cellulose derivatives.

Material pairing directly influences release kinetics, degradation rate, and overall dressing performance.

Influence of Architecture on Wound Healing

The core–shell fiber architecture directly addresses major wound healing challenges:

- **Chronic wounds**: Sustained antibiotic or growth factor delivery supports prolonged healing timelines.
- **Burn wounds**: Controlled moisture environments reduce pain and infection risk.
- **Diabetic ulcers**: Protection of sensitive bioactive prevents rapid degradation in enzyme-rich environments.
- **Post-surgical sites**: Stronger shell layers prevent dressing rupture while ensuring therapeutic support.

This demonstrates a clear continuity with Section 4.1, highlighting how the principles of core–shell structures translate into practical biomedical functionality.

Integration into Modern Dressing Designs

Core–shell fibers can be incorporated into:

- nanofiber mats,
- multilayer composite dressings,
- hydrogel fiber hybrids, and
- stimuli-responsive systems (pH, heat, and enzyme triggered).

These emerging designs form the basis for advanced wound care products that combine protection, therapy, and regeneration within a single platform.

MATERIALS USED IN CORE–SHELL WOUND DRESSINGS

The selection of materials for both the core and shell layers is crucial because it directly influences the wound dressing's mechanical performance, biocompatibility, degradation behavior, and therapeutic efficiency [5]. Core–shell systems rely on strategic pairing of materials, so each layer performs a distinct, complementary function—an extension of the principles discussed in Section 4.2 (Figure 4.3).

Material Selection Criteria

Effective core–shell wound dressings require materials that fulfill specific biomedical, mechanical, and functional roles.

Biocompatibility

Materials must not provoke irritation, inflammation, or cytotoxic reactions. Both layers should support cell adhesion and allow normal wound healing processes.

Controlled Degradation

Since most core–shell systems are designed to degrade or release agents over time:

- The **core** may need quicker degradation to release drugs.
- The **shell** may degrade more slowly to maintain structural integrity.

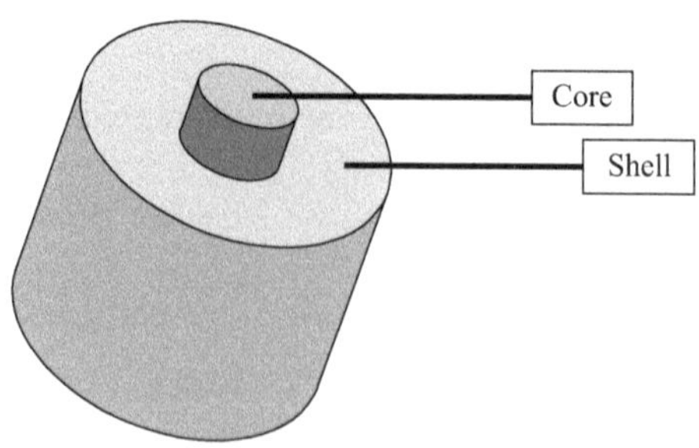

FIGURE 4.3 Core and shell view.

Mechanical Strength

The shell often needs tensile strength and flexibility to withstand stretching, while the core may prioritize absorption or drug encapsulation.

Encapsulation Efficiency

Core materials must effectively encapsulate bioactive compounds without degrading them during fabrication (e.g., during electrospinning or crosslinking).

Core Materials

Core materials typically focus on therapeutic activity, moisture regulation, and controlled release.

Natural Polymers

Natural polymers are common due to their excellent biocompatibility.

- **Chitosan**: It is antimicrobial, hemostatic, and supports cell proliferation. Ideal for drug-loaded cores.
- **Gelatin**: It is biodegradable and supports tissue regeneration.
- **Alginate**: It is highly absorbent and ideal for exudate heavy wounds.
- **Collagen**: It mimics the ECM and promotes cell attachment.

Synthetic Polymers

Synthetic materials offer tunable properties:

- **Poly(vinyl alcohol) (PVA)**: It has excellent film forming ability and biocompatibility.
- **Polyethylene oxide (PEO)**: It is used for encapsulating delicate bioactives because it is water soluble and gentle.
- **Polycaprolactone (PCL)**: It supports sustained release when used in semi-crystalline form.

Hydrogels

Hydrogels (e.g., PEG based, alginate gels) are ideal for:

- keeping wound moist,
- delivering hydrophilic drugs, and
- providing soft, cushion-like support.

Drug and Nanoparticle-Loaded Cores

The core may also include:

- antibiotics (e.g., ciprofloxacin, silver nanoparticles),
- anti-inflammatory agents (e.g., curcumin),
- growth factors (e.g., VEGF, EGF), and
- antioxidant nanoparticles (cerium oxide).

The architecture discussed in Section 4.2 enhances protection and controlled release of these agents.

Shell Materials

Shell materials focus on providing mechanical strength, protection, and controlled penetration of fluids.

Synthetic Polymers

These provide durability and controlled degradation:

- **Poly(lactic acid) (PLA)**: It is biodegradable and forms strong protective shells.
- **Poly(lactic co glycolic acid) (PLGA)**: It offers tunable degradation rates.
- **Polycaprolactone (PCL)**: It is flexible, slow-degrading, and ideal for long-term dressings.

Natural Polymers

These are often used for enhancing biological activity:

- **Cellulose and its derivatives (CMC, HEC)**: These are excellent for moisture control and biocompatibility.
- **Silk fibroin**: It is highly breathable and mechanically robust.
- **Gelatin**: It enhances hydrophilicity and cell adhesion.

Hybrid Composites

Combination materials improve performance:

- Natural/synthetic blends (e.g., PCL gelatin),
- Nanocomposite shells reinforced with clay, graphene, or bioactive glass.

These hybrids strengthen mechanical properties while maintaining bioactivity.

Material Pairing Strategies

The pairing of core and shell materials is one of the most critical decisions in designing a core–shell wound dressing. The selection must support the functional goals identified in Sections 4.1 and 4.3, including controlled release, structural protection, antimicrobial activity, and tissue regeneration.

Fast Releasing Core + Slow-Degrading Shell

This is the most widely used strategy for *controlled and sustained drug delivery.*

- **Core**: It contains rapidly dissolving or water-soluble polymers (e.g., PEO, PVA) loaded with drugs or growth factors.
- **Shell**: It is made of slow-degrading polymers like PCL or PLA.

- **Outcome**:
    - The shell restricts rapid burst release.
    - The drug is delivered over an extended period, ideal for chronic wounds or burns.

Hydrophilic Core + Hydrophobic Shell

This is useful when the core contains hydrophilic or fragile bioactive agents that must be shielded from early degradation.

- **Core**: It includes hydrogels, proteins, hydrophilic polymer blends.
- **Shell**: It includes hydrophobic polymers like PCL or PLGA.
- **Outcome**:
    - Shell acts as a moisture barrier for stability.
    - Water penetration is regulated, ensuring predictable release and protecting sensitive agents.

Antimicrobial Shell + Growth Factor-Loaded Core

This is ideal for dual function dressings where both **infection control** and **tissue regeneration** are required.

- **Shell**: It may incorporate AgNPs, chitosan, or antimicrobial peptides.
- **Core**: It contains growth factors (EGF, VEGF), collagen, or bioactive hydrogels.
- **Outcome**:
    - Prevents surface level infection.
    - Promotes healing through deeper level regenerative activity.

Enzyme-Responsive Shell + Antibiotic Core

This is useful for *smart* wound dressings targeting infected or highly inflamed wounds.

- **Shell**: It is made of enzyme degradable polymers (e.g., gelatin, chitosan).
- **Core**: It contains antibiotics or anti-inflammatory drugs.
- **Outcome**:
    - Shell breaks down faster in infected wounds due to elevated enzyme activity.
    - It releases antibiotic precisely when needed (on-demand therapy).

Rigid Shell + Absorbent Core

This is designed for exudate heavy wounds such as diabetic ulcers.

- **Core**: It includes alginate, hydrogel, and CMC for fluid absorption.
- **Shell**: It includes PCL, PLA, or silk fibroin for durability.
- **Outcome**:
    - Provides structural stability while managing excess moisture.

Multilayer or Multidrug Pairing

Some advanced systems incorporate multiple drugs with staggered release profiles. Example strategies include:

- Antibiotic in shell + antioxidant in core.
- Anti-inflammatory in shell + angiogenic factor in core.

This enables stage-wise healing aligned with the phases discussed in Section 4.1.

Material Compatibility (Expanded)

Material compatibility ensures that the core–shell system remains stable during fabrication, storage, and clinical use. Poor compatibility can lead to layer separation, inconsistent drug release, or toxicity [6].

Solvent Compatibility

A critical factor during techniques such as coaxial electrospinning.

- The shell solvent must **not dissolve** or destabilize the core material.
- Common practice:
  - Use organic solvents for shell (e.g., DCM, DMF for PCL/PLA).
  - Use aqueous systems for core (e.g., PVA, gelatin).

This prevents mixing or diffusion between layers during fabrication.

Viscosity Matching

For stable core–shell fiber formation:

- The viscosity of core and shell polymer solutions must be appropriately balanced.

If the core is too thin or too thick:

- Fiber will collapse or form irregular structures. Matching viscosity ensures uniform fiber morphology.

Chemical Stability

Core-to-shell interactions must not:

- Degrade drugs or biomolecules.
- Trigger unwanted chemical reactions.
- Alter polymer structure.

For example, proteins degrade in harsh organic solvents, so they must be protected inside aqueous core solutions.

Thermal and pH Stability

Some polymers require heating or curing.

- Sensitive agents (enzymes, growth factors) must be paired with shell materials that allow low temperature fabrication.
- pH-sensitive drugs require neutral polymer environments.

Interfacial Adhesion

Strong adhesion between core and shell layers provides:

- structural integrity,
- stable release kinetics, and
- improved mechanical properties.

Polymers with compatible hydrophilicity or hydrogen bonding often form stronger interfaces.

Biocompatibility Matching

Core and shell materials must work **together** without triggering inflammation or cytotoxicity.

- **Example**: PCL shell + gelatin core ensures biocompatibility while maintaining mechanical support.

Sterilization Compatibility

Materials must tolerate standard medical sterilization methods:

- gamma irradiation,
- UV,
- autoclaving (only for heat-stable systems), and
- ethylene oxide (Table 4.1).

TABLE 4.1
Common Materials Used in Core–Shell Wound Dressings

Layer	Material	Type	Key Properties	Typical Applications
Core	Chitosan	Natural polymer	Antimicrobial, hemostatic, biocompatible	Infection control, drug delivery
Core	Gelatin	Natural polymer	ECM like, supports cell adhesion	Growth factor delivery
Core	Alginate	Natural polymer	Highly absorbent, gel forming	Exudate management
Core	Collagen	Natural protein	Excellent for regeneration	Tissue engineering, wound healing
Core	PVA	Synthetic polymer	Hydrophilic, stabilizes drugs	Drug reservoir in core
Core	PEO	Synthetic polymer	Water soluble, gentle on biomolecules	Encapsulation of proteins/enzymes
Core	Hydrogels (PEG, alginate gel)	Composite	Moisture retention, soft structure	Burn dressings, chronic wounds
Core	AgNPs, ZnO NPs	Nanomaterials	Strong antimicrobial action	Infection prone wounds

(Continued)

TABLE 4.1 (*Continued*)
Common Materials Used in Core–Shell Wound Dressings

Layer	Material	Type	Key Properties	Typical Applications
Shell	PCL	Synthetic polymer	Slow degradation, strong and flexible	Long-term wound dressings
Shell	PLA	Synthetic polymer	Biodegradable, protective barrier	Drug-controlled release
Shell	PLGA	Synthetic polymer	Adjustable degradation rate	Precision release control
Shell	Cellulose derivatives (CMC, HEC)	Natural polymer	Excellent moisture control	Hydrophilic shells, comfort
Shell	Silk fibroin	Natural protein	Strong, breathable, biocompatible	Regenerative dressings
Shell	Gelatin	Natural protein	Improves hydrophilicity	Bioactive shell layers
Shell	Graphene oxide composites	Nanomaterial	Antibacterial, mechanical enhancement	High strength dressings
Shell	Chitosan (as shell)	Natural polymer	Antimicrobial, bioadhesive	Infection prevention
Shell	PCL Gelatin blend	Composite	Balanced hydrophilic/hydrophobic behavior	Controlled release systems

FABRICATION TECHNIQUES FOR CORE–SHELL STRUCTURES

The fabrication of core–shell wound dressings depends on technologies capable of producing two-layered (core and shell) architectures with precise control over morphology, material distribution, and functional loading [7,8]. These techniques must maintain the stability of sensitive biomolecules, ensure structural integrity, and meet biomedical requirements such as sterility and biocompatibility (Figure 4.4).

This section builds on the principles established in Sections 4.1 and 4.3, showing how material selection and architecture are translated into real-world engineered wound dressings [9].

Coaxial Electrospinning

Coaxial electrospinning is the most widely used technique for creating core–shell nanofibers [10–12].

Principle

- Two polymer solutions (core and shell) are simultaneously pumped through a **coaxial needle**.
- Under high voltage, a composite jet forms, elongates, and solidifies into a continuous core–shell fiber.

Advantages

- Produces uniform nanofibers resembling the ECM.

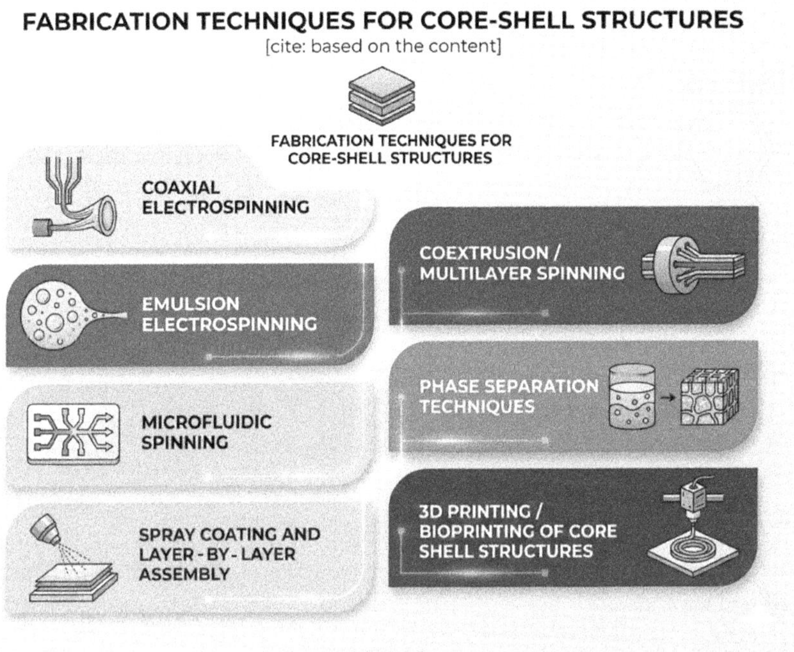

FIGURE 4.4 Fabrication techniques for core–shell structures.

- Allows encapsulation of fragile agents (enzymes, drugs, and growth factors) inside the core without direct exposure to harsh fabrication conditions.
- Enables excellent control over release kinetics by adjusting core/shell thickness.

Limitations

- Requires careful viscosity and solvent compatibility control.
- Organic solvents used in shells may harm sensitive bioactives if not well paired.

Applications

- Drug-loaded dressings.
- Anti-inflammatory wound scaffolds.
- Multidrug sequential release systems.

Emulsion Electrospinning

This method is a simpler alternative to coaxial electrospinning, which relies on an oil-in-water or water-in-oil emulsion [10,13].

Principle

- Core-forming material is dispersed as droplets inside a continuous shell forming polymer phase.

- During electrospinning, phase separation results in fibers with core–shell morphology.

Advantages

- Requires only one nozzle instead of coaxial needles.
- Suitable for encapsulating hydrophilic drugs in hydrophobic shells and vice versa.

Limitations

- Less precise core–shell definition compared to coaxial electrospinning.
- Stability of emulsions must be carefully managed.

Applications

- Antibiotic-loaded nanofibers.
- Growth factor protective wound mats.

Microfluidic Spinning

Microfluidic systems allow precise manipulation of fluid streams to generate well-defined core–shell fibers or microgels [14,15].

Principle

- Core and shell fluids are injected through microchannels with controlled flow rates.
- The system produces microscale fibers, capsules, or beads.

Advantages

- Highly uniform size and structure.
- Extremely gentle on cells and biomolecules—ideal for growth factor or cell-loaded cores.

Limitations

- Produces larger fibers/beads (microscale rather than nanoscale).
- Lower throughput compared to electrospinning.

Applications

- Cell-laden hydrogel dressings.
- Microsphere-based wound healing systems.

Coextrusion/Multilayer Spinning

Coextrusion involves pushing two molten or solution phase polymers through a multilayer die [16,17].

Principle

- Core and shell materials are fed into a die or spinneret that forms a continuous core–shell fiber or sheet.

Advantages

- Suitable for large-scale production.
- Allows fabrication of thicker core–shell fibers or films.

Limitations

- High temperature in melt processing may degrade drugs or proteins.
- Limited to heat-stable polymers unless done in solution phase.

Applications

- Structural wound dressings.
- Slow-release multilayered films.

Spray Coating and Layer-by-Layer Assembly

These techniques build core–shell architecture gradually rather than forming both layers simultaneously [18,19].

Spray Coating

Principle:

- A prefabricated core fiber mat or film is coated with a polymeric shell using spray deposition.

Advantages:

- Shell thickness is easy to control.
- Useful for adding antimicrobial shells or barrier layers.

Limitations:

- Less suitable for encapsulating sensitive core materials.
- Core and shell adhesion must be strong.

Applications:

- Antimicrobial wound surfaces.
- Hydrophobic protective barriers.

Layer-by-Layer (LbL) Self-Assembly

Principle:

- Alternating deposition of positively and negatively charged polymers builds multilayer shells around a core substrate.

Advantages:

- Nanometer level control of shell thickness.
- Allows incorporation of multiple functional layers.

Limitations:

- Time consuming.
- Shell formation depends on electrostatic interactions.

Applications:

- Smart antimicrobial dressings.
- pH or enzyme-responsive shells.

Phase Separation Techniques

These are used to fabricate core–shell microspheres or fibers through controlled demixing of polymers [20].

Principle

- Two polymers separate into core and shell phases during solvent evaporation or thermal treatment.

Advantages

- Simple fabrication.
- Suitable for drug-loaded microspheres used in wound gels.

Limitations

- Limited architectural control.
- Not ideal for highly sensitive bioactive agents.

3D Printing/Bioprinting of Core–Shell Structures

These are emerging technologies that allow direct writing of core–shell filaments [21,22].

Principle

- Dual nozzle printers simultaneously extrude two bioinks to form layered structures.

Advantages

- Enables patient-specific dressings.
- Allows inclusion of living cells or tissue-specific bioinks.
- Tailored porosity and geometry.

Limitations

- Resolution is lower than electrospinning.
- Bioink development remains a major challenge.

Applications

- Regenerative scaffolds.
- Cell instructive wound implants (Table 4.2).

TABLE 4.2
Comparative Summary of Fabrication Techniques

Technique	Scale	Core–Shell Control	Drug Protection	Typical Applications
Coaxial electrospinning	Nano	Excellent	High	Drug-loaded nanofibers
Emulsion electrospinning	Nano micro	Moderate	Moderate	Antimicrobial mats
Microfluidics	Micro	Excellent	Very high	Cell-loaded gels
Coextrusion	Micro macro	High	Low moderate	Structural films
Spray coating	Macro	Moderate	Low	Surface-modified dressings
LbL assembly	Nano	Very high	High	Smart coatings
Phase separation	Micro	Low	Moderate	Drug microspheres
3D bioprinting	Macro	High	High	Regenerative scaffolds

FUNCTIONAL ADVANTAGES IN WOUND HEALING

Core–shell wound dressings provide multiple benefits that directly support the wound healing process by combining controlled delivery, protection, and structural integrity in one integrated system. Their unique architecture developed through material choices (Section 4.3) and fabrication methods (Section 4.4) results in functionalities that surpass conventional wound dressings.

Controlled and Sustained Release of Therapeutics

A major advantage of core–shell systems is the controlled release of drugs, growth factors, and antimicrobial agents. The shell slows down the diffusion of the core materials, preventing rapid drug loss and ensuring prolonged therapeutic levels at the wound site. This is particularly beneficial for chronic wounds, which require long-term treatment. By adjusting the thickness, hydrophilicity, or degradation rate of the shell, the release profile can be precisely managed.

Enhanced Stability and Protection of Bioactive Agents

Many biologically active molecules—such as peptides, proteins, enzymes, and growth factors—are highly sensitive to environmental conditions. The shell acts as a protective shield, reducing exposure to oxygen, moisture, enzymes, or UV light. This helps to retain the biological activity of the core components during both storage and application, improving overall treatment outcomes.

Antimicrobial and Anti-Infective Functionality

Core–shell dressings can effectively prevent or control infection in two ways:

- **Antimicrobial shell**: Materials like chitosan, silver nanoparticles, or zinc oxide incorporated in the shell kill or inhibit bacteria at the wound surface.
- **Antibiotic-loaded core**: Slow release of antibiotics from the core offers deeper and long-lasting antimicrobial action.

This dual approach reduces bacterial colonization, prevents biofilm formation, and supports faster healing.

Moisture Regulation and Exudate Management

A balanced moisture environment is essential for optimal healing. Core–shell dressings achieve this through hydrophilic cores that absorb excess fluid and help maintain moisture, while the shell controls water vapor transmission and prevents external contamination. This prevents issues like maceration and promotes a healthier healing environment.

Mechanical Strength and Structural Support

The shell typically provides mechanical strength and integrity, ensuring that the dressing is durable enough to withstand movement without tearing. Meanwhile, the core can offer flexibility or cushioning. This balance is ideal for wounds located on dynamic body areas such as joints.

Support for Tissue Regeneration

Core–shell nanofibers closely resemble the ECM, giving cells a natural-like environment to attach, migrate, and proliferate. This structure enhances re-epithelialization, collagen deposition, and angiogenesis. Additionally, growth factors or regenerative molecules loaded in the core contribute directly to tissue repair.

Multifunctionality in One System

A key advantage of core–shell dressing design is the ability to combine several therapeutic functions in a single system. For example, the shell may provide antimicrobial protection, while the core releases anti-inflammatory drugs or growth factors. This reduces the need for multiple treatments and contributes to efficient wound management (Figure 4.5; Table 4.3).

CONTROLLED DRUG DELIVERY VIA CORE–SHELL SYSTEMS

Building on the functional advantages discussed in Section 4.5, one of the most significant contributions of core–shell technology to wound healing is **controlled drug delivery**. By separating the therapeutic agents in the core from the protective shell, these systems offer precise spatial and temporal control over drug release, which is critical for effective wound management.

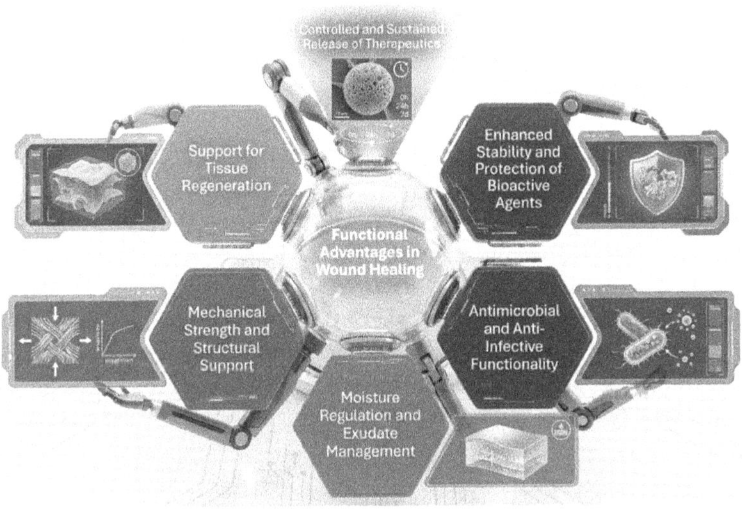

FIGURE 4.5 Functional advantages in wound healing.

TABLE 4.3
Functional Advantages of Core–Shell Wound Dressings

Functional Feature	Role of Core Layer	Role of Shell Layer	Overall Benefit to Wound Healing
Controlled drug release	Stores therapeutic agents and releases them gradually	Regulates diffusion and prevents burst release	Maintains steady drug levels and reduces dosing frequency
Protection of bioactive agents	Holds sensitive molecules (growth factors and enzymes)	Shields from moisture, enzymes, oxygen, and UV light	Preserves the activity of fragile compounds
Antimicrobial activity	Can contain long-term antibiotic reservoirs	Can incorporate antimicrobial agents (AgNPs and chitosan)	Reduces infection risk and prevents biofilm formation
Moisture and exudate control	Absorbs excess fluid and maintains moisture	Controls vapor transmission and acts as barrier	Prevents maceration and supports moist healing environment
Mechanical strength	Provides flexibility and cushioning	Offers tensile strength and durability	Dressing remains intact and comfortable during movement
Tissue regeneration support	Provides growth factors or regenerative molecules	Maintains structure for cell attachment	Enhances cell migration, angiogenesis, and re-epithelialization
Multifunctionality	Delivers therapeutic agents	Provides protection and regulation	Combines antimicrobial, regenerative, and protective functions in one dressing

Principles of Controlled Drug Delivery

Core–shell wound dressings regulate drug release primarily through **diffusion and degradation mechanisms**:

- **Diffusion controlled release**: Drugs migrate from the core through the shell over time. The thickness and porosity of the shell determine the release rate.
- **Degradation controlled release**: Biodegradable shell materials gradually break down in the wound environment, releasing the drug in a sustained or stage-specific manner.
- **Stimuli-responsive release**: Advanced systems incorporate materials that respond to environmental triggers such as pH, temperature, or bacterial enzymes. For example, an enzyme-sensitive shell can release antibiotics only when bacterial activity is high, reducing unnecessary drug exposure.

Advantages of Core–Shell Drug Delivery

Sustained Therapeutic Effect

Encapsulation of drugs in the core allows continuous delivery over extended periods, which is especially beneficial for chronic wounds or burns that require long-term treatment.

Reduced Side Effects

The shell acts as a barrier, limiting initial burst release and minimizing local or systemic toxicity from high drug concentrations.

Protection of Sensitive Drugs

Core–shell systems preserve the bioactivity of labile molecules such as growth factors, peptides, and enzymes by shielding them from moisture, enzymes, and oxidative degradation.

Targeted Delivery

Shell materials can be designed to respond to wound-specific conditions, allowing on-demand release of antibiotics or anti-inflammatory agents at the wound site (Table 4.4).

Examples of Drugs Delivered Via Core–Shell Dressings

- **Antibiotics**: Ciprofloxacin, vancomycin, and gentamicin.
- **Anti-inflammatory agents**: Curcumin and dexamethasone.
- **Growth factors**: VEGF, EGF, and FGF.
- **Antioxidants**: Cerium oxide nanoparticles and vitamin E.
- **Analgesics**: Lidocaine or local anesthetics for pain control.

By controlling the release kinetics, these systems improve drug efficiency, reduce dressing changes, and promote faster wound healing.

TABLE 4.4
Core–Shell Strategies for Drug Delivery

Strategy	Core Material	Shell Material	Therapeutic Goal
Fast releasing core + slow-degrading shell	PVA, gelatin with drug	PCL, PLA	Sustained release over days
Hydrophilic core + hydrophobic shell	Hydrogel with antibiotic	PCL, PLGA	Protects drug from moisture; controls release
Antimicrobial shell + drug-loaded core	Growth factor in core	Chitosan or AgNP-loaded shell	Prevents infection while promoting regeneration
Stimuli-responsive shell	Drug-loaded hydrogel	Enzyme or pH-sensitive polymer	On-demand release in response to infection or inflammation

Summary

Core–shell technology enables **tailored, multifunctional drug delivery systems** in wound care. By carefully selecting core and shell materials and optimizing their architecture, it is possible to achieve:

- Sustained and controlled drug release.
- Protection of sensitive therapeutics.
- Reduced systemic toxicity.
- Targeted, wound-responsive delivery.

This makes core–shell dressings particularly effective for **chronic wounds, burns, infected wounds, and post-surgical sites**, combining therapeutic efficiency with mechanical and protective functionality.

ANTIMICROBIAL AND ANTI-INFLAMMATORY APPLICATIONS

Core–shell wound dressings are particularly effective in **combating infection** and **reducing inflammation**, which are two major barriers to successful wound healing. By combining protective shells with bioactive cores, these systems provide localized therapy while minimizing systemic side effects.

Antimicrobial Functionality

Infection control is a key requirement in wound care. Core–shell dressings achieve antimicrobial activity through:

- **Antimicrobial shells**: Materials such as chitosan, silver nanoparticles (AgNPs), zinc oxide, or antimicrobial peptides are incorporated into the shell. These act at the wound surface to prevent microbial colonization and biofilm formation.

- **Antibiotic-loaded cores**: Core materials can encapsulate antibiotics (e.g., ciprofloxacin, vancomycin) for controlled, sustained release, providing deeper and long-lasting protection.

Advantages

- Reduced infection risk.
- Minimized need for systemic antibiotics.
- Prevention of bacterial resistance through controlled release.

Anti-Inflammatory Functionality

Excessive inflammation slows healing and increases scar formation. Core–shell systems can locally deliver anti-inflammatory agents such as:

- Curcumin,
- Dexamethasone, and
- Nonsteroidal anti-inflammatory drugs (NSAIDs).

Mechanism

- The core contains the anti-inflammatory drug, while the shell protects it from degradation.
- Sustained release ensures modulation of inflammation over days, supporting proper progression through the inflammatory phase of healing.

Combined Antimicrobial and Anti-inflammatory Systems

Advanced designs can combine both functionalities in a single dressing:

- **Example 1**: Antimicrobial shell + anti-inflammatory core.
- **Example 2**: Antibiotic-loaded core + enzyme-responsive shell releasing anti-inflammatory agents during infection.

Benefits

- Simultaneous infection control and inflammation regulation.
- Reduced dressing changes.
- Accelerated healing with minimized tissue damage (Table 4.5).

TABLE 4.5
Advantages Over Conventional Dressings

Feature	Conventional Dressing	Core–Shell Dressing
Drug delivery	Limited or topical only	Sustained and localized release
Antimicrobial protection	Surface level only	Dual layer protection (surface + deep)
Inflammation control	Often systemic drugs	Localized, controlled delivery
Dressing change frequency	Frequent	Reduced due to prolonged activity
Healing efficiency	Moderate	Enhanced by combined therapy

TABLE 4.6
Challenges and Future Perspectives of Core–Shell Wound Dressings

Category	Challenges	Future Perspectives/Solutions
Fabrication	Complex techniques (coaxial electrospinning, microfluidics); difficult scale-up	Develop scalable, automated fabrication methods with uniform fiber/matrix control
Materials	Limited stability of natural polymers; hydrophobicity or slow degradation of synthetic polymers; potential cytotoxicity	Use hybrid materials, biopolymers, and safer nanocomposites for improved biocompatibility and tunable properties
Stability & storage	Bioactive agents may degrade during storage or sterilization; short shelf life	Incorporate protective shells, lyophilization, or smart packaging to extend stability
Cost	High production costs due to advanced materials and fabrication	Optimize materials and manufacturing processes to reduce costs
Regulatory and clinical translation	Multicomponent dressings require extensive safety and efficacy testing; complex approval pathways	Standardize protocols, perform large-scale clinical trials, and streamline regulatory pathways
Functional limitations	Limited responsiveness to wound-specific conditions in current systems	Develop smart, stimuli-responsive dressings (pH, enzyme, temperature) for on-demand therapy
Personalization	Current systems are mostly "one size fits all"	Implement 3D printing and patient-specific designs for tailored therapy

CHALLENGES AND FUTURE PERSPECTIVES

While core–shell wound dressings offer significant therapeutic advantages, several technical, clinical, and regulatory challenges remain. Addressing these challenges is essential to translate laboratory research into widely used clinical products (Table 4.6).

CONCLUSION

Core–shell wound dressings represent a next-generation approach in wound care, combining advanced materials, precise architecture, and multifunctional capabilities. By integrating a protective shell with a bioactive core, these systems provide controlled drug delivery, antimicrobial protection, moisture regulation, mechanical support, and regenerative potential within a single dressing. So, we can conclude that Core–shell wound dressings bridge the gap between conventional wound care and advanced therapeutic systems, offering multifunctional, customizable, and clinically relevant solutions. With continued research on materials, fabrication, and smart delivery systems, these dressings have the potential to redefine wound management, improving outcomes for acute, chronic, and complex wounds.

Key points from this chapter include:

1. **Core–shell architecture**: The separation of core and shell allows independent control of drug release, structural properties, and protection of sensitive agents.
2. **Material selection**: Careful pairing of hydrophilic/hydrophobic polymers, natural/synthetic materials, and bioactive agents ensures compatibility, stability, and biocompatibility.
3. **Fabrication techniques**: Methods such as coaxial electrospinning, microfluidics, emulsion spinning, and 3D printing provide precise control over fiber morphology and functional loading.
4. **Functional advantages**: Core–shell dressings enhance healing by sustaining drug release, preventing infection, modulating inflammation, supporting tissue regeneration, and improving patient comfort.
5. **Controlled drug delivery**: Core–shell systems allow tailored, sustained, and stimuli-responsive delivery of antibiotics, growth factors, anti-inflammatory agents, and other therapeutics.
6. **Antimicrobial and anti-inflammatory applications**: The dual layer design enables simultaneous infection control and inflammation regulation, which accelerates healing and reduces complications.
7. **Challenges and future perspectives**: Issues such as fabrication complexity, material limitations, stability, cost, and regulatory hurdles remain, but advances in smart, responsive, and personalized dressings offer promising solutions.

REFERENCES

1. S. O'Callaghan, P. Galvin, C. O'Mahony, Z. Moore, and R. Derwin, "'Smart' wound dressings for advanced wound care: a review," vol. 29, no. 7, pp. 394–406, Jul. 2020, doi:10.12968/JOWC.2020.29.7.394.
2. E. Rezvani Ghomi, M. Niazi, and S. Ramakrishna, "The evolution of wound dressings: from traditional to smart dressings," vol. 34, no. 2, pp. 520–530, Feb. 2023, doi:10.1002/PAT.5929.
3. S. Ramadhan, A. Riaz, A. Younus, M. Mubin, and M. Ashraf, "Innovations in core–shell nanoparticles: advancing drug delivery solutions and precision medicine," vol. 29, no. 3, pp. 73–86, Mar. 2025, doi:10.1089/OMI.2024.0182.
4. J. Meng, G. Wu, X. Wu, H. Cheng, Z. Xu, and S. Chen, "Microfluidic-architected nanoarrays/porous core–shell fibers toward robust micro-energy-storage," vol. 7, no. 1, Jan. 2020, doi:10.1002/ADVS.201901931.
5. Q. Wei, "The multifunctional wound dressing with core–shell structured fibers prepared by coaxial electrospinning," vol. 10, no. 2, pp. 113–121, Jun. 2016, doi:10.1007/S11706-016-0339-7.
6. Q. Zhang, I. Lee, J. B. Joo, F. Zaera, and Y. Yin, "Core–shell nanostructured catalysts," vol. 46, no. 8, pp. 1816–1824, Aug. 2013, doi:10.1021/AR300230S.
7. R. Ghosh Chaudhuri and S. Paria, "Core/shell nanoparticles: classes, properties, synthesis mechanisms, characterization, and applications," vol. 112, no. 4, pp. 2373–2433, Apr. 2012, doi:10.1021/CR100449N.

8. X. Ma, Y. Li, I. Hussain, R. Shen, G. Yang, and K. Zhang, "Core–shell structured nanoenergetic materials: preparation and fundamental properties," vol. 32, no. 30, Jul. 2020, doi:10.1002/ADMA.202001291.
9. A. S. Yadav, D. T. Tran, A. J. T. Teo, Y. Dai, F. Malekpour Galogahi, C. H. Ooi, and N.-T. Nguyen, "Micromachines, and undefined 2023, "Core–shell particles: from fabrication methods to diverse manipulation techniques," *Micromachines,* vol. 14, no. 3, art. no. 497, Feb. 2023, doi:10.3390/mi14030497..
10. A. Y. P. Cheng, S. Y. L. Wong, and C. W. Kan, "Coaxial electrospinning and emulsion electrospinning of core–shell fibers," vol. 22, no. 3, pp. 310–317, Mar. 2011, doi:10.1002/PAT.1781.
11. J. Yoon, H. S. Yang, B. S. Lee, and W. R. Yu, "Recent progress in coaxial electrospinning: new parameters, various structures, and wide applications," vol. 30, no. 42, Oct. 2018, doi:10.1002/ADMA.201704765.
12. D. Han and A. J. Steckl, "Coaxial electrospinning formation of complex polymer fibers and their applications," vol. 84, no. 10, pp. 1453–1497, Oct. 2019, doi:10.1002/CPLU.201900281.
13. P. McClellan and W. J. Landis, "Recent applications of coaxial and emulsion electrospinning methods in the field of tissue engineering," vol. 5, no. 1, pp. 212–227, Aug. 2016, doi:10.1089/BIORES.2016.0022.
14. M. Zhang, X. Peng, P. Fan, Y. Zhou, and P. Xiao, "Recent progress in preparation and application of fibers using microfluidic spinning technology," vol. 223, no. 5, Mar. 2022, doi:10.1002/MACP.202100451.
15. X. Y. Du, Q. Li, G. Wu, and S. Chen, "Multifunctional micro/nanoscale fibers based on microfluidic spinning technology," vol. 31, no. 52, Dec. 2019, doi:10.1002/ADMA.201903733.
16. E. Garofalo, P. Scarfato, L. Di Maio, and L. Incarnato, "Tuning of co-extrusion processing conditions and film layout to optimize the performances of PA/PE multilayer nanocomposite films for food packaging," vol. 39, no. 9, pp. 3157–3167, Sep. 2018, doi:10.1002/PC.24323.
17. G. Yu, "Progress on the microlayer coextrusion and its derivative technologies," vol. 64, no. 4, pp. 1176–1210, 2024, doi:10.1080/15583724.2024.2372494.
18. J. J. Richardson, J. Cui, M. Björnmalm, J. A. Braunger, H. Ejima, and F. Caruso, "Innovation in layer-by-layer assembly," vol. 116, no. 23, pp. 14828–14867, Dec. 2016, doi:10.1021/ACS.CHEMREV.6B00627.
19. J. J. Richardson, M. Björnmalm, and F. Caruso, "Technology-driven layer-by-layer assembly of nanofilms," vol. 348, no. 6233, Apr. 2015, doi:10.1126/SCIENCE.AAA2491.
20. R. Akbarzadeh, A. Yousefi, "Effects of processing parameters in thermally induced phase separation technique on porous architecture of scaffolds for bone tissue engineering," vol. 102, no. 6, pp. 1304–1315, 2014, doi:10.1002/JBM.B.33101.
21. R. Taymour, N. Chicaiza-Cabezas, M. Groll, and T. Boland, "Core–shell bioprinting of vascularized in vitro liver sinusoid models," https://doi.org/10.1088/1758-5090/ac9019.
22. W. Zhu, H. Cui, B. Boualam, F. Masood, and E. F. Palermo, "3D bioprinting mesenchymal stem cell-laden construct with core–shell nanospheres for cartilage tissue engineering," https://doi.org/10.1088/1361-6528/aaafa1.

5 Challenges in Nanomaterials for Wound Regeneration

Sadia Razzaq, Rubab Fatima, Syeda Rubab Batool, and Muhammad Anwaar Nazeer

INTRODUCTION

The largest organ in the human body is known as the skin, which comprises three layers: dermis, epidermis, and dermal appendages. It protects the body from the external environment and performs different functions like maintaining moisture level in the body, regulating body temperature, fostering emotions, regulating body fluids, and providing defense against infections [1]. But sometimes, the skin encounters diseases and accidents. This action will lead to the formation of wounds. Internal and external physical stress can cause a wound, compromising the body's integrity, normal anatomical structure, and tissue function. Wounds are a challenging therapeutic issue with several repercussions that raise morbidity and mortality rates. This has become a big issue with regular occurrences and effects. The complicated biological process of wound healing is divided into four distinct phases: hemostasis, proliferation, inflammatory processes, and skin remodeling [2]. Its main point is to restore the skin's structure and functionality to preserve its integrity and optimal performance. When the body is unable to restore anatomical and functional integrity through regular and timely repair practices, chronic wounds develop. These wounds often result in lower mobility, persistent pain, and an increased risk of infection. Chronic wounds that fail to heal impose a significant burden on healthcare systems due to increased health complications, prolonged hospital stays, and more frequent medical interventions [3].

Nanomaterials (NMs) have attracted significant interest and demonstrated considerable potential in the challenging area of wound healing. Their unique physicochemical properties and functionalities have led to their widespread application in wound care [4]. These components help to improve the stability, target, and dissolution of medications, as well as their antibacterial and pro-wound healing effects, and better adapt to complex and variable wounds because they can be precisely controlled in terms of size, shape, and chemical properties. They have attracted a lot of consideration due to their distinct chemical, physical, and biological characteristics that aid in the wound healing process at various phases [5].

DOI: 10.1201/9781003616726-6

An intriguing emerging field is nanotechnology, which has multiple applications in skin regeneration. Nanofibers have received special interest in the field of skin regeneration because of their structural similarity to the extracellular matrix (ECM) [6]. In addition to promoting tissue healing, nanofibrous materials can function as growth factors, proteins, medications, and other molecular delivery systems. Specific wound healing conditions can also be attained by regulating morphology, biodegradability, and other properties of nanofibrous substances. Various nanostructured drug delivery systems have been utilized to improve wound healing at different stages of the recovery process, such as liposomes, nanoparticles (NPs), micelles, and nanoemulsions [7].

NMs still hold a lot of potential for future development, and they have a tremendous ability to stimulate wound healing. However, it is important to note that the intact skin does not protect the incision site, leaving it exposed to external elements. The biological safety of the products should be considered before application because the NPs will come into close contact with the wound's tissue [8]. NMs have been demonstrated to help in wound healing at every phase of the procedure. However, the expense of the formulations remains the main barrier to the clinical usage of NMs in wound healing. The cost of the formulations can be decreased by reducing the dosage of NMs. Two effective approaches to improve therapeutic consequences are integrating cost-effective adjuvants and developing composite NMs for better execution [9].

IMPORTANCE OF ADDRESSING THE CHALLENGES/ TACKLING CHALLENGES: A CRITICAL STEP

Nano-drug delivery systems (Nano-DDSs) have a huge potential to increase the therapeutic efficacy of medications since they can sustain drug release and stop drug degradation. A growing number of nano-DDSs with therapeutic compounds are being developed and used to enhance skin regeneration and wound healing, maximizing the potential of synthetic and biological molecules [10]. These drug carriers extend drug release, protect drugs from degradation, and enhance skin retention, helping to reduce or eliminate wound bacterial loads and promote re-epithelialization [11]. Additionally, various combinations of nano-DDSs are used as complementary delivery platforms, with some mimicking and providing the ideal physiological environment for the healing process. Despite the development of promising biomaterials and nanotechnology-based solutions for wound healing, their application in clinical practice remains limited [12].

The field of NP formulations has reached a mature state in the last 10 years, and a notable growth in the complexity, sophistication, and therapeutic potential of the coming generations of NPs is anticipated, given the commercial and clinical success of various nano compounds. There is an increasing need to get ready for the growing demand for and production of nanotherapeutics as the field of NPs develops and grows [13]. However, researchers are compelled to completely employ nano-DDSs, overcome technological barriers, and offer tangible advantages to wound sufferers. Nano-DDSs will surely be one of the most effective and affordable ways to encourage wound healing and skin regeneration.

POTENTIAL CHALLENGES

Nanomaterial-based wound rehabilitation therapies provide many benefits, but there are a few issues that need to be resolved. These include concerns about toxicity, legal issues, production scalability, and the enduring stability of NMs [14]. Intensive research is required to optimize their design and composition regarding NMs. Cost-effectiveness, scalability, safety concerns, and regulatory limitations are some of these challenges. Chronic wounds are becoming more common due to some issues, including counting the age of our population and the number of people with diabetes. Promising biomaterials and nanotechnology-based applications for wound healing have yet to translate scientific knowledge into commercially viable solutions. Although many nanotechnologies with unique properties address specific issues in wound healing, their practical adoption remains limited [15]. Figure 5.1 illustrates the challenges associated with using nanotechnology in wound healing.

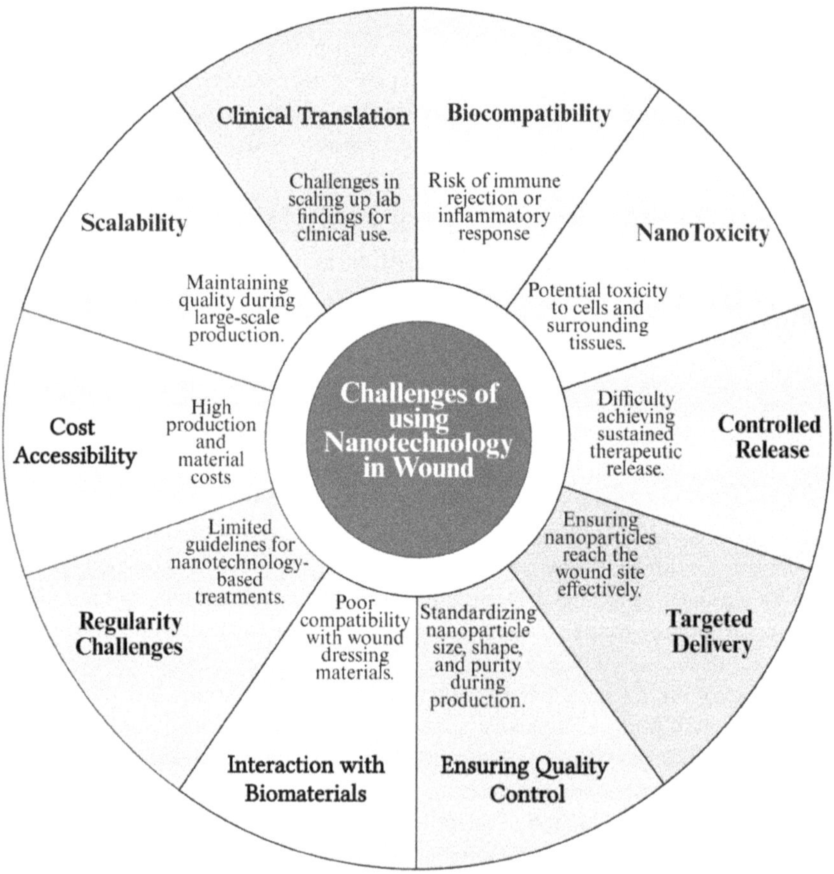
Challenges of using Nanotechnology in Wound
Clinical Translation
Challenges in scaling up lab findings for clinical use.
Biocompatibility
Risk of immune rejection or inflammatory response
NanoToxicity
Potential toxicity to cells and surrounding tissues.
Controlled Release
Difficulty achieving sustained therapeutic release.
Targeted Delivery
Ensuring nanoparticles reach the wound site effectively.
Ensuring Quality Control
Standardizing nanoparticle size, shape, and purity during production.
Interaction with Biomaterials
Poor compatibility with wound dressing materials.
Regularity Challenges
Limited guidelines for nanotechnology-based treatments.
Cost Accessibility
High production and material costs
Scalability
Maintaining quality during large-scale production.

FIGURE 5.1 Challenges of using nanotechnology in wound.

BIOCOMPATIBILITY

The application of nano- or micro-hybrid materials has demonstrated significant capability in the treatment of complex wounds, including chronic and ischemic ulcers. A clear distinction must be made between the properties of novel NMs and conventional materials used in wound healing therapies. Silver nanoparticles (AgNPs) and zinc oxide nanoparticles (ZnO NPs) pose biocompatibility challenges in wound healing, despite their antimicrobial advantages. AgNPs can produce reactive oxygen species (ROS), causing cytotoxicity in keratinocytes and fibroblasts, while ZnO NPs may activate inflammation if inappropriately formulated, highlighting the requirement of better safety methods in their uses [16]. More preclinical research is required to fully use the potential of these tiny particles in tissue regrowth. This research should focus on finding and testing new NMs that can speed up the healing procedure of chronic wounds [17]. In the future, this area might make progress in creating biocompatible and biodegradable NMs that can control all stages of wound healing. These NMs will pose significant characteristics like adhesion, antibacterial, and self-healing. These advanced materials will be the emerging approach, employed in clinical applications due to their effectiveness [18]. NMs can interact with cells by binding to specific membrane receptors, which may start signaling routes or permit the NMs to be taken into the cells. Some NMs stimulate positive signaling pathways, while others can be functionalized with ligands or antibodies to target receptors and moderate these pathways [19].

TOXICITY ISSUES

NMs can revolutionize wound healing by stimulating tissue regeneration and decreasing infection rates. Metal NPs have remarkable antimicrobial and anticancer properties. Numerous investigations have shown that the same processes that drive their cytotoxicity can also interact adversely with healthy cells, resulting in toxicity and damage. However, numerous studies have shown that NPs are safe when tested on normal cells but effective against germs and cancer. The lack of conclusive proof on either issue, even 20 years after their inception in biomedical research, is likely also a result of the complexity of making sense of the inconsistencies between the various outcomes [20]. While NMs can enhance wound healing, they can also induce toxicity. Their toxicity profile can be affected by size, shape, surface chemistry, and exposure duration. However, concerns have been raised about the safe utilization of gold-based nanocosmeceuticals because it has been demonstrated that small sheets of gold (Au) in cosmetic creams can quantitatively permeate into the skin's epidermis, dermis, and subcutaneous layer during a ten-day cutaneous exposure [21]. The same study also demonstrated that although Au nanosheets cannot enter the bloodstream, they can reduce keratinocyte cell viability and cause keratinocyte and skin dermal fibroblast cell necrosis at a low level. These results bring up the question of NP safety once more. However, it appears that AuNPs that are biosynthesized might be more biocompatible and have fewer negative effects [22].

Undoubtedly, the remarkable characteristics of particles in the biomedical field, especially those associated with skin treatments, are crucial to the creation of innovative, state-of-the-art materials for a variety of applications. Though there have been no definitive results, concerns regarding the toxicity of NPs have been studied in recent decades. Owing to their small size, NPs can interact with matter in a way that is entirely diverse from that of comparable bulk resources. As a result, they can have unanticipated impacts on people and other living things. The size of NPs enables efficient interactions with both prokaryotic and eukaryotic cells [23]. There are several factors influencing NPs' toxicity, making it impossible to establish a reliable standard that would enable a meaningful comparison and good conclusions. However, a general tendency has emerged, with particles that are excessively small (10 nm) and highly effective against germs and cancer. It is necessary to carefully consider and thoroughly research the nanotoxicity of wound dressing formulations and nanocosmetics because injured skin, such as that found in burns and wounds, is more permeable to NPs than healthy skin. Furthermore, it is crucial to remember that the potent effect of NPs may have a negative impact on even healthy skin when discussing innovative topical treatments [24]. An immunological reaction triggered by NMs may result in inflammation and possible tissue damage. NM-induced immunomodulation is a complicated method that depends on different factors like, size, surface chemistry, molecule structure, and chemical content. This process has been studied previously, but only for a subset of parameters. For example, the focus on immune adjuvants and their therapeutic impacts. Figure 5.2 demonstrates different factors that affect the immune response of NPs.

Thus, there is a risk of transdermal toxicities associated with NPs, which might irritate the skin and create hypersensitivity. This suggests that before applying NMs for wound healing, their biological safety needs to be considered. The concentration, stability, size, and form of the particles, as well as their size, all influence how dangerous NMs are [25]. To reduce the toxicity to the skin and create new NMs that aid in wound healing, it is important to alter the chemical and physical properties of NPs. Several stabilizers, such as metal shells, polymers, surfactants, covalent adsorption, electrochemical synthesis, and particle size control technology, should also be used

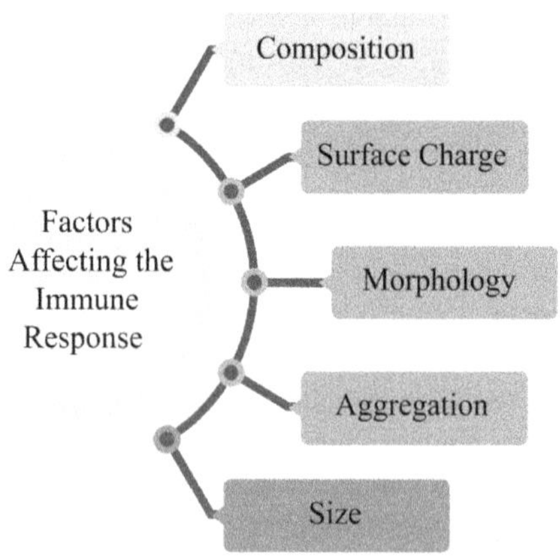

FIGURE 5.2 Diagrammatical representation of factors affecting the immune response of nanoparticles.

to decrease skin irritation. Another challenge is that different chronic wounds have different properties, which limits the ability of NMs to self-heal and regenerate [26].

Future research should emphasize examining the long-term influences of NPs on the body and developing practices to relieve risks. The development of clear recommendations and regulations for the safe use of NPs in wound healing is also important. Collaboration among scientists/researchers, healthcare professionals, and regulatory organizations is crucial for determining NMs advantages and consequences. We can carefully harness the full possibility of NMs to speed up and advance wound healing by addressing these challenges [27]. The development and utilization of reliable NMs in wound healing have the potential to revolutionize the field and improve the results for patients. Examining the consequences of long exposure to NMs on both the environment and patients is crucial. The regulations and specifications can be altered due to the continuous assessment, which will facilitate any risks or adverse effects. This commitment will improve patients' health and open the way for advanced innovations in wound recovery. For example, researchers may use NMs to develop smart bandages that examine wound healing in real time and alert medical professionals instantly if they detect any symptoms of infection. In addition to significantly improving patient results, this proactive approach would decrease the possibility of long-term troubles [28].

SCALABILITY

A nanotechnology system must have a feasible clinical adaptability and market transfer potential, which requires streamlining the development challenge. Furthermore, it is still challenging to produce and scale biopolymeric nanoformulations. One of the main obstacles to large-scale manufacture from laboratory-scale synthesis is the complexity of manufacturing processes. The development of scalable and repeatable manufacturing processes that can guarantee the reliable manufacture of superior nanoformulations should be the main goal of future research. This could involve creating continuous production processes, optimizing formulation parameters, and integrating process analytical tools for monitoring and control [29]. Variations in manufacturing approaches can affect the quality and efficacy of NPs. Variations in production practices can also affect the execution and safety of NPs. It can be challenging to improve the production of NPs while sustaining their reliability and repeatability in terms of their characteristics. The versatility of NP production is one of the major hurdles to wound treatment. Although these items can potentially improve tissue regeneration and drug delivery, their large-scale production remains challenging. A comprehensive context of manufacturers, scientists, and regulatory bodies can help settle this obstacle by regulating the advancement procedures for NPs, checking a consistent supply, and improving the procedures for manufacturing [30].

Furthermore, this can decrease the barriers to the commercialization of NP-based wound healing medications by accelerating the approval practice. It is feasible to improve the efficacy and safety of wound healing medicines based on NPs by developing standards and approaches for their assessment. Scientists and medical experts may now evaluate and compare different formulations, leading to more efficient treatments.

When we proceed from the bench to the bedside, scale-up becomes a considerable obstacle. It is valuable to continue the unique properties of NMs while developing them in large amounts. This ensures they meet the requirements of global healthcare manufacturing without compromising their effectiveness [31]. One of the primary issues is optimizing the kinetics of drug release. Biopolymeric nanoformulations can encapsulate a wide range of medical compounds, containing growth hormones, antibiotics, and anti-inflammatory drugs. However, these drugs need to have the appropriate delivery mechanism to efficiently cure wounds [32].

TARGETED DRUG DELIVERY

To correspond with the dynamic healing phases, the regulated release of therapeutic chemicals from these NPs presents a substantial challenge. Another problem is that NPs might affect multisystem abnormalities via scattering throughout the body and into separate organs. After entering the bloodstream, the number of NPs decreases significantly in comparison to their original concentration and may partially degrade in urine and feces. Death and weight loss have been observed in animal experiments. Nevertheless, there isn't any solid proof that using NPs in real life will cause cancer or organ harm [33].

Additionally, future extended exposure studies are needed to determine whether continuous contact with NPs by skin accumulation and transdermal techniques will have a substantial effect. After entering the body, NPs cause hemolysis because they come into direct touch with blood cells through injured blood arteries in lesions or enter the bloodstream. It has been demonstrated that a few metal NPs, including AgNPs and ZnO NPs, can stimulate hemolysis [34,35]. The physicochemical characteristics can be changed to get around the above-mentioned issue, or biologically active materials like phospholipids and polysaccharides can be affected by the surface of NP [36]. It is difficult to make sure that NPs exclusively transport their payload to the injury site and not to neighboring tissues. The development of NPs with the ability to bind to wound tissues selectively or react to environmental cues is necessary for effective targeting. It binds to injured tissues or responds to stimuli in its surroundings. A significant challenge is making sure that NPs only target injured areas and not healthy tissues. This accuracy is important to avoid accidental consequences, such as toxicity or inflammation, which can develop when NPs interact with healthy cells. This demands the development of advanced delivery systems, such as functionalized NPs designed to recognize and attach to specific markers on wounded tissue. Moreover, managing the release of therapeutic agents to prevent unnecessary accumulation in healthy areas is necessary for stating safety and efficiency. Overcoming these issues will facilitate more effective and targeted methods of wound healing. Sophisticated NP design and functionalization are necessary for effective targeting [37].

CONTROLLED RELEASE

Getting consistent and reliable therapeutic medication release rates using nanocarriers can be difficult. Variations in the size, form, and surface properties of NPs can cause unequal medication release, which can affect how well wounds heal.

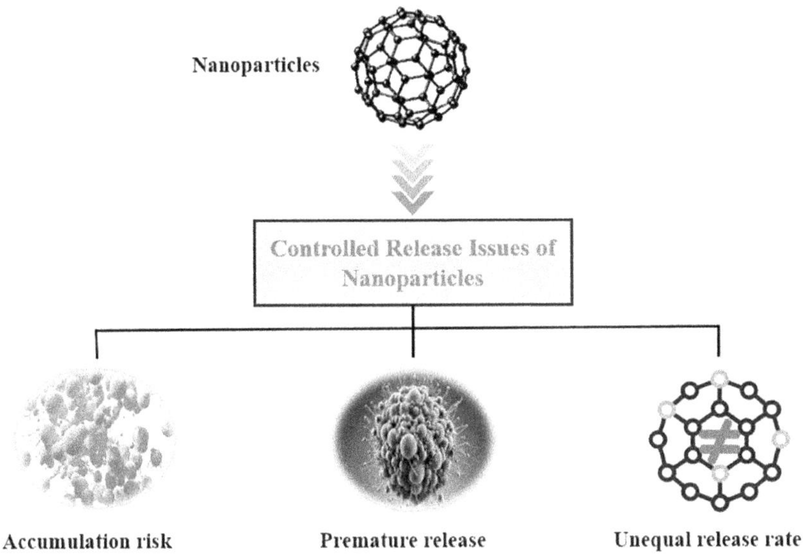

FIGURE 5.3 Showcasing of problems in controlled release of nanoparticles.

The complex biological environment and wide range of NP properties make it challenging to obtain controlled and sustainable release of therapeutic medicines from nanocarriers [38]. The pace of breakdown and removal of nanocarriers needs to be controlled to support therapeutic objectives. Rapid breakdown may cause premature release, accumulation risks, and unequal release rates. Premature release can happen because of the uncertainty in biological conditions, reducing therapeutic agents before getting to the target area and producing side effects. Accumulation risk develops when NPs assemble in non-target sites, causing toxicity/inflammation. Unequal release rates indicate inconsistent drug concentrations, causing damage to the neighboring tissues. Improved designs are required to ensure controlled release for effective and safe treatments [39]. Figure 5.3 shows controlled release of NPs in wound healing, which faces some issues that can affect their efficiency.

Stability of Nanoparticles

Ensuring the long-term stability of NPs under physiological and storage circumstances is necessary. NP stability is crucial for their efficiency in wound healing and is influenced by several factors [40]. Figure 5.4 shows key factors of NPs influencing their stability. Temperature plays a critical role: high heat can cause thermal degradation, while low temperatures may cause structural differences. Biodegradation needs to be controlled carefully to ensure good drug release, as cracking down too early can affect the treatment's outcomes. Aggregation of NPs can decrease their surface area, making it challenging for them to work efficiently with target areas. Proper storage of NPs is also important to regulate their stability, such as storing them in the right temperature, humidity, and light. A short shelf life can also restrict their utilization in large-scale uses. The pH variations in the body can cause NPs to break down,

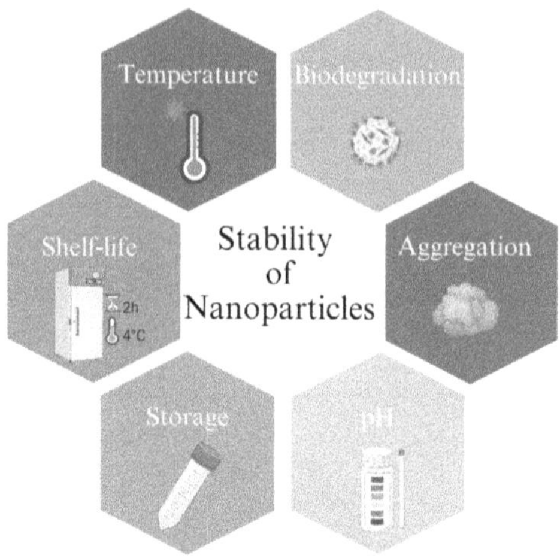

FIGURE 5.4 Key factors of nanoparticles influencing the stability.

decreasing their therapeutic efficiency. Directing these challenges via advanced formulations and optimized methods is necessary to ensure NP stability [41].

INTERACTIONS WITH BIOLOGICAL MATERIALS

Complex interactions between NPs and biological fluids can affect the distribution, behavior, and properties of release. The physicochemical characteristics of a nanomaterial, such as its size, charge, or surface characteristics, impact its interaction with a biological system. These interactions then dictate the biological performance, stability, biocompatibility, and side effects of the nanomaterial. In this way, the relationships between the structure and activity of NMs would give a conceptual basis for the rational development and responsible application of personalized nanomedicines [39].

When proteins adhere to NMs, they change and may become less effective in interacting with injured cells. The absorption of NMs by cells can be affected by various factors, including the type of cell, the properties of the nanomaterial, and the wound environment. To encourage tissue regeneration, NMs need to engage in an interaction with the ECM [42]. For example, nanofibrous scaffolds made of biodegradable components can resemble the ECM, giving support for cells to attach, move, and develop. This raw material can also carry growth factors or cytokines to further help in healing. The interaction between NPs and the ECM is significant for establishing a healing environment that aids both immune and non-immune cells in tissue. For long-term success, NPs must be capable of incorporating into tissue with time. This includes how they break down, how the immune system clears them, and ensuring that they support tissue growth without affecting long-term inflammation. Proper design permits NPs to help both in the short-term immune response and in the long-term healing development [43].

REGULARITY CHALLENGES OF NANOPARTICLES

Using NPs in wound healing offers possible benefits but also presents regulatory challenges. Extensive testing is essential to ensure safety, efficacy, production, labeling, and usage must all follow strict recommendations and regulations. Regulatory bodies must also report concerns over these NPs' possible toxicologic and environmental impacts. It is necessary to strike a balance between innovation and patient safety [30]. It is necessary to acquire techniques for pursuing and measuring the long-term outcomes of NP-based treatments to recognize any adverse effects or problems. A comprehensive approach to regulation involves cooperation between researchers, industry stakeholders, and regulatory agencies [44]. There will be a prompt resolution of any problems if researchers, government agencies, and medical experts interact openly. The extensive utilization of these advanced treatments in clinical settings will be made possible by the strict limitations that result from this cooperative technique, which places a high priority on patient safety and environmental sustainability. Frequent evaluation and feedback can reduce risks and increase the effectiveness of healthcare personnel. In addition to helping patients, creating a detailed structure that encourages openness and cooperation expedites the creation and accessibility of innovative drugs for a range of situations [28].

The cytotoxic effects of nanostructures on wound healing pose significant regulatory challenges due to the potential risks associated with NMs. Medical devices incorporating NPs are categorized as high risk under the European regulatory framework unless the exposure potential is minimal or nonexistent. Nanotoxicity is a significant concern, especially in wound healing applications, as hemolysis is influenced by factors such as surface properties, size, shape, and other characteristics of NMs. Because of their unique characteristics, the absence of standardized testing procedures, and the paucity of epidemiological data demonstrating toxicity, engineered nanomaterials (ENMs) present challenges for regulatory bodies seeking to establish protective frameworks that don't impede production. For NPs to be widely used, clinical trial results proving their effectiveness are necessary. Determining the viability of nanomaterial-based wound therapies requires assessing their cost-effectiveness [45]. Since NMs are still relatively new, regulatory agencies could need a lot of testing and paperwork to make sure using them for wound care is safe. Examples include environmental impact analyses, biocompatibility assessments, and toxicity studies. Obtaining regulatory approval is often costly and time-consuming, delaying market entry and increasing development expenses. This challenge is particularly pronounced for smaller companies with limited budgets. Additionally, securing insurance reimbursement for nanomaterial-based therapies can be difficult, especially when treatments are considered experimental or off-label [46].

COSTS ACCESSIBILITY

Advanced technologies and techniques are often required for the development of NMs, which drives up production costs. The exceptional properties of NPs often require the use of specialist materials, which can be expensive. Because of the significant variation in nanomaterial qualities, it might be difficult to ensure consistent quality and performance. To understand the behavior of NMs and make sure their safety, precise characterization is crucial, but it can be expensive and technically complex [47]. Advanced technologies and techniques are often required for the synthesis and manufacturing of NMs, which drives up production costs. For instance, complicated processes like sol-gel or chemical vapor deposition are needed when using the bottom-up approach to create NMs from single atoms or molecules. For example, different types of carbon nanotubes require different carbon sources and purifying techniques. The cost-effectiveness of NPs in electrochemical devices is still another disadvantage. While some NMs can be made at a low cost, others may need more expensive methods [48].

Furthermore, the economic viability of electrochemical devices may be restricted due to the increased cost of incorporating NMs compared to standard materials. The development of novel synthesis techniques and increased scalability are essential for lowering the price of producing NMs. To fully execute the economic potential of NMs, it will also be critical to identify applications where the execution benefits exceed the extra expense. Applications of green nanotechnology can reduce greenhouse gas emissions and hazardous waste, clean up contaminated areas including air and water, and stop climate change. How green nanotechnology will eventually lead to environmental sustainability is still a mystery. Green nanotechnology solutions must advance to reduce these concerns [49].

QUALITY CONTROL CHALLENGES

"Nano analysis" checks the atomic structure of NMs for quality control. Companies need to identify their product's unique "fingerprint" and track it over time. Generally, screening and quality assurance procedures are created with simple, unaltered medications in mind. The quality assessment process must standardize on procedures and equipment. Furthermore, various manufacturing processes and preparations may induce diversity in the preparations' physicochemical qualities, necessitating the use of particular testing techniques for each. Furthermore, the NLC system's development of preparations requires the addition of additional materials, procedures, and energy, all of which raise production costs and ultimately result in higher product pricing [50].

To keep the final product appealing and within the reach of the target market, developers are forced to carefully balance cost and efficacy. The performance of the finished product can be significantly impacted by even minor variations because no two NMs are alike. The development of standardized methods for characterizing NMs is essential for reproducibility and comparison of research findings. The surface characteristics of NMs can affect their interaction with biological tissues and wound environments. Controlling surface chemistry is crucial for biocompatibility and efficiency. Modifications can affect biocompatibility, drug delivery, and wound healing consequences [51]. Measurements of nanomaterial characteristics like size, shape, surface charge, and porosity require accurate and trustworthy characterization methods. It is difficult to standardize these measurement methods across many manufacturers and labs. Standardized procedures and guidelines are required for the characterization of NMs, as they are frequently absent or inconsistent among various regulatory and research organizations. Safety and effectiveness depend on maintaining the purity of NMs and reducing impurity contamination. The development of scalable manufacturing techniques is essential for the commercial manufacture and broad application of wound dressings based on NMs. Reproducibility in manufacturing processes is crucial for guaranteeing that every batch of NMs fulfills the requirements. Controlled release of medications or growth factors from NMs is crucial for the best possible wound healing. The performance of NMs may be impacted by degradation or changes in their properties over time. For practical use, it is essential to guarantee their stability and shelf life. To retain their qualities, adequate storage conditions need to be established and kept up. Furthermore, it can be difficult to navigate the changing regulatory frameworks for nanomaterial applications in medicine [52].

CLINICAL APPLICATIONS

Several logistical challenges prevent the wide adoption of cell-based regeneration therapies. Clinical translation of NMs for wound regeneration entails bridging the gap between laboratory studies and clinical applications. Conventional 2D static cultures are the starting point for many cell-based therapies. These cultures distinguish a limited number of cells through a labor-intensive, time-consuming, and labor-intensive procedure that needs clinical grade [53].

Designing clinical trials to evaluate the safety and efficiency of NMs for wound regeneration can be complex due to alterations in wound types and patient symptoms. It is essential to address the right considerations, such as consent and patient safety, in these trials. Additionally, addressing public concerns and misconceptions about NMs is key to their acceptance in clinical use. Understanding patient preferences and concerns about nanomaterial-based wound dressings is also crucial for successful execution [54]. Nanotechnology may be subject to medical device regulations if it involves biological materials or nanomedicine techniques. Clinical trials may be required to evaluate the safety and efficacy of nanotechnology-based treatments for angiogenesis if these treatments are still in the developmental stage. Usually, regulations are in place for these experiments to guarantee participant safety and moral behavior [55]. There may be safety and environmental issues when using NPs in angiogenesis applications. There are regulations concerning the removal of NPs and their potential environmental impact. However, current regulations are insufficient and not well-suited to address the unique aspects of nanotechnology-based products, particularly their toxicity. While NMs have entered the global market, further research is needed to understand their environmental fate, therapeutic uses, and effects on other consumer goods. Efforts are underway in the United States, European Union, and other countries to assess the safety of NMs. Addressing these translation challenges requires collaboration between scientists, clinicians, regulatory bodies, and industry. By developing standardized methods, conducting rigorous clinical trials, and addressing ethical concerns, the potential of NMs for wound regeneration can be fully realized [56]. Table 5.1 outlines the major challenges associated with nanotechnology in wound healing.

TABLE 5.1
Challenges in Nanotechnology for Wound Healing and Their Solutions

Challenges	Problems	Recommendations	Technologies/ Techniques	Reference
Biocompatibility	Tissue rejection	• Utilization of biodegradable and non-toxic components • Conduct biocompatibility testing	• Biodegradable polymers, e.g., PLA • Surface modification	[57,58]
Nano toxicity	Tissue accumulation and oxidative stress	• Optimization of NP size, shape, and surface characteristics	• Size optimization (PEG, chitosan)	[59,60]
Controlled release	Inconsistent drug delivery, burst occurrence	• Design smart release systems	• pH-sensitive • Drug encapsulation	[7,61]
Targeted delivery	Complications in targeting	• Functionalize with ligands	• Surface functionalization	[11,38]
Quality control	Irregularity in nanoparticle characteristics	• Utilization of accurate characterization approaches	• TEM, DLS • Standardized manufacturing	[51]
Interaction with biomaterials	Integration challenges	• Design NPs compatible with ECM and biomaterials	• Nanofibrous scaffolds • Biocompatible composites	[39]
Regulatory challenges	Developing regulatory environment	• Involvement of regulators in the initial stage • Establishment of safety profiles	• FDA guidelines	[30]
Cost accessibility	High manufacturing costs	• Optimize production methods	• Green chemistry	[49]
Scalability	Problems in large-scale production	• Improve scalable methods	• Microfluidics and sol-gel	[29,58]
Clinical translation	Challenges in clinical trials	• Conduct large-scale trials	• Regulatory compliance tools	[56]

CONCLUSIONS

Developments in nanotechnology are transforming wound healing by leveraging the distinctive characteristics of NMs to enhance antimicrobial activity, promote cell growth, and control inflammation. Nanostructured lipid carriers (NLCs) show capability for chronic wounds by permitting continuous drug release, but future research is required to increase their application to a wide range of drugs and confirm their safety, biocompatibility, and long-term results, mainly in burns, diabetic ulcers, and chronic wounds. Developing adaptable nanomaterial-based medications is crucial, as different wound types require tailored advances. However, clinical research faces challenges due to the complications of wounds and injuries, which hinder the development of clear goals and standards. Despite these obstacles, the growing body of research on multifunctional nanosystems fuels optimism that is essential for their safe and effective clinical application, including nanotherapeutic interventions, by addressing knowledge gaps in their physicochemical properties, behavior, and toxicity.

FUTURE ASPECTS

NMs hold great promise for advancing wound healing by enabling controlled, replicable platforms that minimize adverse effects. However, key amendments in synthesis, characterization, and site-specific targeting are required, as well as severe observance of FDA guidelines on systemic absorption and materials. It is anticipated that this field will use a variety of nanomaterial combinations in the future. Because metal NPs can target many metabolic processes in bacteria, they present an appealing option to stop the development of antimicrobial resistance (AMR) in a wound. Thus, metals are combined with different NMs and polymer types to create effective wound dressing manufacturing methods. Even though research on bio-nanocomposites is still in its infancy, new products should come from this subject in the next 10 years.

Lack of knowledge about non-material-controlled wound healing applications in vivo models is another problem. Most published studies on the application of NMs for wound healing either are based mostly on single-target bacteria or are conducted in vitro. Therefore, a comprehensive study using skin microbiota, Gram-positive organisms, and negative bacterial strains is required when considering in vivo wound healing applications. Future research should focus on improving site specification and directing efficiencies for more effective wound healing products, based on the nanomaterial that is being used.

NMs in wound regeneration hold great promise, but ongoing research is needed to overcome current challenges. As scientists refine their applications, breakthroughs are expected to transform wound care and improve patient outcomes, making NMs a key part of future healing technologies. This technology can be used in the future to construct electronic skin monitoring systems for signaling pathway proteins, pH, humidity, and inflammatory variables. This will help the physician in precisely operating wound care and selecting the right NPs in response to the current conditions. Now, researchers have successfully used NPs to prevent hurting and aid in wound healing. Furthermore, nanotechnology holds significant assurance for improving unusual pigmentation, regulating paresthesia, and restoring hair follicles.

ACKNOWLEDGMENTS

The schematics are made by using the paid version of BioRender® (https://BioRender.com). The authors acknowledge the funding from the Higher Education Commission of Pakistan under Grant No. TTSF-195 for completing this work.

REFERENCES

1. A. A. E. Ibrahim, B. R. Smoller, C. Reyes-Baron, and N. Bagherani, "Functions of the skin," In: M. F. Murphy & D. A. Carr (Eds.), *Skin Anatomy, Physiology, and Pathophysiology* (pp. 1–11). Springer, 2021, doi:10.1007/978-3-319-45134-3_4-1.
2. H. N. Wilkinson and M. J. Hardman, "Wound healing: Cellular mechanisms and pathological outcomes," *Open Biol.,* vol. 10, no. 9, Art. no. 200223, 2020, doi:10.1098/rsob.200223.
3. V. Falanga *et al.*, "Chronic wounds," *Nat. Rev. Dis. Prim.,* vol. 8, no. 1, pp. 1–21, 2022, doi:10.1038/s41572-022-00377-3.
4. W. Fu *et al.,* "Opportunities and challenges of nanomaterials in wound healing: Advances, mechanisms, and perspectives," *Chem. Eng. J.*, vol. 495, p. 153640, 2024, doi:10.1016/J.CEJ.2024.153640.
5. W. Fatima, S. R. Batool, F. Mushtaq, M. Aslam, Z. A. Raza, and M. A. Nazeer, "Controlled release of doxorubicin from gelatin-based nanoparticles: Theoretical and experimental approach," *Mater. Adv.*, vol. 5, no. 6, pp. 2347–2358, 2024.
6. T. Alberti *et al.,* "Nanotechnology: A promising tool towards wound healing," *Curr. Pharm. Des.*, vol. 23, no. 24, 2017, doi:10.2174/1381612823666170503152550.
7. A. Sultana, M. Zare, V. Thomas, T. S. S. Kumar, and S. Ramakrishna, "Nano-based drug delivery systems: Conventional drug delivery routes, recent developments and future prospects," *Med. Drug Discov.*, vol. 15, p. 100134, 2022, doi:10.1016/J.MEDIDD.2022.100134.
8. M. A. Subhan and T. Subhan, "Safety and global regulations for application of nanomaterials," In: M. Rai and T. A. Nguyen (Eds.), *Nanomaterials Recycling* (pp. 83–107). Elsevier, 2022, doi:10.1016/B978-0-323-90982-2.00005-6.
9. S. Tanuku, D. Velisila, D. Thatraju, and A. Kumar Vadaga, "Nanoemulsion formulation strategies for enhanced drug delivery," *J. Pharma Insights Res.*, vol. 2, no. 4, pp. 125–138, 2024, doi:10.69613/3F8M9151.
10. R. Tenchov *et al.,* "Transforming medicine: Cutting-edge applications of nanoscale materials in drug delivery," *ACS Nano.*, 2025, doi:10.1021/ACSNANO.4C09566.
11. S. R. Batool, M. A. Nazeer, D. Ekinci, A. Sahin, and S. Kizilel, "Multifunctional alginate-based hydrogel with reversible crosslinking for controlled therapeutics delivery," *Int. J. Biol. M*acromol., vol. 150, pp. 315–325, 2020, doi:10.1016/j.ijbiomac.2020.02.042.
12. D. Liu, F. Yang, F. Xiong, and N. Gu, "The smart drug delivery system and its clinical potential," *Theranostics*, vol. 6, no. 9, p. 1306, 2016, doi:10.7150/THNO.14858.
13. R. K. Thapa and J. O. Kim, "Nanomedicine-based commercial formulations: Current developments and future prospects," *J. Pharm. Investig.*, vol. 53, no. 1, pp. 19–33, 2023, doi:10.1007/S40005-022-00607-6.
14. A. Naskar and K. S. Kim, "Recent advances in nanomaterial-based wound-healing therapeutics," *Pharmaceutics*, vol. 12, no. 6, p. 499, 2020, doi:10.3390/PHARMACEUTICS12060499.
15. G. Han and R. Ceilley, "Chronic wound healing: A review of current management and treatments," *Adv. Ther.*, vol. 34, no. 3, p. 599, 2017, doi:10.1007/S12325-017-0478-Y.

16. A. Pormohammad, N. K. Monych, S. Ghosh, D. L. Turner, and R. J. Turner, "Nanomaterials in wound healing and infection control," *Antibiot.,* vol. 10, no. 5, p. 473, 2021, doi:10.3390/ANTIBIOTICS10050473.
17. M. Sajid, "Nanomaterials: Types, properties, recent advances, and toxicity concerns," *Curr. Opin. Environ. Sci. Heal.*, vol. 25, p. 100319, 2022, doi:10.1016/J.COESH.2021.100319.
18. J. J. Andrew and H. N. Dhakal, "Sustainable biobased composites for advanced applications: Recent trends and future opportunities: A critical review," *Compos. Part C*, vol. 7, p. 100220, 2022, doi:10.1016/J.JCOMC.2021.100220.
19. T. R. Kyriakides *et al.,* "Biocompatibility of nanomaterials and their immunological properties," *Biomed. Mater.*, vol. 16, no. 4, pp. 1088–1748, 2021, doi:10.1088/1748-605X/ABE5FA.
20. E. Sánchez-López et al., "Metal-based nanoparticles as antimicrobial agents: An overview," *Nanomaterials*, vol. 10, no. 2, pp. 1–39, 2020, doi:10.3390/nano10020292.
21. A. Sukhanova, S. Bozrova, P. Sokolov, M. Berestovoy, A. Karaulov, and I. Nabiev, "Dependence of nanoparticle toxicity on their physical and chemical properties," *Nanoscale Res. Lett.,* vol. 13, no. 1, pp. 1–21, 2018, doi:10.1186/S11671-018-2457-X.
22. M. A. Saifi, A. Khurana, and C. Godugu, Nanotoxicology: Toxicity and risk assessment of nanomaterials. In: M. P. Shaikh and A. K. Mishra (Eds.), *Nanomaterials in Chromatography: Current Trends in Chromatographic Research Technology and Techniques* (pp. 437–465). Elsevier, 2018, doi:10.1016/B978-0-12-812792-6.00017-0.
23. X. Zhang, G. Ma, and W. Wei, "Simulation of nanoparticles interacting with a cell membrane: Probing the structural basis and potential biomedical application," *NPG Asia Mater.,* vol. 13, no. 1, pp. 1–18, 2021, doi:10.1038/s41427-021-00320-0.
24. K. A. Altammar, "A review on nanoparticles: Characteristics, synthesis, applications, and challenges," *Front. Microbiol.*, vol. 14, p. 1155622, 2023, doi:10.3389/FMICB.2023.1155622.
25. S. Patel, S. Srivastava, M. R. Singh, and D. Singh, "Mechanistic insight into diabetic wounds: Pathogenesis, molecular targets and treatment strategies to pace wound healing," *Biomed. Pharmacother.*, vol. 112, p. 108615, 2019, doi:10.1016/J.BIOPHA.2019.108615.
26. P. Kolimi, S. Narala, D. Nyavanandi, A. A. A. Youssef, and N. Dudhipala, "Innovative treatment strategies to accelerate wound healing: Trajectory and recent advancements," *Cells*, vol. 11, no. 15, 2022, doi:10.3390/cells11152439.
27. M. A. Shalaby, M. M. Anwar, and H. Saeed, "Nanomaterials for application in wound healing: Current state-of-the-art and future perspectives," *J. Polym. Res.,* vol. 29, no. 3, pp. 1–37, 2022, doi:10.1007/S10965-021-02870-X.
28. J. Nandhini, E. Karthikeyan, and S. Rajeshkumar, "Nanomaterials for wound healing: Current status and futuristic frontier," *Biomed. Technol.*, vol. 6, pp. 26–45, 2024, doi:10.1016/J.BMT.2023.10.001.
29. M. J. Getahun, B. B. Kassie, and T. S. Alemu, "Recent advances in biopolymer synthesis, properties, & commercial applications: A review," *Process Biochem.*, vol. 145, pp. 261–287, 2024, doi:10.1016/J.PROCBIO.2024.06.034.
30. F. Ali, K. Neha, and S. Parveen, "Current regulatory landscape of nanomaterials and nanomedicines: A global perspective," *J. Drug Deliv. Sci. Technol.*, vol. 80, p. 104118, 2023, doi:10.1016/J.JDDST.2022.104118.
31. E. Hemmrich and S. McNeil, "Strategic aspects for the commercialization of nanomedicines," *J. Control.* Release, vol. 369, pp. 617–621, 2024, doi:10.1016/J.JCONREL.2024.04.003.
32. T. Zaheer *et al.,* "Key challenges and scopes of biomaterials commercialization: Therapeutic delivery," In: K. Pal (Ed.), *Bio-Manufactured Nanomaterials: Perspectives and Promotion* (pp. 321–337). Springer, 2021, doi:10.1007/978-3-030-67223-2_15.

33. Y. Feng *et al.*, "A systematic review of the impacts of exposure to micro- and nano-plastics on human tissue accumulation and health," *Eco-Environ. Heal.*, vol. 2, no. 4, pp. 195–207, 2023, doi:10.1016/J.EEHL.2023.08.002.
34. T. Bruna, F. Maldonado-Bravo, P. Jara, and N. Caro, "Silver nanoparticles and their antibacterial applications," *Int. J. Mol. Sci.*, vol. 22, no. 13, p. 7202, 2021, doi:10.3390/IJMS22137202.
35. F. M. Husain *et al.*, "Biosynthesized zinc oxide nanoparticles disrupt established biofilms of pathogenic bacteria," *Appl. Sci.*, vol. 12, no. 2, p. 710, 2022, doi:10.3390/APP12020710.
36. P. Nie, Y. Zhao, and H. Xu, "Synthesis, applications, toxicity and toxicity mechanisms of silver nanoparticles: A review," *Ecotoxicol. Environ. Saf.*, vol. 253, p. 114636, 2023, doi:10.1016/J.ECOENV.2023.114636.
37. S. Hamdan *et al.*, "Nanotechnology-driven therapeutic interventions in wound healing: Potential uses and applications," *ACS Cent. Sci.*, vol. 3, no. 3, p. 163, 2017, doi:10.1021/ACSCENTSCI.6B00371.
38. F. Moradi Kashkooli, M. Soltani, and M. Souri, "Controlled anti-cancer drug release through advanced nano-drug delivery systems: Static and dynamic targeting strategies," *J. Control. Release*, vol. 327, pp. 316–349, 2020, doi:10.1016/J.JCONREL.2020.08.012.
39. Y. Ji *et al.*, "Beyond the promise: Exploring the complex interactions of nanoparticles within biological systems," *J. Hazard. Mater.*, vol. 468, p. 133800, 2024, doi:10.1016/J.JHAZMAT.2024.133800.
40. S. Singh and H. S. Nalwa, "Nanotechnology and health safety--toxicity and risk assessments of nanostructured materials on human health," *J. Nanosci. Nanotechnol.*, vol. 7, no. 9, pp. 3048–3070, 2007, doi:10.1166/JNN.2007.922.
41. W. Najahi-Missaoui, R. D. Arnold, and B. S. Cummings, "Safe nanoparticles: Are we there yet?," *Int. J. Mol. Sci.*, vol. 22, no. 1, p. 385, 2020, doi:10.3390/IJMS22010385.
42. A. Zhang *et al.*, "Absorption, distribution, metabolism, and excretion of nanocarriers in vivo and their influences," *Adv. Colloid Interface Sci.*, vol. 284, p. 102261, 2020, doi:10.1016/J.CIS.2020.102261.
43. K. C. Gupta, A. Haider, Y. R. Choi, and I. K. Kang, "Nanofibrous scaffolds in biomedical applications," *Biomater. Res.*, vol. 18, no. 1, pp. 1–11, 2014, https://doi.org/10.1186/2055-7124-18-5.
44. M. Alberto Pérez-Díaz *et al.*, "Nanoparticle and nanomaterial involvement during the wound healing process: An update in the field," *J. Nanoparticle Res.*, vol. 25, no. 2, pp. 1–23, 2023, doi:10.1007/S11051-023-05675-9.
45. M. Afshar *et al.*, "Nanomaterial strategies in wound healing: A comprehensive review of nanoparticles, nanofibres and nanosheets," *Int. Wound J.*, vol. 21, no. 7, p. e14953, 2024, doi:10.1111/IWJ.14953.
46. P. O. Isibor, "Regulations and policy considerations for nanoparticle safety," In: P. O. Isibor, G. Devi, and A. A. Enuneku (Eds.), *Environmental Nanotoxicology: Combatting the Minute Contaminants* (pp. 295–316). Springer, 2024, doi:10.1007/978-3-031-54154-4_14.
47. S. Kumari *et al.*, "A comprehensive review on various techniques used for synthesizing nanoparticles," *J. Mater. Res. Technol.*, vol. 27, pp. 1739–1763, 2023, doi:10.1016/J.JMRT.2023.09.291.
48. M. Negahdary and S. Mabbott, "Automated synthesis and processing of functional nanomaterials: Advances and perspectives," *Coord. Chem. Rev.*, vol. 523, p. 216249, 2025, doi:10.1016/J.CCR.2024.216249.
49. L. Pokrajac *et al.*, "Nanotechnology for a sustainable future: Addressing global challenges with the international network4sustainable nanotechnology," *ACS Nano*, vol. 15, no. 12, pp. 18608–18623, 2021, https://doi.org/10.1021/acsnano.1c10919.

50. J. P. MacDuffie, K. Sethuraman, and M. L. Fisher, "Product variety and manufacturing performance: Evidence from the international automotive assembly plant study," *Manage. Sci.*, vol. 42, no. 3, pp. 350–369, 1996, doi:10.1287/MNSC.42.3.350.
51. S. Sharifi, N. N. Mahmoud, E. Voke, M. P. Landry, and M. Mahmoudi, "Importance of standardizing analytical characterization methodology for improved reliability of the nanomedicine literature," *Nano-Micro Lett.*, vol. 14, no. 1, pp. 1–15, 2022, https://doi.org/10.1007/s40820-022-00922-5.
52. M. Kalivaand M. Vamvakaki, "Nanomaterials characterization," *Polym. Sci. Nanotechnol. Fundam. Appl.*, pp. 401–433, 2020, doi:10.1016/B978-0-12-816806-6.00017-0.
53. J. Tian et al., "Regulatory perspectives of combination products," *Bioact. Mater.*, vol. 10, p. 492, 2021, doi:10.1016/J.BIOACTMAT.2021.09.002.
54. S. T. Haque, S. K. Saha, M. E. Haque, and N. Biswas, "Nanotechnology-based therapeutic applications: In vitro and in vivo clinical studies for diabetic wound healing," *Biomater. Sci.*, vol. 9, no. 23, pp. 7705–7747, 2021, doi:10.1039/D1BM01211H.
55. F. DeGrazio and D. Paskiet, "Injectable combination product development: Facilitating risk-based assessments for efficiency and patient centric outcomes," *J. Pharm. Sci.*, vol. 109, no. 7, pp. 2101–2115, 2020, doi:10.1016/J.XPHS.2020.03.020.
56. M. A. Younis, H. M. Tawfeek, A. A. H. Abdellatif, J. A. Abdel-Aleem, and H. Harashima, "Clinical translation of nanomedicines: Challenges, opportunities, and keys," *Adv. Drug Deliv. Rev.*, vol. 181, 2022, doi:10.1016/J.ADDR.2021.114083.
57. S. Razzaq, S. Shahid, and Y. Nawab, "Applications and environmental impact of biodegradable polymers in textile industry: A review," *Int. J. Biol. M*acromol., vol. 282, p. 136791, 2024, https://doi.org/10.1016/j.ijbiomac.2024.136791.
58. K. Saeed, and I. Khan, "Nanoparticles: Properties, applications and toxicities," *Arab. J. Chem.*, vol. 12, no. 7, pp. 908–931, 2019, doi:10.1016/J.ARABJC.2017.05.011.
59. A. Ramanathan, "Toxicity of nanoparticles challenges and opportunities," *Appl. M*icrosc., vol. 49, no. 1, 2019, doi:10.1007/S42649-019-0004-6.
60. S. R. Batool, M. A. Nazeer, E. Yildiz, A. Sahin, and S. Kizilel, "Chitosan-anthracene hydrogels as controlled stiffening networks," *Int. J. Biol. M*acromol., vol. 185, pp. 165–175, 2021, doi:10.1016/j.ijbiomac.2021.06.023.
61. O. C. Onder, S. R. Batool, and M. A. Nazeer, "Self-assembled silk fibroin hydrogels: From preparation to biomedical applications," *Mater. Adv.*, vol. 3, no. 18, pp. 6920–6949, 2022, doi:10.1039/d2ma00568a.

Section II

Wound Dressings

6 Evolution of Wound Healing

Tooba Jabri and Abdul Salam

INTRODUCTION

Natural forces within us are the true healers of disease.

Hippocrates (460–356 BC)

Through the evolutionary history, human skin has developed into a protective and highly adaptive organ, serving as the body's first line of defence against the physical threats and continuous exposure to chemical and ultraviolet stressors [1–3]. Despite its protective function, skin remains particularly vulnerable due to its constant interaction with the external environment, rendering it highly susceptible to injury. When exposed to traumatic stimuli, the skin's structural integrity is compromised, resulting in tissue damage and the formation of wound [4]. This damage initiates a complex cascade of biological processes aimed at restoring skin function, promoting tissue regeneration and preventing further complications [1,5].

The practice of wound care is as ancient as human existence [6–8]. Although its precise origins are difficult to trace, it is plausible that the early humans, in the absence of scientific knowledge instinctively used natural material like leaves to cover wounds, clay, animal fats or water to cleanse them, unknowingly initiating the foundation steps in the long and evolving journey of medical and surgical practices [8].

The evolution of the wound healing reflects a significant transition from instinctive to ritualistic practices to sophisticated, evidence-based medical therapies. Early approaches were rooted in mystical tradition, magical incantations, sorcery, exorcism and herbal potions [9]. Over time, systemic framework emerged, notably through the contribution of pioneer scholars such as Sushruta, Hippocrates and Celsus, who documented early surgical techniques and principles of wound management [7,10]. As civilizations progressed—particularly in Egypt, China, India and Africa—distinctive bodies of written knowledge and practical methodologies in wound care were established [11]. These traditions integrated plant-based remedies, spiritual philosophies and rudimentary surgical and battlefield medicines. However, for many centuries, the advancement of wound care was hindered by limited anatomical understanding and the absence of germ theory, which constrained the scientific progress in this domain [12,13].

A pivotal transformation wound care field occurred during the 19th and 20th centuries with the introduction of surgical sterility, antiseptics and advances

DOI: 10.1201/9781003616726-8

in microbiology. These breakthroughs catalysed progress in tissue biology, nanotechnology, immunology and biochemistry [14–16]. Notably, Joseph Lister, a Professor of Surgery in London, pioneered the use of antiseptics in wound, marking a milestone in reducing infections and improving clinical outcomes. This era also enabled scientist to delineate the distinct phases of wound healing, elucidate the roles of inflammation and tissue regeneration and develop targeted therapeutic intervention to enhance and accelerate the process [17].

Modern wound care encompasses advanced modalities such as hyperbaric oxygen therapy, laser and ultrasound treatments, negative pressure wound therapy and biosurgery. Recent innovations in nanotechnology [18,19], molecular biology, gene therapy [20] and regenerative medicine—including the use of as stem cells and growth factors [21]—have revolutionized therapeutic strategies for managing chronic and complex wounds. This ongoing progression from traditional healing methods to cutting-edge biomedical innovations highlights the intricate, dynamic and multidisciplinary nature of wound healing science.

This chapter covers the historical evolution of wound management, outlines the fundamental biological mechanisms underlying wound healing and examines the recent advancement in the field.

Historical Perspective of Wound Healing

Traditional wound healing practices have continuously evolved over time, forming the foundational basis of medical knowledge long before the advent of modern medicine [22]. These indigenous approaches, ranging from shamanic rituals to the structured medical systems of ancient civilizations and Hippocratic medicine, reflect a progression of empirical understanding. The development of these early practices has had a lasting impact on contemporary healthcare, significantly shaping medical philosophies, therapeutic strategies and clinical approaches to wound management [23]. The evolution of wound healing from the ancient civilization to date is summarized in Table 6.1.

Role of Shamanism and Spiritual Healing in Wound Care

The word "shamanism," which comes from the Tungus people of Siberia, one of the earliest known healing systems, played a crucial role in early care wound regimens among indigenous cultures [23,24]. It refers to a variety of spiritual and therapeutic techniques used by people all over the world. Shamanism rooted their belief in the concepts that physical wounds were often signs of spiritual imbalances or evil forces [25]. It created a bridge between the spiritual and physical world to heal people. Although the precise date of the origin of shamanism is unknown, archaeological findings indicate that it may have originated more than 30,000 years ago, amid the Upper Palaeolithic period [26]. The core element of shamanism is the shaman, a person thought to have unique abilities in divination, healing and spirit-world connection [11].

For the treatment of wound care, Shamans used a blend of natural and spiritual rituals. Healing ceremonies typically included drumming, chanting and the application

TABLE 6.1
Historical Development of Wound Healing

Time Period	Wound Healing Techniques/Methods
Shamanic periods	Spiritual rituals and natural remedies (holy plants like tobacco, peyote and ayahuasca)
Mesopotamian	Clay tablets, cleanse wounds with wine or beer and used sesame infusion
Egyptian	Honey, animal fats, lint, ointments, resins, garlic, potassium alum and salts
Indians	Herbal remedies such as *Curcuma longa* and *Aloe vera*
Chinese medicine	Tinctures, acupuncture, wine and tea leaves
Greece	Mineral-based treatments, Hippocrates relied on the dry healing
Rome	Innovation of Surgical instruments and wound dressings
19th century	Introduction of lister, hygiene methods and aseptic environment
20th century	Wound classification, improvised surgical procedures and antibiotics
Modern	New wound dressings (hydrocolloids, hydrogels), Nanomaterials, tissue engineering, Regenerative therapies, etc.

of plant-based poultices, resins and animal fats to cleanse and seal wound [27,28]. These treatments were believed both to promote physical healing and to drive out evil forces. Shamans used to perform ceremonies to cure and diagnose soul loss like soul retrieval (restores the lost pieces of the soul) and spirit removal (dissolving of bad energies) [29]. Along with soul healing, shamans often employ symbolic actions, herbal treatments and ceremonial cleansing to improve mental, emotional and spiritual well-being. Shamanic culture had various sacred plants including tobacco, peyote and ayahuasca due to their medicinal properties and their potential to induce altered states of consciousness that encourage spiritual awakening and transformation [30].

Shamanism thrives to evolve and flourish throughout the world despite centuries of colonization, suppression of culture and modernization. Shamanic wisdom is being preserved, studied and respectfully incorporated into modern healing frameworks by organizations like the Society for Shamanic Practice and the Foundation for Shamanic Studies [31].

Ancient Civilization's: Pre-Hippocratic and Hippocratic Periods of Wound Healing

Before the advent of Hippocratic medicine in ancient Greece, wound healing practices were mostly regulated by spiritual beliefs, empirical observations and ancestral practices transmitted from generation to generation [32,33]. To treat wounds, prehistoric cultures like the Mesopotamia, Egypt, India and China used a range of natural products, such as honey, resins, plant extracts, clay and animal fats. Although these early techniques lacked knowledge of contemporary pathology and microbiology, they established the groundwork for empirical approaches to healing that were based on experience and observation [34].

This timeframe marks a turning point in the development of wound care, when cultural customs and intuitive reasoning, rather than scientific theory, influenced treatment approaches. These early interventions laid the foundation for the methodical and logical ideas that Hippocratic medicine would eventually establish.

Still, traditional medicine is an important component of healthcare for an enormous percentage of the world's population. The World Health Organization (WHO) estimates that between 60% and 80% of people in underdeveloped nations still get their primary medical care from traditional healers and indigenous remedies. This continued dependence highlights traditional medical strategies' enduring significance and continuing importance in contemporary health systems. The WHO estimates that traditional practitioners provide their daily medical care [12].

Mesopotamian

Ancient Mesopotamia, often referred to as birthplace of civilizations, emerged some of the ancient advanced civilizations, including the Sumerians, Akkadians, Babylonians and Assyrians [35]. These cultures laid the foundation for future medical procedures through their significant contributions to early medicine, especially in wound treatment. One of the first known documented medical treatments, which dates to approximately 2200 BCE, was Sumerian clay tablet. It described the methodical approach to wound care that includes three essential steps: (i) cleaning the wound, (ii) putting a dressing on it and (iii) covering it with a bandage [9].

According to historical reports, antiseptic compounds like wine and beer were used to disinfect wounds, demonstrating an early awareness of infection control. In addition, the seeds were ground into a paste and purified to create sesame infusions, often mixed with beer, which were then administered to wounds for their healing properties. Due to its widespread therapeutic properties, beer is regarded as one of the earliest known medicines used to cure wounds [8,36,37]. Despite lacking the scientific integrity of modern medicine, Mesopotamian medicine had a significant impact on early healthcare models and showed an impressive empirical understanding of wound care for their period.

Ancient Egyptian

The Egyptian civilization is regarded as the earliest and most significant to mankind history. It had made numerous achievements in the art and science including medicine. Around 6000 BCE, Egyptians therapeutic techniques were closely connected to spiritual beliefs [9]. Treatments involved incantations, exorcisms and magical ceremonies, and illness and injuries were usually ascribed to supernatural forces. Imhotep, a highly regarded physician and priest, was eventually worshipped as the God of healing. Later, the temple built after his devotion served as a first centre of therapy [38].

Even though Egyptian surgical methods were simple, mainly confined to ceremonial treatments like circumcision, the medical understanding and expertise of Egyptian was advanced for that medical papyri including important information about their practices such as the Edwin Smith Papyrus (1700 BCE) [7], the Ebers Papyrus (1550 BCE) and the Kahun Papyrus (2000–1800 BCE) [9].

The Edwin Smith Papyrus, which is recognized as one of the first written surgical manuals, included diagnosis, prognoses and remedies for 48 different wound kinds. The Ebers Papyrus describes how to treat wounds using natural materials like honey, animal fat and plant-based lint. Egyptian healers palpated tissues to assess infection and applied ointments and balms containing ingredients such as fig (*Ficus carica*), aloe (*Aloe barbadensis*), benzoin resin (*Styrax benzoin*), garlic (*Allium sativum*), potassium alum and various salts [7]. According to evidence, the ancient Egyptian may be accountable to employ bandages for the first time in history, maybe because of their embalming techniques. Gum-coated linen strips applied as an adhesive dressing, aiding in the proximity of wound margins [10,39].

Ancient literature also emphasizes topical treatments made from unusual concoctions, such as milk, plant gum and even milk from a lady who had just given birth to a baby boy [40]. Additionally, Sumerian and Egyptian literature included early medical terms like "UMMU" and "SHEMEMET," which are now understood to relate to inflammation. Egyptian medicine distinguished between "good" and "bad" wounds, emphasizing their observational approach to prediction and healing results [8].

Ancient Indian (Ayurvedic)

In wound management, ancient Indian practices, especially in the context of Ayurvedic system, proved to be the most conventional yet advanced effective treatment [38]. Ayurveda rooted date back to 5,000 years ago in Hinduism's intellectual and spiritual traditions culture. It is referred to as "science of life", achieving balance and harmony among the body, mind and spirit to improve overall wellness and health [41].

Ayurvedic medicine, including dietary guidelines, surgical procedures and the use of therapeutic plants, is thoroughly explained in extensive literature like the *Sushruta Samhita* and the *Charaka Samhita* [42].

The former literature was assembled by the ancient surgeon Sushruta, especially relevant for wound care. It comprises two chapters regarding wound healing and cites more than 100 plant-based treatments. The latter highlights the importance of complete debridement before suturing wounds, suggesting that foreign materials including stones, hair, clots and detritus be removed. Vrana Shodhana and Vrana Ropana were the names attributed to the cleaning and healing processes of wounds, respectively [7].

Classical Ayurvedic scholars like Sushruta, Charaka, Vagbhata and Jivaka documented numerous medicinal plants under the category *Vranaropaka* (wound healers), including *Cynodon dactylon*, *Ficus benghalensis*, *Symplocos racemosa*, *Rubia cordifolia*, *Centella asiatica*, *Berberis aristata*, *Curcuma longa* (turmeric) and *Aloe vera* [11]. Consequently, several phytochemicals owing to their antibacterial, anti-inflammatory and regenerating properties have been proven by science. The current ongoing research on nutraceuticals and phytochemicals has proven the effectiveness in accelerating wound healing. Curcumin, one key component of turmeric has proven to be the potential candidate for wound healing [43]. As a result, conventional wound care established by ancient Indian Ayurvedic practices continues to influence contemporary integrative medical techniques.

Traditional Chinese Medicine

For more than 2,500 years, people in China and other East Asian countries have been using Traditional Chinese Medicine (TCM), a complete medicinal system. With its roots in ancient philosophical and cultural frameworks, especially Daoism, TCM combines several therapeutic techniques to cure disease, prevent sickness and boost health [23].

The primary concept behind TCM is the theory of *Qi* (pronounced "chee"). It explains the concept of essential life energy, which permeates the body and keeps all living things alive. It was thought that the illness was caused by the disturbance and imbalance in *Qi*, whereas health depends on its harmonious balance and unhindered flow. This ideology was closely related to the Yin-Yang theory, initially introduced by Fu Hsi, which accounts for the dynamic interaction of opposing but harmonious forces inside the body and is intimately associated with this philosophy. While their discord leads to disease, Yin and Yang must be in balance for good health [9,44].

Some historical personalities contributed to wound care and surgical methods. Hua Tuo and Huang Di (Yellow Emperor) were pioneers of Chinese surgical and herbal experts. They have recorded early surgical techniques and wound treatment methods in foundational books like the Huangdi Neijing (Inner Canon of the Yellow Emperor) [26]. Although there was limited surgical practice, many people used herbal remedies. In wound management, tincture from tea leaves was usually administered to wounds due to their antibacterial properties. However, recent scientific studies evidence the utilization of tannic acid present in tea leaves for its efficient wound healing and antimicrobial characteristics. These outcomes highlight the significant approach of Chinese healers and their contribution to wound management [45].

Ancient Greece and Hippocrates

A key turning point in medical history culminated in ancient Greece, when scientific and observational methods replaced mystical explanations of illness. The most famous instance of this philosophical change may be found in the writings of Hippocrates, who is often referred to as the "Father of Medicine." He and his followers' teachings are gathered in the Hippocratic Corpus, a collection of more than 60 writings that established the principles of logical and methodical medicine [44,45].

Hippocrates and his colleagues made revolutionary advances in wound treatment by differentiating between acute ("fresh") and chronic ("non-healing") wounds, classifying into different stages, which are still used today. They demonstrated the crucial steps that require wound cleansing, which involves the use of vinegar or wine due to their alleged antibacterial qualities. Hippocrates advocated avoiding greasy ointments and keeping the wound bed dry to promote healing. However, after being cleaned, fig leaves are also mentioned in some instances as being used as wound dressings [45].

Throughout history, Greek medicines have revolutionized and introduced the fundamental concepts of pharmacology and the incorporated plant-based treatments that focused on diet and minerals. Although, in Greek medical period, the scientific approach works parallel with their rites. They carved the non-venomous snakes in the temples of Asklepios, which are thought to promote healing [46]. According to contemporary views, this might be connected to growth factors found in serpent saliva, which may have helped to heal wounds. Therefore, the innovation in the Greek period, especially that was influenced by Hippocratic thoughts, leads to the fusion of observation-based wound care and scientific approach [46].

Graeco-Roman

The earliest documented Greek (Unani) physician to reside in Rome was Archagathus (219 BCE), who was recognized to practice Greek medicine for the first time. His proficiency in surgical and therapeutic methods thrilled the Roman society, strengthening Greek medical philosophy's acceptability in Roman culture. He had expertise in wound care and surgery, and he often embraced Roman military expeditions to treat injured troops. His presence sparked more interest and research among Roman practitioners and indicated the beginning of the gradual incorporation of Greek/ Unani medicine into Roman healthcare [9].

After the emergence of Greek medicine in Rome, Roman physicians gained recognition for their scientific discoveries. Roman achieved significant advancement in wound healing, such as the application of silver nitrate as an antibiotic in medicine. Among the most significant Roman medical writers, Aulus Cornelius Celsus compiled the treatise *De Medicina*, which describes the core surgical techniques and basic surgical procedures; he is also known for establishing the four cardinal indicators of inflammation: rubor (redness), tumour (swelling), calor (heat) and dolor (pain) [47]. In 1478 CE, this book became one of the first medical texts to be published. Additionally, Celsus reported the application of a variety of topical therapies for wound care, such as styptics, astringents, escharotics and erodents [48].

Galen of Pergamum is another prominent Greek physician who worked as the personal physician for Roman gladiators from 120 to 201 CE. He laid the groundwork for surgical anatomy and clinical care through significant advancements in the treatment of severe injuries and haemorrhage management [49].

At that time, Roman's breakthrough achievements in military medicine have also marked significant development. They invented emergency surgical procedures like tracheotomies, which are utilized for combatants with airway blockage or hypoxia after battle injuries. All these developments demonstrate how the fusion of Roman invention and Greek medical philosophy led to tremendous breakthroughs in ancient surgical and wound care techniques [50,51].

Classical to Medieval Transition

During the first century AD, Dioscorides (also called Doskareedos in Urdu) became well-known in Rome for using single-drug treatments made from minerals, plants and animals [52]. His methods were compiled in the influential text *De Universa Medicina*. By the fourth century AD, the centre of Greco-Roman medicine had shifted to Byzantium (modern-day Turkey), where Nestorian scholars translated Galenic medical texts into Syriac, facilitating the transmission of classical medical knowledge into the Islamic world. Key medical compilers such as Paulus Aegineta,

Aetius of Amida, Alexander of Tralles and Oribasius preserved and expanded on Galenic wound management strategies. Aegineta's encyclopaedic work, *Epitome*, later translated into Arabic, systematically classified wound treatments into erodents, astringents, styptics and cleansing agents [53,54].

By the 10th century, Arabic medical scholarship had matured, heavily drawing from Greek and Roman foundations. Ali Ibn Abbas Majoosi and Ibn Sina (Avicenna) offered comprehensive classification of wounds and treatment protocols in their seminal works *Liber Regius* and *Al-Qanoon Fit Tib*, respectively. Meanwhile, Rhazes (Zakaria Raazi) contributed significantly through his emphasis on bloodletting and cauterization [55]. Additional contributions from physicians such as Abu Sahl Masihi further enriched the medical literature with detailed wound care strategies [56].

In Islamic Spain, the intellectual and medical focus shifted to Cordoba, where Albucasis (Abul Qasim Zohrawi) distinguished himself as a pioneer in surgical innovation. He underlined anatomical knowledge and used ointments, which triggered suppuration to promote wound healing. His reputable research documented in 18 clinical instances, 11 of which addressed wound care, and he suggested several haemostatic techniques, such as ligatures, cauterization, vessel division and styptics [57].

The discipline was further developed by later physicians Ali Ibn Isa, Ibn Zuhr (Avenzoar), Isma'il Jurjani and Ibn Baytar, who used cutting-edge surgical methods and novel pharmaceuticals. They performed specialized operations including ocular surgery, used plaster casting and recorded treatments with natural chemicals. The fundamentals of contemporary wound care and pharmacological research were established by collective efforts [58].

Modern Treatment

The field of wound management has been explored since the existence of mankind to heal site of injury. Throughout history, humans continuously explored the newer and better methods of healing. According to the literature, it has been evident that the development in wound care eventually progressed from shamanic rites to the empirical approach of Hippocratic medicines. The development in scientific research and clinical findings revealed several novel approaches to cure different types of wounds and injuries. It has still gained the scientific attention to improve practical implementation with patient compliance.

In 19th century, Joseph Lister, a prominent professor of surgery, discovered antiseptics to combat with infections. He sterilized wounds and reduced the risk of infection by applying carbolic acid to open fractures. Furthermore, he also highlights the importance of preserving a sterile environment. Then, in 1880, he introduced the sterilization instruments along with the adoption of handwashing and proper surgical gowns and gloves [59,60].

A new era in wound care emerged with the discovery of antibiotics, especially penicillin, in the 1940s. However, antibiotics have proven to reduce the sepsis, but infections were not completely eradicated due to the growth of bacterial resistance and evolution of surgical instruments. Today, the focus remains on preventive measures, including systemic antibiotic administration and surgical debridement to remove necrotic tissue and prevent complications [61].

Modern treatments for chronic or non-healing wounds incorporate advanced modalities such as laser therapy, hydrotherapy, electrotherapy and psoralen combined with ultraviolet light A (PUVA). Other techniques include biosurgery using sterile maggots for debridement, hyperbaric oxygen therapy to enhance oxygen supply to hypoxic tissues and intermittent pneumatic compression (IPC) for treating chronic venous ulcers [62].

With an improved understanding of the pathophysiology of chronic wounds, advancements in nanotechnology, molecular biology and functional genomics have led to the development of novel therapies such as growth factors and tissue-engineered constructs. These innovations continue to enhance current wound management approaches, reflecting ongoing progress in both clinical and scientific fields [63].

Biological Aspects of Wound Healing

Wound healing process has four distinct and differentiated phases, as illustrated in Figure 6.1, which constitutes a highly coordinated biological process: haemostasis, inflammation, proliferation and remodelling. These phases demonstrate how well cellular and molecular reactions interact to repair the structural and functional integrity of the affected tissue [64]. Other factors that can also affect wound healing may include nature of wound, pathological status, extent of tissue perfusion, oxygenation and microbial contamination [65]. These phases of wound healing and the factors

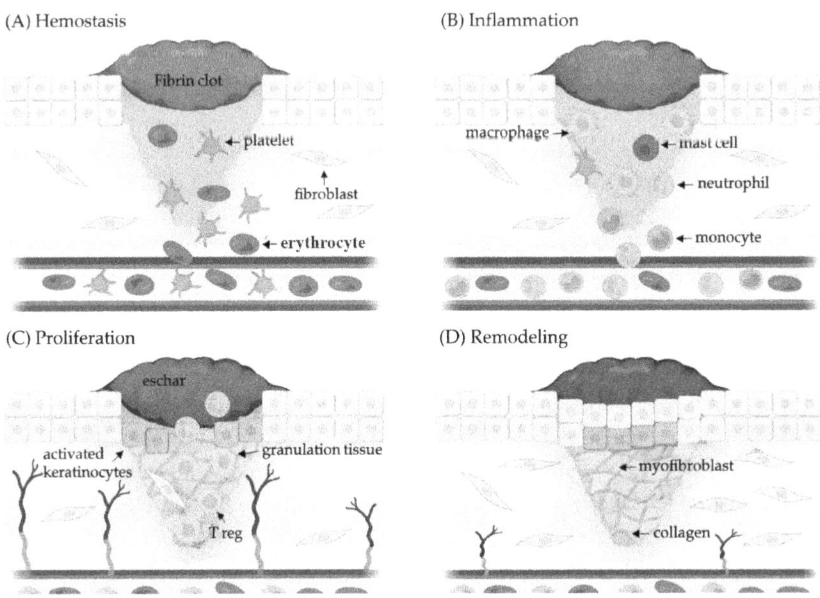

FIGURE 6.1 Phases of wound healing: A) Hemostasis, B) Inflammation, C) Proliferation, and D) Remodeling. (Reproduced from [66] under the terms and conditions of the Creative Commons Attribution (CC BY) licence (https://creativecommons.org/licenses/by/4.0/).)

that influence these physiological aspects of wound healing are described briefly in this section.

Homeostasis

The initial response of homeostasis to the injury is rapid vasoconstriction at the site of vascular disruption. This further leads to the formation of fibrin-rich clot and stops the excessive blood loss [67]. The glycoprotein VI surface receptors mediate the accumulation of platelets on the subendothelial matrix and binds to extracellular matrix (ECM) components including collagen, fibronectin and von Willebrand factor, resulting in adhesion of platelets at the wounded site. Thrombin further stimulates this activation by inducing the conformational changes in platelets and triggering the production of alpha and dense granules [68,69]. These granules contain a variety of pro-coagulant and signalling molecules that enhance the clotting cascade. As a result, insoluble clot (eschar) is formed, which is composed of fibrin, fibronectin, vitronectin and thrombospondin that serves as a primary barrier to blood loss. Besides its mechanical function, this eschar also provides secondary role, which serves as a provisional matrix, a protective barrier against microbial invasion, a scaffold for cell migration and delivering cytokines and growth factors (e.g., epidermal growth factor (EGF), basic fibroblast growth factor (bFGF), platelet-derived growth factor (PDGF) and transforming growth factors β (TGF-β)) and cytokines (e.g., tumour necrosis factor-α (TNF-α) and interleukin 1β (IL-1β)), which are essential for initiating the early phases of wound repair [70,71].

Inflammation

The innate inflammatory phase constitutes a crucial component of the host defence response following tissue injury to counteract microbial invasion and initiate repair. This process is triggered by molecular cues released from damaged or necrotic cells, including the damage-associated molecular patterns (DAMPs), as well as pathogen-associated molecular patterns (PAMPs) originating from invading microorganisms [72]. These molecular sequences are recognized by pattern recognition receptors (PRRs) expressed on immune cells such as Langerhans cells, macrophages, mast cells and T lymphocytes. Activation of these receptors triggers intracellular signalling pathways that lead to the production and release of pro-inflammatory cytokines and chemokines [73,74].

These mediators contribute to vasodilation and enhance the vascular permeability, facilitating the immune cell trafficking. Simultaneously, endothelial cells increase the expression of adhesion molecules, particularly E- and P-selectins, which mediate leukocyte tethering, rolling and extravasation into the damaged tissue. The essential roles of E- and P-selectins in leukocyte recruitment have been well established through genetic and pharmacologic studies, where their inhibition correlates with decreased immune cell infiltration and delayed wound resolution [64,75,76].

Neutrophils are the first immune cells to infiltrate the wound site, where they act to eliminate pathogens by phagocytosis, generation of reactive oxygen species (ROS) and secretion of proteolytic enzymes. As the inflammatory phase progresses, circulating monocytes are recruited and differentiate into macrophages within the wound environment. These macrophages play a pivotal role in clearing apoptotic cells and modulating the local inflammatory milieu, thereby facilitating the transition from the inflammatory phase to tissue regeneration and repair [64].

Proliferative Phase

Following the inflammatory phase, the proliferative phase of wound healing initiates around the third day post-injury and typically spans up to 2–3 weeks [77]. Here, in this phase, fibroblasts, endothelial cells and keratinocytes coordinated to new ECM deposition, which leads to neovascularization and re-epithelialization. The migration of fibroblast into the injured tissue leads to the synthesis of necessary ECM components like hyaluronic acid, fibronectin, proteoglycans, glycosaminoglycans and different types of collagens. These components enhance the rate of tissue regeneration and give structural support to the injured tissue [78,79].

Subsequently, actin stress fibres influence the differentiation of fibroblasts into myofibroblasts, which can generate contractile forces at the site of injury through interactions with ECM proteins such as collagen and fibronectin. Simultaneously, the oxygen supply towards the wounded area improved through angiogenesis, where new blood vessels sprout from pre-existing vasculature, which also supply nutrients to support the metabolic activity of injured tissues [80].

Epidermal keratinocytes proliferate across the injured tissue to re-grow the epidermal barrier, and the whole process is called re-epithelialization. These cells are responsible to maintain the strength and integrity of affected tissues and protect them from microbial infections and external injuries. Physiologically, the proliferative phase is divided into three subsequent steps: ECM synthesis and remodelling by fibroblasts, neovascularization through endothelial proliferation and epithelial regeneration via keratinocyte activity [73,81].

Remodelling

Remodelling refers to the final stage of wound healing where newly regenerated cells reformed skin architecture and its physiological function. Remodelling leads to the controlled clearance of growth factors and clotting factors like vascular endothelial growth factor, macrophages, fibroblasts and endothelial cells, which further leads to the reduction in angiogenesis and excess vasculature. Finally, type III collagen initiates structural rearrangement into a stable triple helix structure after depositing in the ECM [82,83].

Endothelial cells and apoptotic fibroblasts secrete an enzyme, matrix metalloproteinases (MMP), which helps in remodelling of ECM by cleaving collagen molecules [84,85]. This process is critical to eradicate irregular matrix components and evolve the ECM to its mature form. Then, the elasticity and tensile strength of matrix are enhanced by crosslinking of collagen fibres. Finally, these physiological processes altogether enhanced the biomechanical characteristics of neotissue, making it more like healthy tissues and the overall skin, ultimately restoring tissue homeostasis [86,87].

Advanced Wound Treatment

Here, we will investigate various categories of wound dressings and advanced treatment methods that have been developed to efficiently treat wounds. Additionally, we will also focus on recently published techniques and innovations in the field wound healing.

Wound Dressings

The classical approach to wound healing had gradually evolved from rites to remedies. The design and development of wound dressings were limited to those wounds that were dry, clean and have minimal exudate [88,89]. Conventionally, various types of dressing materials were utilized like cotton, wool, plasters, lint, bandages and gauze dressings [90]. However, these wound dressings were periodically changed to prevent the maceration of healthy tissues. Despite the fact that gauze prevents external exposure, it adheres to the injured site and is not appropriate to patient, making it painful while removing and potentially damaging regenerating tissue. Additionally, excessive absorption can lead to desiccation of the wound, potentially delaying the healing process [91,92].

Traditional bandages are typically composed of natural cotton or synthetic fibres such as polyamides or cellulose. Cotton-based bandages are commonly employed for compression or to secure primary dressings in place. Over time, conventional materials have been chemically enhanced to improve flexibility and functionality. Despite these modifications, traditional dressings are increasingly being supplanted by advanced wound care products designed to maintain an optimal moisture balance—crucial for promoting efficient healing [93,94]. As a result, a variety of modern wound dressings have been developed to meet specific clinical needs and enhance patient compliance, as illustrated in Figure 6.2.

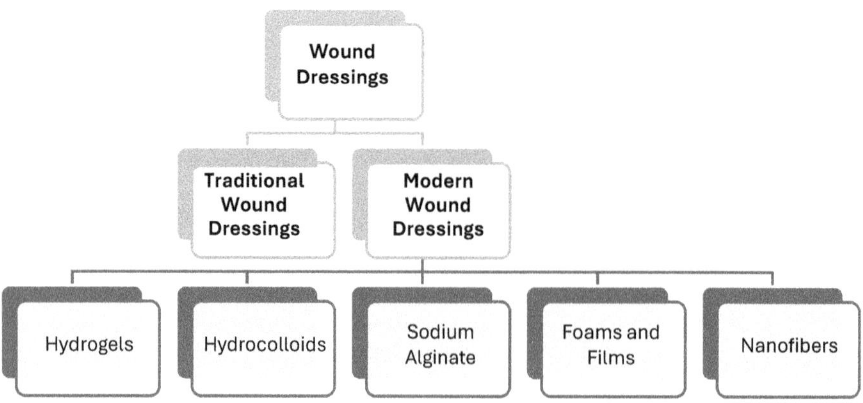

FIGURE 6.2 Classification of wound dressing.

Hydrogels

Hydrogels are made of hydrophilic materials and have a three-dimensional structure. As they are water insoluble, they absorb water at a rate that ranges from 10% to thousands of times their weight [95,96]. Because of their superior moisturising properties, hydrogels help to reduce necrotic tissue and keep the wound moist. Moreover, because the hydrogels are usually transparent, a wound can be monitored through covered dressing. These properties make hydrogels ideal for treatment on burns, radiation dermatitis, pressure ulcers, surgical wounds, etc. They can be appropriate for the wounds with little to moderate exudate [97,98]. The hydrogel rate of degradation can be tuned, which makes it suitable to incorporate biologically active materials and drug carriers.

Hydrocolloids

Hydrocolloids are occlusive, gel-forming wound dressings composed of biocompatible and biodegradable materials such as pectin, carboxymethyl cellulose, gelatin, alginate, elastomers and medical-grade adhesives [99]. These dressings are available in various forms, including powders, sheets and pastes. Moreover, they are appropriate for shock injuries, small burns, bruises and surface ulcers. However, these dressing materials are not suitable for deeper wounds, particularly those with infections that require oxygen to speed up healing. Like hydrogels, hydrocolloids can absorb small to moderate amount of wound exudate. Due to its occlusive nature, hydrocolloid dressings prevent oxygen, bacteria and water from penetrating into the wound. Additionally, hydrocolloids lower the pH of wound environment, resulting in inhibition of microbial growth [3]. These dressings have ease in applicability and have appropriate skin adhesion.

Sodium Alginate-Based Wound Dressings

Sodium alginate (SA) is a naturally occurring anionic biopolymer obtained from brown seaweed. It is non-toxic, biocompatible and widely accessible. Alginate-based wound dressings have two primary advantages for wound healing: (i) they provide a moist environment and (ii) they reduce the microbial invasion. Wound dressings from alginate can be synthesized either by crosslinking their solution with calcium, magnesium, cobalt, cadmium, lead, zinc, strontium, etc. to form a gel or by forming a porous sheet through lyophilized fibrous scaffolds, hydrogels or foams [100]. Alginate dressings can absorb dry wound fluid and create gels that can minimize bacterial infections, give the dry wound a physiologically moist environment and accelerate the formation of granulation tissue and re-epithelialization. Some of the commercially available wound dressings are Algicell™ (SA with 1.4% silver), AlgiSite M™ and SeaSorb® (calcium alginate), Comfeel Plus™ (calcium alginate with carboxymethyl cellulose), Kaltostat™ and Tegagen™ (SA), Algivon® (calcium alginate with Manuka honey), Tromboguard® (SA, calcium alginate, chitosan, polyurethane and silver cations), etc. [93].

Foam Dressings

Foam dressings were invented in the mid-20th century; they are layered hydrophobic and hydrophilic materials that have the capability to absorb the wound exudate and create a protective barrier against the bacterial growth. The development of foam dressing modified from single-layered to multilayered dressing, ensuring to maintain the moist environment while also improving adhesion and accelerating healing. Moreover, some foam dressings are designed with silicone-based adhesive borders that strengthen the mechanical strength of wound dressings. In addition, these dressings have been applied in wound care to absorb exudate, minimize the bacterial environment, improve patient compliance and reduce the skin rupture while applying and removing the dressing [101].

Nanofibres

Nanofibrous scaffolds have gained the scientific interest in skin tissue engineering due to its unique properties and the ability to customize the wound dressings. In clinical settings, nanofibrous dressings achieve a reproducible, non-invasive, biocompatible and cost-effective therapeutic approach that is practically approved for scarless wound healing. The porous architecture of nanofibres provides breathability and helps to regulate the moist environment, which enables the airflow and reduces the microbial growth. Its large surface-to-volume ratio improves cell adhesion, proliferation and accelerates tissue regeneration [102]. Nanofibrous wound dressings are comprised of biocompatible synthetic or natural materials such as chitosan and collagen, which circumvent the adverse effects. Moreover, these polymeric scaffolds incorporate different therapeutic agents that promote the healing efficiently [103,104].

Nanomaterials in Wound Healing

Nanotechnology has revolutionized and has achieved tremendous growth in healing wounds, owing to its unique physiochemical characteristics such as high surface-area-to-volume ratio at nanoscale size [105]. Moreover, it can tailor the surface chemistry and can incorporate the active pharmaceutical ingredients or therapeutic agents to facilitate drug delivery. These nanomaterials have proven to promote healing at cellular and molecular levels.

Nanomaterials utilized in wound therapy can be broadly classified into two categories: those with intrinsic wound healing properties and those that serve as carriers for therapeutic agents. Over the past two decades, there has been a significant increase in the development and use of advanced nanomaterials, such as nanoparticles specifically designed for infection control and wound repair [106].

Nanoparticle-based scaffolding has emerged as a promising strategy for improving wound dressings, garnering substantial interest. Antimicrobial nanomaterials, available in various formulations, incorporate polymers like cellulose, mesoporous silica and lipid-based structures such as liposomes, acting as delivery vehicles for antibacterial agents and wound healing compounds. This advancement underscores the pivotal role of nanotechnology in enhancing the effectiveness of modern wound care solutions.

Bioactive Dressings

Bioactive dressings represent an advanced class of wound care materials composed of natural or synthetic biomaterials that are designed to enhance the healing process. Common constituents include collagen, hyaluronic acid, chitosan, alginate and elastin—materials recognized for their biocompatibility, biodegradability and non-toxicity. These polymers may be used individually or in combination, tailored to the specific type and condition of the wound. To further accelerate wound healing, bioactive dressings are often supplemented with growth factors or antimicrobial agents [94].

Bioengineered Skins

To promote wound healing, skin substitutes have been intensively investigated as one of the successful approaches. Skin substitutes are a diverse collection of biologic, synthetic or biosynthetic materials that are utilized to both temporarily and permanently replace the functions of skin in wound healing and closure [107,108].

Bioengineered skin substitutes have the potential to aid in tissue regeneration in addition to acting as protective bandages [109]. Their main goals are to lessen fluid loss and the quantity of bacteria that enter and colonize the wound. Fibroblasts, keratinocytes, endothelial cells, neutrophils and macrophages enter the wound bed when the wound is covered by a skin substitute. Then, these cells release growth factors and cytokines, which promote angiogenesis, ECM deposition and re-epithelialization process.

Skin substitutes can be classified into three categories according to its structure, as shown in Table 6.2. Synthetic and biological (biodegradable and non-biodegradable) replacements are separated based on the kind of biomaterial utilized in the building. Also, autologous, allogenous or xenogenous cells can be

TABLE 6.2
Classification of Various Skin Substitutes

Class	Skin Substitute Product	Material Used	Role
Class 1	TransCyte™—(Dermagraft™)	Two-layered dressing (fibroblast on nylon mesh with porcine collagen)	Used for second- and third-degree burn wounds
	DermoFilm	Single-layered hydrocolloid patch/spray	Graft wounds and ulcers, radiotherapy skin lesions
	Opsite	Polyurethane membrane	Used for burns and after surgical wounds
	Epigard	Microporous foil and soft polyurethane matrix	Burns, grafting
	TegaDerm	Transparent polyurethane film	Radiotherapy, surgical wounds, catheter

(Continued)

TABLE 6.2 (*Continued*)
Classification of Various Skin Substitutes

Class	Skin Substitute Product	Material Used	Role
Class 2	Epicel	Cultured autologous keratinocytes on non-stick gauze	Chronic ulcers, burns
	LaserSkin®	Benzyl hyaluronan scaffold with autologous keratinocytes	Full-thickness burns, chronic ulcers
	BioSeed®	Autologous keratinocytes cultured in fibrin sealant	Chronic leg ulcers
	MatriDerm	Bovine collagen + elastin	Full-thickness wounds, burns, tumour excision sites
	Apligraf	Neonatal fibroblasts + bovine collagen matrix + keratinocytes	Diabetic foot ulcers, venous ulcers
	HyloMatrix PA	Benzyl ester of hyaluronic acid + semipermeable silicone membrane	Burns, chronic/postoperative wounds
	Permacol™	Cross-linked porcine dermal collagen	Hernia repair, abdominal wall, reconstructive surgery
Class 3	Biobrane®	Cell-free dermal substitute	Nylon mesh with collagen and ultra-thin silicone
	OASIS Wound Matrix	Acellular dermal substitute	Porcine jejunum ECM (single or triple layer)
	Nevelia	Multilayered dermal–epidermal substitute	Stabilized bovine type I collagen + semipermeable silicone membrane
	OrCel	Cellular dermal–epidermal (biological dressing)	Allogeneic keratinocytes and fibroblasts on bovine collagen sponge

employed as substitutes. The benefit of using biological alternatives is that the ECM's structure is mostly unaltered [110,111].

Hyperbaric Oxygen

Experimental evidence suggests that increasing the concentration of inspired oxygen positively influences both collagen deposition and wound tensile strength. In a 1981 study, Knighton et al. demonstrated that ambient or inspired oxygen levels could modulate angiogenesis during wound healing [112]. Later, in 1985, Sheffield reported that certain chronic diabetic foot ulcers exhibited significant hypoxia and responded favourably to changes in the partial pressure of inspired oxygen, as measured using polarographic electrodes [113]. These findings contributed to the transition of hyperbaric oxygen therapy (HBOT) from an experimental approach to an established adjunctive treatment. Subsequent case reports laid the groundwork for future clinical trials. Notably, Hammarlund and Sundberg demonstrated that HBOT significantly improved healing outcomes in chronic leg ulcers when used as an adjunct therapy. Although large-scale double-blind trials remain limited, short-term HBOT and localized application of oxygen are gaining attention for their potential to enhance wound healing while minimizing systemic side effects [114].

Lasers

In addition to standard wound dressings, low-level laser therapy (LLLT) delivering energy at 10 J/cm^2 has been explored as a treatment for chronic ulcers. This approach is based on the hypothesis that exposure of wound tissues to photon energy from LLLT may stimulate cellular regeneration and proliferation, thereby enhancing the healing process. Gas lasers such as helium-neon (HeNe) and gallium arsenide (GaAs) have been applied in wound care for this purpose [115]. However, a thorough review of randomized controlled trials involving laser therapy for ulcer treatment has revealed insufficient evidence to establish definitive clinical guidelines.

Future Perspective

Gene Therapy

Gene therapy involves the introduction of specific genes into target cells to modify cellular function. While initially developed for treating genetic disorders and certain cancers, the skin has recently emerged as a promising therapeutic target for gene-based interventions [116]. In the context of wound healing, gene therapy has demonstrated encouraging potential by influencing cellular behaviour to enhance tissue repair. Depending on the method and vector used, gene transfer can lead to either transient or stable modifications in cellular physiology, initiating cascades that support wound regeneration. A deeper understanding of growth factors and cell biology is enabling more precise and effective gene-based strategies for tissue repair [117,118].

Despite these advancements, ongoing research is essential to further elucidate the molecular and cellular mechanisms driving wound repair. It's also crucial to emphasize that while gene therapy holds great promise, it should complement and do not replace the foundational principles of conventional wound care.

Cell-Based Therapies (Stem Cells)

Recent progress in wound care, especially the use of platelet-derived products and growth factors, has enabled the integration of various stem cells into wound dressings. Stem cells such as adipose-derived mesenchymal stem cells (AMSCs), bone marrow-derived mesenchymal stem cells (BMMSCs), umbilical cord mesenchymal stem cells (UCMSCs), human amniotic fluid-derived stem cells (AFMSCs), human gingival-derived mesenchymal stem cells (GMSCs), peripheral blood stem cells (PBSCs), placenta-derived mesenchymal stem cells (PMSCs), embryonic stem cells

(ESCs), epidermal stem cells (EpSCs) and induced pluripotent stem cells (iPSCs) have shown great promise in enhancing wound healing and skin regeneration [119,120]. These stem cells accelerate healing by self-renewing, differentiating into skin-related cell types and releasing growth factors and cytokines that support key processes such as tissue granulation, new blood vessel formation, re-epithelialization and collagen production [5,121].

CONCLUSION

Wound management has been practiced since ancient times and has gradually evolved throughout history. Each culture contributed unique techniques and methods that laid the foundation for modern wound care. These early approaches have been refined and improved over time, leading to the development of advanced treatments supported by scientific research today. In the modern era, extensive research and clinical trials continue to enhance the effectiveness of wound healing therapies.

REFERENCES

1. Almadani, Y.H., J. Vorstenbosch, P.G. Davison, and A.M. Murphy. Wound healing: a comprehensive review. *Seminars in Plastic Surgery*, 2021. 35: p. 141–144.
2. Peate, I., The skin: largest organ of the body. *British Journal of Healthcare Assistants*, 2021. **15**(9): p. 446–451.
3. Rezvani Ghomi, E., S. Khalili, S. Nouri Khorasani, R. Esmaeely Neisiany, and S. Ramakrishna, Wound dressings: current advances and future directions. *Journal of Applied Polymer Science*, 2019. **136**(27): p. 47738.
4. Su, J., C. Liu, A. Sun, J. Yan, F. Sang, Y. Xin, Y. Zhao, S. Wang, and Q. Dang, Hemostatic and antimicrobial properties of chitosan-based wound healing dressings: a review. *International Journal of Biological Macromolecules*, 2025. 306: p. 141570.
5. Borena, B.M., A. Martens, S.Y. Broeckx, E. Meyer, K. Chiers, L. Duchateau, and J.H. Spaas, Regenerative skin wound healing in mammals: state-of-the-art on growth factor and stem cell based treatments. *Cellular Physiology and Biochemistry*, 2015. **36**(1): p. 1–23.
6. Sarabahi, S. and V. Tiwari, *Principles and Practice of Wound Care*. JP Medical Ltd, 2012.
7. Bhattacharya, S., Wound healing through the ages. *Indian Journal of Plastic Surgery*, 2012. **45**(2): p. 177–179.
8. Thomas, J., Topical antibacterial agents; growth factors. In: A Shai and H. I. Maibach (Eds.), *Wound Healing and Ulcers of the Skin: Diagnosis and Therapy—The Practical Approach*. Springer, 2005, pp. 185–191. ISBN: 3540 2127520470 848987.
9. Ahmad, W., Z. Aquil, and S.S. Alam, Historical background of wound care. *Hamdan Medical Journal*, 2020. **13**(4): p. 189–195.
10. George Broughton, I., J.E. Janis, and C.E. Attinger, A brief history of wound care. *Plastic and reconstructive surgery*, 2006. **117**(7S): p. 6S–11S.
11. Cantwell, M.F., Map of the spirit: diagnosis and treatment of spiritual disease. *Advances in Mind-body Medicine*, 2008. **23**(2): p. 6–16.
12. Dorai, A.A., Wound care with traditional, complementary and alternative medicine. *Indian Journal of plastic surgery*, 2012. **45**(02): p. 418–424.
13. Manring, M., A. Hawk, J.H. Calhoun, and R.C. Andersen, Treatment of war wounds: a historical review. *Clinical Orthopaedics and Related Research*, 2009. **467**: p. 2168–2191.

14. Phillips, T.J., New skin for old: developments in biological skin substitutes. *Archives of dermatology*, 1998. **134**(3): p. 344–349.
15. Forrest, R.D., Development of wound therapy from the Dark Ages to the present. *Journal of the Royal Society of Medicine*, 1982. **75**(4): p. 268–273.
16. Han, S.-K., *Innovations and Advances in Wound Healing*. Springer Nature, 2023.
17. Cozen, L.N., Military orthopedic surgery. *Clinical Orthopaedics and Related Research*, 1985. **200**: p. 50–53.
18. Alberti, T., D. S Coelho, A. Voytena, H. Pitz, M. de Pra, L. Mazzarino, S. Kuhnen, R. M Ribeiro-do-Valle, M. Maraschin, and B. Veleirinho, Nanotechnology: a promising tool towards wound healing. *Current Pharmaceutical Design*, 2017. **23**(24): p. 3515–3528.
19. Ullah, A., M. Ullah, G.-J. Lee, and S.I. Lim, A review of recent advances in nanotechnology for the delivery of therapeutics in wound healing. *Journal of Pharmaceutical Investigation*, 2025. **55**(1): p. 33–54.
20. Pang, C., K.S. Fan, L. Wei, and M.K. Kolar, Gene therapy in wound healing using nanotechnology. *Wound Repair and Regeneration*, 2021. **29**(2): p. 225–239.
21. Tsai, H.-W., P.-H. Wang, and K.-H. Tsui, Mesenchymal stem cell in wound healing and regeneration. *Journal of the Chinese Medical Association*, 2018. 81: p. 223–224.
22. Cohen, I.K., Lessons from the history of wound healing. *Clinics in Dermatology*, 2007. **25**(1): p. 3–8.
23. Cook, H.J., The history of medicine and the scientific revolution. *Isis*, 2011. **102**(1): p. 102–108.
24. Elendu, C., The evolution of ancient healing practices: from shamanism to Hippocratic medicine: A review. *Medicine*, 2024. **103**(28): p. e39005.
25. McClenon, J., Shamanic healing, human evolution, and the origin of religion. *Journal for the Scientific study of Religion*, 1997: p. 345–354.
26. Cassell, E.J., The nature of suffering and the goals of medicine. *Loss, Grief & Care*, 1998. **8**(1–2): p. 129–142.
27. Winkelman, M., Shamanism and the evolutionary origins of spirituality and healing. *NeuroQuantology*, 2011. **9**(1): p. 54–71.
28. McVay, M.R., Medicine and spirituality: a simple path to restore compassion in medicine. *South Dakota Journal of Medicine*, 2002. **55**(11): p. 487–491.
29. Claridge, J.A. and T.C. Fabian, History and development of evidence-based medicine. *World Journal of Surgery*, 2005. **29**(5): p. 547–553.
30. Woolf, S.H., R. Grol, A. Hutchinson, M. Eccles, and J. Grimshaw, Potential benefits, limitations, and harms of clinical guidelines. *BMJ*, 1999. **318**(7182): p. 527–530.
31. Georgescu, A.M., C. Banescu, R. Azamfirei, A. Hutanu, V. Moldovan, I. Badea, S. Voidazan, M. Dobreanu, I.R. Chirtes, and L. Azamfirei, Evaluation of TNF-α genetic polymorphisms as predictors for sepsis susceptibility and progression. *BMC Infectious Diseases*, 2020. **20**: p. 1–11.
32. Montoya-Ruiz, C., F.A. Jaimes, M.T. Rugeles, J.Á. López, G. Bedoya, and P.A. Velilla, Variants in LTA, TNF, IL1B and IL10 genes associated with the clinical course of sepsis. *Immunologic Research*, 2016. **64**: p. 1168–1178.
33. Hinohara, S., Medicine and religion: spiritual dimension of health care. *Humane Health Care*, 2001. **1**(2): p. E2–E2.
34. Žuškin, E., J. Lipozenčić, J. Pucarin-Cvetković, J. Mustajbegović, N. Schachter, B. Mučić-Pučić, and I. Neralić-Meniga, Ancient medicine-a review. *Acta Dermatovenerologica Croatica*, 2008. **16**(3): p. 0–0.
35. Hamburg, M.A. and F.S. Collins, The path to personalized medicine. *New England Journal of Medicine*, 2010. **363**(4): p. 301–304.
36. Levey, M., *Early Arabic Pharmacology: An Introduction based on Ancient and Medieval Sources*. Brill Archive, 1973.

37. Shah, J.B., The history of wound care. *The Journal of the American College of Certified Wound Specialists*, 2011. **3**(3): p. 65–66.
38. Mueller, P.S., D.J. Plevak, and T.A. Rummans. Religious involvement, spirituality, and medicine: implications for clinical practice. *Mayo Clinic Proceedings*, 2001. 76: p. 1225–1235.
39. Forrest, R.D., Early history of wound treatment. *Journal of the Royal Society of Medicine*, 1982. **75**(3): p. 198–205.
40. Shah, J., The history of wound care. *The Journal of the American College of Certified Wound Specialists,* 2011. 3: 65.
41. Daaleman, T.P. and B. Frey, Prevalence and patterns of physician referral to clergy and pastoral care providers. *Archives of Family Medicine*, 1998. **7**(6): p. 548.
42. Kandwal, A., R.K. Mamgain, and P. Mamgain, Comparative evaluation of turmeric gel with 2% chlorhexidine gluconate gel for treatment of plaque induced gingivitis: a randomized controlled clinical trial. *AYU (An International Quarterly Journal of Research in Ayurveda)*, 2015. **36**(2): p. 145–150.
43. Akbik, D., M. Ghadiri, W. Chrzanowski, and R. Rohanizadeh, Curcumin as a wound healing agent. *Life Sciences*, 2014. **116**(1): p. 1–7.
44. Wardlaw, M.P., American medicine as religious practice: care of the sick as a sacred obligation and the unholy descent into secularization. *Journal of Religion and Health*, 2011. **50**: p. 62–74.
45. Shalev, D., K. Brenner, R.L. Carlson, D. Chammas, S. Levitt, P.E. Noufi, G. Robbins-Welty, and J.A. Webb, Palliative care psychiatry: building synergy across the spectrum. *Current Psychiatry Reports*, 2024. **26**(3): p. 60–72.
46. Shai, A. and H. Maibach, *Wound Healing and Ulcers of the Skin: Diagnosis and Therapy—The Practical Approach.* Marion Philipp, 2005.
47. Rosenthal, T., Aulus Cornelius Celsus: his contributions to dermatology. *Archives of Dermatology*, 1961. **84**(4): p. 613–618.
48. Talamonti, G., G. D'Aliberti, and M. Cenzato, Aulus cornelius celsus and the head injuries. *World Neurosurgery*, 2020. **133**: p. 127–134.
49. Fullerton, J.B. and M.E. Silverman, Claudius Galen of Pergamum: authority of medieval medicine. *Clinical Cardiology*, 2009. **32**(11): p. E82.
50. McCallum, J.E., *Military Medicine: From Ancient Times to the 21st Century.* 2008, Bloomsbury.
51. Morris, M.J., Acute respiratory distress syndrome in combat casualties: military medicine and advances in mechanical ventilation. *Military Medicine*, 2006. **171**(11): p. 1039–1044.
52. Riddle, J.M., Dioscorides on Pharmacy and Medicine. University of Texas Press, 1985.
53. Gäbel, R., *Aetius of Amida on Diseases of the Brain: Translation and Commentary of Libri Medicinales 6.1–10 with Introduction.* Walter de Gruyter GmbH & Co KG, Vol. 13, 2022.
54. Gurunluoglu, R. and A. Gurunluoglu, Paul of Aegina: landmark in surgical progress. *World Journal of Surgery*, 2003. **27**: p. 18–25.
55. Khan, A.A., M. Zulkifle, A.H. Ansari, and K.N.A. Hai, Persian contribution to Greco-Arab medicine: a review. *Journal of the International Society for the History of Islamic Medicine,* 2008. **2007**: p. 107.
56. Taghavi-Shirazi, M., R. Ghods, F. Hashem-Dabaghian, and A. Zargaran, Abu-Sahl al-Masihi (died circa 1010 AD): the Persian physician in the early medieval era. *Journal of Medical Biography*, 2020. **28**(3): p. 132–135.
57. Al-Benna, S., Albucasis, a tenth-century scholar, physician and surgeon: his role in the history of plastic and reconstructive surgery. *European Journal of Plastic Surgery*, 2012. **35**(5): p. 379–387.

58. Azar, H.A., *Ibn Zuhr (Avenzoar), "Supreme in the Science of Medicine Since Galen": The Translation of His Work into Latin and his Image in Medieval Europe.* The University of North Carolina at Chapel Hill, 1998.
59. Pitt, D. and J.-M. Aubin, Joseph Lister: father of modern surgery. *Canadian Journal of Surgery*, 2012. **55**(5): p. E8.
60. Michaleas, S.N., K. Laios, A. Charalabopoulos, G. Samonis, M. Karamanou, and S. Michaleas, Joseph Lister (1827–1912): a pioneer of antiseptic surgery. *Cureus*, 2022. **14**(12).
61. Durand, G.A., D. Raoult, and G. Dubourg, Antibiotic discovery: history, methods and perspectives. *International Journal of Antimicrobial Agents*, 2019. **53**(4): p. 371–382.
62. Fan, W.P.L., M. Rashid, and S. Enoch, Current advances in modern wound healing. *Wounds UK*, 2010. **6**(3): p. 22–36.
63. Zielińska, A., J. Karczewski, P. Eder, T. Kolanowski, M. Szalata, K. Wielgus, M. Szalata, D. Kim, S.R. Shin, and R. Słomski, Scaffolds for drug delivery and tissue engineering: the role of genetics. *Journal of Controlled Release*, 2023. **359**: p. 207–223.
64. Schultz, G.S., G.A. Chin, L. Moldawer, and R.F. Diegelmann, Principles of wound healing. In: R. Fitridge and M. Thompson (Eds.), *Mechanisms of Vascular Disease: A Reference Book for Vascular Specialists.* University of Adelaide Press, 2011, pp. 423–450.
65. Singer, A.J. and R.A. Clark, Cutaneous wound healing. *New England Journal of Medicine*, 1999. **341**(10): p. 738–746.
66. Srivastava, G.K., S. Martinez-Rodriguez, N.I. Md Fadilah, D. Looi Qi Hao, G. Markey, P. Shukla, M.B. Fauzi, and F. Panetsos, Progress in wound-healing products based on natural compounds, stem cells, and microRNA-based biopolymers in the European, USA, and Asian markets: opportunities, barriers, and regulatory issues. *Polymers*, 2024. **16**(9): p. 1280.
67. Wang, G., F. Yang, W. Zhou, N. Xiao, M. Luo, and Z. Tang, The initiation of oxidative stress and therapeutic strategies in wound healing. *Biomedicine & Pharmacotherapy*, 2023. **157**: p. 114004.
68. Furie, B. and B.C. Furie, Mechanisms of thrombus formation. *New England Journal of Medicine*, 2008. **359**(9): p. 938–949.
69. Enoch, S. and D.J. Leaper, Basic science of wound healing. *Surgery (Oxford)*, 2008. **26**(2): p. 31–37.
70. Shoji, T., T. Nakasa, M. Yoshizuka, T. Yamasaki, Y. Yasunaga, N. Adachi, and M. Ochi, Comparison of fibrin clots derived from peripheral blood and bone marrow. *Connective Tissue Research*, 2017. **58**(2): p. 208–214.
71. Dargaville, T.R., B.L. Farrugia, J.A. Broadbent, S. Pace, Z. Upton, and N.H. Voelcker, Sensors and imaging for wound healing: a review. *Biosensors and Bioelectronics*, 2013. **41**: p. 30–42.
72. Nurden, A.T., Molecular basis of clot retraction and its role in wound healing. *Thrombosis Research*, 2023. **231**: p. 159–169.
73. Sorg, H. and C.G. Sorg, Skin wound healing: of players, patterns, and processes. *European Surgical Research*, 2023. **64**(2): p. 141–157.
74. Wang, Z., F. Zhao, C. Xu, Q. Zhang, H. Ren, X. Huang, C. He, J. Ma, and Z. Wang, Metabolic reprogramming in skin wound healing. *Burns & Trauma*, 2024. **12**: p. tkad047.
75. Frenette, P.S. and D.D. Wagner, Adhesion molecules—Blood vessels and blood cells. *New England Journal of Medicine*, 1996. **335**(1): p. 43–45.
76. Frenette, P.S. and D.D. Wagner, Adhesion molecules. *New England Journal of Medicine*, 1996. **334**(23): p. 1526–1529.

77. Landén, N.X., D. Li, and M. Ståhle, Transition from inflammation to proliferation: a critical step during wound healing. *Cellular and Molecular Life Sciences*, 2016. **73**: p. 3861–3885.
78. Criollo-Mendoza, M.S., L.A. Contreras-Angulo, N. Leyva-López, E.P. Gutiérrez-Grijalva, L.A. Jiménez-Ortega, and J.B. Heredia, Wound healing properties of natural products: mechanisms of action. *Molecules*, 2023. **28**(2): p. 598.
79. Abazari, M., A. Ghaffari, H. Rashidzadeh, S.M. Badeleh, and Y. Maleki, A systematic review on classification, identification, and healing process of burn wound healing. *International Journal of Lower Extremity Wounds*, 2022. **21**(1): p. 18–30.
80. Fernández-Guarino, M., M.L. Hernández-Bule, and S. Bacci, Cellular and molecular processes in wound healing. *Biomedicines*, 2023. **11**(9): p. 2526.
81. Stone, R.C., I. Pastar, N. Ojeh, V. Chen, S. Liu, K.I. Garzon, and M. Tomic-Canic, Epithelial-mesenchymal transition in tissue repair and fibrosis. *Cell and Tissue Research*, 2016. **365**: p. 495–506.
82. Diegelmann, R.F., Analysis of collagen synthesis. In: L. A. DiPietro and A. L. Burns (Eds.), *Wound Healing: Methods and Protocols*. Humana Press, 2003, pp. 349–358.
83. Carlson, M.A. and M.T. Longaker, The fibroblast-populated collagen matrix as a model of wound healing: a review of the evidence. *Wound Repair and Regeneration*, 2004. **12**(2): p. 134–147.
84. Visse, R. and H. Nagase, Matrix metalloproteinases and tissue inhibitors of metalloproteinases: structure, function, and biochemistry. *Circulation Research*, 2003. **92**(8): p. 827–839.
85. Caley, M.P., V.L. Martins, and E.A. O'Toole, Metalloproteinases and wound healing. *Advances in Wound Care*, 2015. **4**(4): p. 225–234.
86. Das, P., S. Manna, S. Roy, S.K. Nandi, and P. Basak, Polymeric biomaterials-based tissue engineering for wound healing: a systemic review. *Burns & Trauma*, 2023. **11**: p. tkac058.
87. Xiao, H., X. Chen, X. Liu, G. Wen, and Y. Yu, Recent advances in decellularized biomaterials for wound healing. *Materials Today Bio*, 2023. **19**: p. 100589.
88. Sun, X., Y. Zhang, J. Cui, C. Zhang, C. Xing, H. Bian, J. Lv, D. Chen, L. Xiao, and J. Su, Advanced multilayer composite dressing with co-delivery of gelsevirine and silk fibroin for burn wound healing. *Composites Part B: Engineering*, 2023. **253**: p. 110549.
89. Malik, S., K. Muhammad, and Y. Waheed, Emerging applications of nanotechnology in healthcare and medicine. *Molecules*, 2023. **28**(18): p. 6624.
90. Nguyen, H.M., T.T.N. Le, A.T. Nguyen, H.N.T. Le, and T.T. Pham, Biomedical materials for wound dressing: recent advances and applications. *RSC Advances*, 2023. **13**(8): p. 5509–5528.
91. Tiwari, N., D. Kumar, A. Priyadarshani, G.K. Jain, G. Mittal, P. Kesharwani, and G. Aggarwal, Recent progress in polymeric biomaterials and their potential applications in skin regeneration and wound care management. *Journal of Drug Delivery Science and Technology*, 2023. **82**: p. 104319.
92. Sharma, A., D. Sharma, and F. Zhao, Updates on recent clinical assessment of commercial chronic wound care products. *Advanced Healthcare Materials*, 2023. **12**(25): p. 2300556.
93. Boateng, J.S., K.H. Matthews, H.N. Stevens, and G.M. Eccleston, Wound healing dressings and drug delivery systems: a review. *Journal of Pharmaceutical Sciences*, 2008. **97**(8): p. 2892–2923.
94. Dhivya, S., V.V. Padma, and E. Santhini, Wound dressings—a review. *BioMedicine*, 2015. **5**(4): p. 22.
95. Khandan, A., H. Jazayeri, M.D. Fahmy, and M. Razavi, Hydrogels: types, structure, properties, and applications. In: M. Razavi (Ed.), *Biomaterials for Tissue Engineering*. Bentham Science Publishers, 2017, pp. 143–169.

96. Singh, N., S. Agarwal, A. Jain, and S. Khan, 3-Dimensional cross linked hydrophilic polymeric network "hydrogels": an agriculture boom. *Agricultural Water Management*, 2021. **253**: p. 106939.
97. Gounden, V. and M. Singh, Hydrogels and wound healing: current and future prospects. *Gels*, 2024. **10**(1): p. 43.
98. Liang, Y., J. He, and B. Guo, Functional hydrogels as wound dressing to enhance wound healing. *ACS Nano*, 2021. **15**(8): p. 12687–12722.
99. Finnie, A., Hydrocolloids in wound management: pros and cons. *British Journal of Community Nursing*, 2002. **7**(7): p. 338–345.
100. Aderibigbe, B.A. and B. Buyana, Alginate in wound dressings. *Pharmaceutics*, 2018. **10**(2): p. 42.
101. Hargis, A., M. Yaghi, N.M. Bermudez, and A. Gefen, Foam dressings for wound healing. *Current Dermatology Reports*, 2024. **13**(1): p. 28–35.
102. Shariatzadeh, F.J., S. Currie, S. Logsetty, R. Spiwak, and S. Liu, Enhancing wound healing and minimizing scarring: a comprehensive review of nanofiber technology in wound dressings. *Progress in Materials Science*, 2024. 147: p. 101350.
103. Sylvester, M.A., F. Amini, and C.K. Tan, Electrospun nanofibers in wound healing. *Materials Today: Proceedings*, 2020. **29**: p. 1–6.
104. Chen, S., B. Liu, M.A. Carlson, A.F. Gombart, D.A. Reilly, and J. Xie, Recent advances in electrospun nanofibers for wound healing. *Nanomedicine*, 2017. **12**(11): p. 1335–1352.
105. Baig, N., I. Kammakakam, and W. Falath, Nanomaterials: A review of synthesis methods, properties, recent progress, and challenges. *Materials Advances*, 2021. **2**(6): p. 1821–1871.
106. Nandhini, J., E. Karthikeyan, and S. Rajeshkumar, Nanomaterials for wound healing: current status and futuristic frontier. *Biomedical Technology*, 2024. **6**: p. 26–45.
107. Halim, A.S., T.L. Khoo, and S.J.M. Yussof, Biologic and synthetic skin substitutes: an overview. *Indian Journal of Plastic Surgery*, 2010. **43**(S 01): p. S23–S28.
108. Kelangi, S.S., G. Theocharidis, A. Veves, W.G. Austen, R. Sheridan, J. Goverman, and M. Bei, On skin substitutes for wound healing: current products, limitations, and future perspectives. *Technology*, 2020. **8**(01n02): p. 8–14.
109. Metcalfe, A.D. and M.W. Ferguson, Bioengineering skin using mechanisms of regeneration and repair. *Biomaterials*, 2007. **28**(34): p. 5100–5113.
110. te W, D., Classification of skin substitutes. *Burns*, 2008. **34**: p. 148–149.
111. Ferreira, M.C., A.O. Paggiaro, C. Isaac, N. Teixeira Neto, and G.B.d. Santos, Skin substitutes: current concepts and a new classification system. *Revista Brasileira de Cirurgia Plástica*, 2011. **26**: p. 696–702.
112. TK, H., The effect of varying ambient oxygen tensions on wound metabolism and collagen synthesis. *Surgery, Gynecology & Obstetrics*, 1972. **135**: p. 561–567.
113. PJ, S., Tissue oxygen measurements with respect to soft tissue wound healing with normobaric and hyperbaric oxygen. *HBO Rev*, 1985. **6**: p. 18–46.
114. Hammarlund, C. and T. Sundberg, Hyperbaric oxygen reduced size of chronic leg ulcers: a randomized double-blind study. *Plastic and Reconstructive Surgery*, 1994. **93**(4): p. 829–833.
115. Flemming, K., N. Cullum, and E. Nelson, A systematic review of laser therapy for venous leg ulcers. *Journal of Wound Care*, 1999. **8**(3): p. 111–114.
116. Sayed, N., P. Allawadhi, A. Khurana, V. Singh, U. Navik, S.K. Pasumarthi, I. Khurana, A.K. Banothu, R. Weiskirchen, and K.K. Bharani, Gene therapy: comprehensive overview and therapeutic applications. *Life Sciences*, 2022. **294**: p. 120375.
117. Karimzadeh, F., E.S. Fard, A. Nadi, R. Malekzadeh, F. Elahian, and S.A. Mirzaei, Advances in skin gene therapy: utilizing innovative dressing scaffolds for wound healing, a comprehensive review. *Journal of Materials Chemistry B*, 2024. 12: p. 6033–6062.
118. Branski, L., C. Pereira, D. Herndon, and M. Jeschke, Gene therapy in wound healing: present status and future directions. *Gene Therapy*, 2007. **14**(1): p. 1–10.

119. Wang, M., X. Xu, X. Lei, J. Tan, and H. Xie, Mesenchymal stem cell-based therapy for burn wound healing. *Burns & Trauma*, 2021. **9**: p. tkab002.
120. Kureel, S.K., R. Maroto, K. Davis, and M. Sheetz, Cellular mechanical memory: a potential tool for mesenchymal stem cell-based therapy. *Stem Cell Research & Therapy*, 2025. **16**(1): p. 159.
121. Nourian Dehkordi, A., F. Mirahmadi Babaheydari, M. Chehelgerdi, and S. Raeisi Dehkordi, Skin tissue engineering: wound healing based on stem-cell-based therapeutic strategies. *Stem Cell Research & Therapy*, 2019. **10**: p. 1–20.

7 Application of Nanomaterials in Wound Dressings

Ling Wang, Simeng Liu, Muhammad Nauman Sarwar, Gopiraman Mayakrishnan, Ji Ha Lee, and Azeem Ullah

INTRODUCTION

Wound healing remains a complex and multifaceted biological process involving sequential and overlapping phases of hemostasis, inflammation, proliferation, and remodeling [1–3]. Despite advances in conventional wound care, the management of acute and chronic wounds continues to pose significant clinical challenges, particularly due to complications such as microbial infections, biofilm formation, and impaired tissue regeneration [3,4]. Chronic wounds, prevalent especially among diabetic and immunocompromised patients, not only increase morbidity and healthcare costs but also impose a considerable burden on patients' quality of life [4,5].

Nanotechnology offers promising solutions to these challenges by enabling the design of wound dressings with enhanced functionalities that can actively participate in the healing process [1,2,4]. Nanomaterials, due to their unique physicochemical properties including high surface-area-to-volume ratios, tunable surface chemistry, and intrinsic bioactivity, have demonstrated multifaceted roles in promoting wound repair. These include antimicrobial effects, modulation of inflammation, stimulation of cell proliferation and angiogenesis, and targeted delivery of therapeutic agents [1,2,4,5].

Various classes of nanomaterials such as metal and metal oxide nanoparticles (e.g., silver, gold, and zinc oxide), polymeric nanocarriers, nanofibrous scaffolds, and composite nanomaterials have been extensively explored for incorporation into advanced wound dressings [1,2,4,5]. These nanostructured dressings are engineered to maintain a moist wound environment, facilitate gas exchange, and provide controlled release of bioactive compounds, thereby overcoming the limitations of traditional passive dressings [1,3]. Furthermore, nanoscale architecture can mimic the extracellular matrix (ECM), supporting cellular activities crucial for tissue regeneration [1,4].

Although the clinical translation of nanomaterial-based wound dressings is advancing, challenges related to biocompatibility, toxicity, and standardization remain [1,4,5]. Continued interdisciplinary research is essential to optimize nanomaterial formulations for safe, cost-effective, and efficacious wound care solutions.

DOI: 10.1201/9781003616726-9

This chapter provides a comprehensive overview of the current landscape and emerging trends in the application of nanomaterials for wound dressings, highlighting their mechanisms of action, material design strategies, and therapeutic potential in improving wound healing outcomes.

OVERVIEW OF NANOMATERIALS FOR WOUND HEALING

Wound healing is a highly complex, dynamic, and well-orchestrated biological process involving a series of overlapping phases: hemostasis, inflammation, proliferation, and remodeling. Each phase is critical for restoring the integrity and functionality of the damaged tissue and can last from days to months depending on the type of wound and patient conditions.

Hemostasis is the immediate response to injury, where vascular constriction and platelet aggregation occur to prevent excessive blood loss. The formation of a fibrin clot not only seals the wound but also provides a temporary matrix that facilitates the migration of immune cells and fibroblasts essential for the subsequent healing stages [1,6].

Inflammation follows hemostasis and is characterized by the recruitment of immune cells such as neutrophils and macrophages to the wound site. These cells work to clear pathogens, remove cellular debris, and release signaling molecules such as cytokines and growth factors, which orchestrate the healing cascade. The inflammatory phase typically manifests clinically as redness, swelling, and pain around the wound area [1,6].

During the *proliferation* phase, fibroblasts become activated and begin synthesizing ECM components, primarily collagen, which is vital for tissue strength and integrity. Concurrently, angiogenesis is the formation of new blood vessels that supply oxygen and nutrients essential for tissue regeneration. Re-epithelialization also occurs in this phase as keratinocytes migrate to cover the wound surface, restoring the skin barrier [1,6].

The final *remodeling* phase can last from several weeks up to a year, wherein the newly formed tissue is reorganized and strengthened. Collagen fibers are realigned, and excess cells undergo apoptosis, resulting in scar formation and functional recovery of the skin tissue [1,6].

The wound microenvironment, including oxygen levels, moisture, and microbial presence, significantly influences the healing trajectory. Chronic wounds, often associated with infections and biofilm formation, result from disruptions in one or more of these phases, leading to prolonged inflammation, impaired angiogenesis, and defective matrix deposition. Advances in biomaterials and nanotechnology aim to support each phase by providing dressings that maintain optimal moisture, prevent infection, and deliver bioactive agents to stimulate cell proliferation and tissue remodeling, ultimately improving healing outcomes [1].

Understanding the fundamental differences between chronic and acute wounds is crucial for appreciating the complexities of the wound healing process. While acute wounds typically follow a well-regulated and timely sequence of healing phases such as hemostasis, inflammation, proliferation, and remodeling, chronic wounds exhibit disrupted or stalled progression through these stages. The impaired healing in chronic wounds often results from persistent inflammation, poor vascularization, and cellular dysfunction, which contrast with the balanced and coordinated cellular activities seen in acute wounds. This distinction underscores the importance of tailoring therapeutic strategies according to wound type, as interventions must address the unique biological challenges present in each category to effectively restore tissue integrity.

Chronic wounds are those that fail to proceed through the normal stages of healing in a timely manner, often due to underlying metabolic or vascular disorders. These wounds are characterized by a prolonged inflammatory phase, impaired cell proliferation, and disrupted ECM remodeling, which collectively delay tissue repair. Common types of chronic wounds include venous or vascular ulcers, diabetic ulcers, pressure ulcers, and ischemic wounds. Venous ulcers usually affect the lower legs due to poor venous circulation, while diabetic ulcers arise from neuropathy and compromised immunity, making even minor injuries difficult to heal. Pressure ulcers result from sustained pressure that impairs blood flow, often seen in immobilized patients. Ischemic wounds occur due to restricted blood supply, causing oxygen and nutrient deprivation, which further complicates healing [7].

Acute wounds, in contrast, typically result from sudden external trauma such as cuts, abrasions, burns, or surgical incisions. These wounds usually follow an orderly healing process, progressing through hemostasis, inflammation, proliferation, and remodeling phases within a predictable timeframe. Acute wounds can be classified as traumatic wounds, including abrasions, lacerations, avulsions, crush injuries, and missile wounds—or surgical wounds created intentionally during medical procedures. Because acute wounds generally have balanced cellular activity and intact physiological responses, they tend to heal faster and with fewer complications than chronic wounds provided appropriate care is given. Understanding whether a wound is acute or chronic is essential for determining the most effective treatment approach [7].

Nanomaterials employed in wound dressings encompass a diverse array of substances engineered at the nanoscale to exploit their unique physicochemical and biological properties for enhanced healing. Commonly utilized nanomaterials include inorganic nanoparticles such as silver (AgNPs), zinc oxide (ZnO NPs), titanium dioxide (TiO_2 NPs), and gold nanoparticles (AuNPs), which are prized for their potent antimicrobial effects and ability to modulate inflammation. Polymeric nanomaterials, including nanofibers fabricated by electrospinning techniques from biocompatible polymers like polycaprolactone (PCL) and chitosan, are designed to mimic the ECM, providing structural support that promotes cell adhesion, proliferation, and angiogenesis. Composite nanomaterials, such as nanobioglass-incorporated hydrogels, offer multifunctional platforms combining hemostatic, antimicrobial, and regenerative capabilities. Additionally, nanomaterials can serve as carriers for controlled release of bioactive agents including antibiotics, growth factors, and anti-inflammatory drugs, thereby enhancing the therapeutic efficacy of wound dressings. Emerging innovations also focus on "smart" nanomaterials capable of real-time wound monitoring and precision drug delivery, reflecting the growing intersection of nanotechnology and bioelectronics in advanced wound care. Overall, the tailored application of these nanomaterials aims to overcome limitations of traditional dressings by accelerating wound closure, preventing infection, and supporting tissue regeneration through multiple synergistic mechanisms [8].

Polymeric nanofibers have gained significant attention in wound dressing applications due to their structural similarity to the native ECM, high surface-area-to-volume ratio, and tunable physical and chemical properties. Electrospinning is the most widely used technique for producing polymeric nanofibers, allowing the incorporation of various bioactive agents such as antimicrobial nanoparticles, antibiotics, and growth factors directly into the fibrous matrix to enhance wound healing efficacy. Both synthetic polymers like PCL, poly(lactic acid) (PLA), and polyvinyl alcohol (PVA), as well as natural biopolymers such as chitosan, collagen, and hyaluronic acid, are utilized either individually or in blends to optimize biocompatibility, mechanical strength, and biodegradability for wound care. These nanofibrous dressings maintain a moist wound environment, protect against microbial invasion, and support cellular adhesion, proliferation, and migration essential for tissue regeneration. Furthermore, the porous structure of electrospun nanofibers facilitates gas exchange and exudate absorption, which are crucial for effective wound management. Recent advancements include multifunctional nanofibers with controlled drug release profiles achieved via blend, coaxial, or emulsion electrospinning, enabling sustained delivery of therapeutics at the wound site to reduce infection and accelerate healing. Such developments underscore the potential of polymeric nanofibers as versatile platforms in advanced wound dressings, offering enhanced antimicrobial activity, biocompatibility, and tailored mechanical properties for diverse wound types [9–12].

Metallic nanoparticles (MNPs), MXene nanosheets, and metal-organic frameworks (MOFs) represent emerging classes of nanomaterials with significant potential in advanced wound dressing applications due to their unique physicochemical and biological properties. MNPs, including silver, gold, copper, and zinc oxide nanoparticles, exhibit potent antimicrobial activity against a broad spectrum of pathogens, which is critical for preventing infection and biofilm formation in wounds. Beyond their antimicrobial effects, MNPs also promote wound healing by modulating inflammation, stimulating angiogenesis, and enhancing collagen deposition. However, challenges such as potential cytotoxicity and instability require the integration of MNPs into biocompatible matrices like hydrogels to improve their safety and efficacy. MXenes, a family of two-dimensional transition metal carbides and nitrides, offer excellent electrical conductivity, mechanical strength, and biocompatibility, which make them suitable scaffolds that support cell adhesion, proliferation, and tissue regeneration. Their large surface area and hydrophilic nature facilitate interactions with biological tissues, further enhancing wound repair. MOFs, composed of metal ions coordinated to organic ligands, provide highly porous structures with tunable chemical functionality, enabling controlled and sustained delivery of therapeutic agents such as antibiotics, growth factors, and anti-inflammatory drugs directly at the wound site. This controlled-release capability addresses issues of drug stability and bioavailability, contributing to improved healing outcomes. Collectively, the incorporation of MNPs, MXenes, and MOFs into wound dressings creates multifunctional platforms that combine antimicrobial protection, enhanced healing kinetics, and smart delivery systems, thus offering promising solutions for both acute and chronic wound management [13–16].

Carbon-based nanomaterials (CBNs), including graphene and its derivatives, carbon nanotubes (CNTs), fullerenes, carbon quantum dots, and activated carbon, have emerged as highly promising materials for wound healing applications due to their unique physicochemical and biological properties. Their high surface-area-to-volume ratios, excellent mechanical strength, electrical conductivity, and inherent antibacterial, antioxidant, and anti-inflammatory activities enable them to actively promote multiple stages of the wound healing process. For instance, graphene-based materials (GBMs) enhance cell adhesion, proliferation, and migration, while also stimulating angiogenesis and modulating inflammatory responses, which are crucial for tissue regeneration. CNTs provide structural support resembling the ECM and facilitate fibroblast growth and collagen synthesis, thus accelerating wound closure. Fullerenes, known for their strong antioxidant capacity, reduce oxidative stress at the wound site, mitigating chronic inflammation. Activated carbon dressings, derived from biomass, offer high adsorption capacity for wound exudates and bacterial toxins, thereby creating a favorable healing environment. Moreover, CBNs can serve as effective carriers for targeted drug delivery, enabling controlled release of antibiotics and growth factors to infected or chronic wounds. Despite their promising potential, biocompatibility and toxicity concerns require thorough investigation to ensure safe clinical translation. Collectively, the multifunctional properties of CBNs hold great promise for developing advanced wound dressings that combine antimicrobial defense, tissue regeneration, and efficient wound management [17–20].

The nanomaterials presented in this overview including polymeric nanofibers, metallic nanoparticles, MXenes, MOFs, and CBNs constitute a diverse and rapidly evolving toolkit for enhancing wound healing outcomes. Their distinct physicochemical properties and biological functionalities enable targeted interventions across various stages of the wound repair process, addressing key challenges such as infection control, inflammation modulation, and tissue regeneration. In the following sections, these materials will be examined in greater depth, with detailed analyses of their fabrication methods, biological interactions, and integration into wound dressing platforms. Such comprehensive evaluation aims to elucidate the current state of the art and future directions in the application of nanomaterials for advanced wound care.

POLYMERIC NANOFIBERS IN WOUND DRESSING

Polymeric nanofibers, particularly those fabricated via electrospinning, have emerged as a transformative material platform for advanced wound dressings due to their exceptional structural and functional properties. These nanofibers closely mimic the architecture of the natural ECM, providing an ideal microenvironment that supports cellular adhesion, proliferation, and migration, which are essential for effective tissue regeneration [21–23]. The high porosity and large surface area of electrospun nanofibers facilitate efficient oxygen and nutrient exchange while maintaining optimal moisture balance, which is critical parameters for accelerated wound healing [21,23]. Moreover, polymeric nanofibers can be engineered from a variety of synthetic and natural polymers such as PCL, PVA, chitosan, collagen, and alginate offering tunable mechanical strength, biodegradability, and biocompatibility to meet the diverse requirements of different wound types [23–25].

Beyond structural support, polymeric nanofibers serve as versatile carriers for therapeutic agents including antimicrobial nanoparticles, growth factors, and anti-inflammatory drugs, enabling localized and sustained delivery to the wound site [21,23,26]. Recent advances in electrospinning techniques—such as coaxial, emulsion, and multi-fluid electrospinning—allow the fabrication of complex nanofiber architectures capable of multifunctional performance, including infection control and enhanced tissue regeneration [21,22,26]. These attributes position electrospun polymeric nanofibers as a highly promising class of biomaterials in wound management, especially for chronic wounds that demand tailored healing strategies. This section explores the synthesis, properties, and biomedical applications of polymeric nanofibers in wound dressings, emphasizing recent developments and prospects for improving wound healing outcomes.

Nanofibers are fabricated through various advanced techniques, with electrospinning, centrifugal spinning, and melt spinning being the most prominent methods owing to their ability to produce fibers with nanoscale diameters and tunable morphology. Among these, electrospinning remains the most extensively studied and utilized due to its versatility, control over fiber properties, and suitability for incorporating diverse polymers and bioactive agents.

The conventional electrospinning setup consists of four primary components: a high-voltage power supply, a syringe pump, a spinneret (needle), and a grounded collector. The polymer solution is pumped through the spinneret, and a high voltage applied between the spinneret and collector induces the formation of a charged polymer jet. This jet undergoes stretching and solvent evaporation before depositing as continuous nanofibers on the collector. Fiber diameters typically range from 100 to 500 nm, with the process parameters such as voltage, solution viscosity, flow rate, and distance between the needle and collector directly influencing fiber morphology and diameter [27–29].

To address limitations like low production rate, needle clogging, and fiber alignment control, several variations of electrospinning have been developed:

- **Coaxial electrospinning**: This utilizes a concentric spinneret to simultaneously electrospin two different polymer solutions, producing core–shell nanofibers. This enables encapsulation and controlled release of bioactive molecules within the core while maintaining structural integrity with the shell [27–29].
- **Needleless electrospinning**: This replaces a single needle with a free liquid surface or rotating drum as the spinneret, enabling higher throughput by producing multiple jets simultaneously, which is advantageous for scaling up production [29].
- **Near-field electrospinning (NFES)**: This reduces the spinneret-to-collector distance to a few millimeters, suppressing the jet's whipping instability and enabling direct writing of precise, patterned nanofibers suitable for tissue engineering scaffolds [27,28].
- **Melt electrospinning**: Instead of polymer solutions, melts are electrospun, eliminating the use of solvents. Melt electrospinning produces thicker fibers due to higher viscosity but offers better environmental compatibility.

The process requires precise temperature control to maintain polymer fluidity without degradation [27,28].

- **Magnetic field-assisted and airflow-assisted electrospinning**: These incorporate external fields to manipulate jet behavior for aligned fiber production and improved fiber uniformity [28].

These modifications expand electrospinning's capabilities, enabling fabrication of nanofibers with tailored architecture, composition, and functionality for specific biomedical applications such as wound dressings.

Centrifugal spinning (also called rotary jet spinning or Forcespinning™) uses high-speed rotation of a spinneret containing polymer solution or melt. The centrifugal force overcomes surface tension, ejecting polymer jets that solidify into fibers upon solvent evaporation or cooling. This method achieves production rates hundreds of times higher than traditional electrospinning and does not require high voltage, offering enhanced safety and scalability. Centrifugal spinning can process a broad range of polymers, though controlling fiber uniformity and avoiding bead formation can be challenging. The technique is increasingly explored for mass production of nanofibers in wound dressing and drug delivery systems [28,30].

Melt spinning involves melting thermoplastic polymers and extruding them through spinnerets to form fibers. Melt electrospinning applies an electric field to the polymer melt, combining benefits of solvent-free processing with fiber diameter control, though the resulting fibers are generally larger than solution electrospun fibers. Melt electro-writing, a derivative technique, allows precise fiber depositions enabling 3D scaffold fabrication important for tissue engineering applications. Melt spinning offers an environmentally friendly alternative with good scalability but is limited by polymer thermal stability and relatively coarse fiber diameters [28,30].

The diverse fabrication techniques for nanofibers including electrospinning, centrifugal spinning, and melt spinning provide versatile platforms to tailor fiber morphology, composition, and functionality to meet specific biomedical needs. The ability to control fiber diameter, porosity, and surface chemistry during manufacturing directly influences the biological performance of nanofibers when applied as wound dressings. For instance, electrospinning's fine control over fiber architecture enables the creation of scaffolds that closely mimic the ECM, promoting cell adhesion and tissue regeneration. Meanwhile, centrifugal spinning offers scalable production of nanofibers suitable for antimicrobial-loaded dressings with enhanced mechanical stability. Melt spinning allows solvent-free fabrication of biocompatible fibers ideal for sustained drug delivery. By harnessing these advanced production methods, researchers can design nanofibrous wound dressings with optimized properties such as moisture retention, gas permeability, antimicrobial activity, and controlled therapeutic release, addressing critical challenges in both acute and chronic wound management.

Electrospun nanofibers have been extensively investigated as advanced wound dressings due to their ECM-mimicking structure, high porosity, and excellent drug-loading capability. Kazeminava et al. [31] fabricated electrospun nanofibers composed of carboxymethyl cellulose (CMC) and PVA, crosslinked with citric acid-based quantum dots (CA-QDs) and loaded with the antibiotic colistin to impart antimicrobial properties. The nanofibers exhibited appropriate mechanical strength and hydrophilicity, and in vitro cytocompatibility tests showed over 80% cell viability against human foreskin fibroblasts. Antibacterial testing demonstrated significant zones of inhibition against pathogens including *Staphylococcus aureus*, *Escherichia coli*, *Klebsiella pneumoniae*, and *Pseudomonas aeruginosa*, suggesting the potential utility of these nanofibers as effective antimicrobial wound dressings.

In another study, Nezhad-Mokhtari et al. [32] developed hybrid electrospun nanofibers composed of PCL, sulfonated chitosan (SPCS), zeolite imidazolate framework-8 nanoparticles (ZIF-8 NPs), and *Matricaria chamomilla* essential oil (MCEO). The addition of ZIF-8 NPs and MCEO provided enhanced antibacterial activity against *S. aureus* and *E. coli*, with inhibition zones exceeding 30 mm. The nanofiber mats also showed improved cytocompatibility and mechanical properties. In vitro cell studies revealed enhanced adhesion and proliferation of normal human foreskin fibroblasts (HFF-2), highlighting the multifunctional potential of these composite nanofibers in accelerating wound healing.

Wang et al. [33] reported a core–shell electrospun membrane composed of poly(lactic-co-glycolic acid) (PLGA) loaded with dual bioactive agents: zinc oxide nanoparticles (ZnO NPs) for antimicrobial action and vascular endothelial growth factor (VEGF) to promote angiogenesis. The scaffold exhibited smooth nanofiber morphology, effective antibacterial properties, and biocompatibility with in vitro cell viability maintained at high levels. In vivo animal experiments demonstrated enhanced wound contraction and improved tissue organization, confirming the synergistic effects of ZnO NPs and VEGF in promoting vascularization and wound repair.

Furthermore, Zhang et al. [34] designed a multifunctional Janus electrospun nanofiber dressing with one hydrophobic layer encapsulating polyoxometalates (POMs) and oxacillin to inhibit methicillin-resistant *Staphylococcus aureus* (MRSA), and a hydrophilic layer containing a pH-sensitive dye for real-time wound monitoring. This dressing effectively drained excess biofluid while providing antibacterial action and promoting skin repair. In vivo studies showed accelerated wound healing and good biocompatibility, demonstrating a promising integrated approach to wound management combining antimicrobial activity, fluid control, and wound status monitoring.

Beyond this, Ren et al. [35] reported stereocomplexed electrospun nanofibers integrating PLA with quaternized chitosan, which showed enhanced thermal and mechanical properties and antibacterial activity. In vivo wound healing tests demonstrated full wound closure within 15 days, outperforming controls and illustrating the promise of biomass-derived multifunctional nanofibers for disinfectant wound dressings (Figure 7.1). Hwang et al. [36] fabricated polycaprolactone-ulvan (PCL-ULV) electrospun composite mats, where ulvan, a sulfated polysaccharide, improved hydrophilicity and promoted fibroblast proliferation and gene expression linked to scarless wound healing. These mats mimicked ECM microstructure and enhanced dermal regeneration in vitro, highlighting the potential of marine polysaccharides in nanofiber wound dressings.

In another example, Amani et al. [37] developed pH-sensitive bilayer electrospun nanofibrous mats combining ethyl cellulose and Eudragit S-100 loaded with gentamicin sulfate and diclofenac sodium (DS) for burn wound treatment. The mats

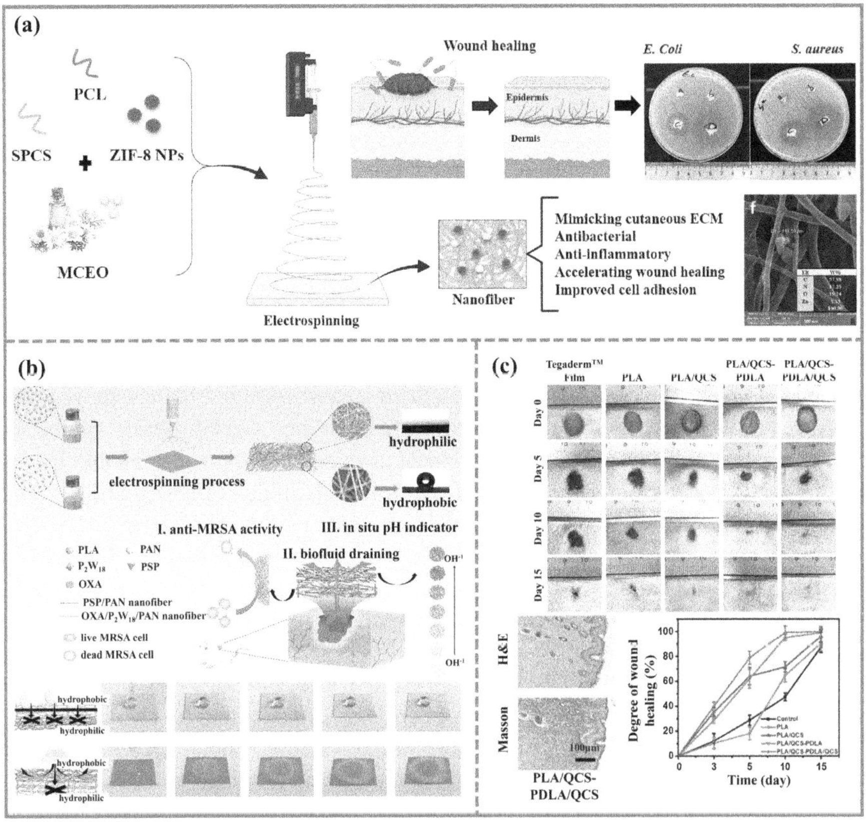

FIGURE 7.1 Schematic diagram of the fabrication and application of (a) MCEO-loaded ZIF-8/PCL/SPCS NFs [32]. (b) Multifunctional Janus electrospun nanofiber dressing and the droplet interacting with the Janus electrospun nanofiber dressing [34]. (c) The differential therapeutic efficacy of various membrane treatments in promoting the healing of *S. aureus*-infected full-thickness dermal wounds, with progressive tissue regeneration observed over time [35].

exhibited controlled dual-drug release responsive to wound pH, showed excellent cytocompatibility, and accelerated burn wound healing in vivo by reducing inflammation and infection risk.

Gelatin is a widely studied natural biopolymer for the fabrication of electrospun nanofiber wound dressings due to its excellent biocompatibility, biodegradability, and intrinsic similarity to collagen, a major component of the ECM in skin tissue. Electrospinning gelatin produces nanofibrous mats with high porosity and interconnected pore structures, closely mimicking the native ECM to support cell adhesion, proliferation, and migration, which are essential for efficient wound healing. However, pure gelatin exhibits poor mechanical strength, rapid solubility in aqueous environments, and challenges in electrospinning due to strong hydrogen bonding and gelation at room temperature. To overcome these limitations, various approaches such as blending with synthetic or natural polymers (e.g., PCL, chitosan, hyaluronic acid) and chemical or physical crosslinking techniques have been developed to enhance the mechanical stability, water resistance, and biological performance of gelatin-based nanofiber mats.

Innovative electrospinning strategies including blend electrospinning, emulsion electrospinning, and coaxial electrospinning have enabled the incorporation of bioactive agents such as antimicrobial compounds, growth factors, and anti-inflammatory drugs into gelatin nanofibers, imparting multifunctional properties to the dressings. For example, bi-layered gelatin-based nanofiber dressings combining gelatin with keratin or PCL have demonstrated accelerated wound closure, enhanced angiogenesis, and reduced inflammation in vivo. Moreover, 3D gelatin nanofiber sponges fabricated via modified electrospinning and crosslinking exhibit superior hemostatic properties and high blood absorption capacity, facilitating rapid hemorrhage control in acute wounds.

Recent advancements include in situ electrospinning of gelatin-based nanofiber mats directly onto wound sites using handheld electrospinning devices, enabling conformal dressings that improve patient comfort and treatment efficacy. Collectively, gelatin-based electrospun nanofibers, especially when modified or loaded with therapeutic agents, offer a highly promising platform for wound dressing applications, addressing critical challenges in both acute and chronic wound management due to their biomimetic structure, biological compatibility, and multifunctional therapeutic capabilities [38].

Polyacrylonitrile (PAN) is a synthetic polymer widely investigated for electrospun nanofiber wound dressings due to its excellent mechanical strength, chemical resistance, and ease of fabrication via electrospinning. PAN nanofibers typically exhibit uniform morphology with fiber diameters in the nanometer range, offering high surface area and porosity beneficial for gas exchange and exudate absorption in wound care. Despite their promising properties, pure PAN nanofibers are hydrophobic and have limited biocompatibility, which may hinder cell adhesion and proliferation. To address this, surface modifications such as chemical treatments introducing hydrophilic functional groups (e.g., amine, hydroxyl) and biomineralization with proteins like bovine serum albumin have been employed to improve wettability and cellular response. Additionally, blending PAN with natural polymers such as gelatin, chitosan, or synthetic polymers like PVA enhances hydrophilicity and bioactivity of the resulting nanofibers.

Drug loading is a significant advantage of PAN nanofibers in wound dressings. Various therapeutic agents including anti-inflammatory drugs (e.g., DS), antibiotics (e.g., gentamicin sulfate), plant extracts (e.g., *Moringa oleifera*), and nitric oxide donors have been successfully incorporated into PAN fibers via blend or coaxial electrospinning to achieve controlled and sustained release profiles. For instance, dual-drug core–shell nanofibers with diclofenac and gentamicin exhibit biphasic release, providing initial antimicrobial protection followed by prolonged anti-inflammatory effects. Furthermore, PAN nanofibers functionalized with antimicrobial agents like silver sulfadiazine or quaternary ammonium salts display enhanced antibacterial activity against common pathogens including MRSA. Advanced composite structures such as Janus and multilayer nanofibers enable multifunctional wound dressings with properties including unidirectional exudate drainage, real-time monitoring, and multidrug delivery. Collectively, these developments highlight PAN electrospun nanofibers as a versatile and promising material platform for next-generation wound dressings, capable of addressing complex wound healing challenges through tailored physical, chemical, and biological functionalities [39].

Cellulose-based nanofibers have garnered significant interest as wound dressing materials owing to their excellent biocompatibility, biodegradability, and structural similarity to the natural ECM of skin tissue. These nanofibers can be fabricated primarily through electrospinning, which enables the production of highly porous, interconnected fibrous mats with large surface areas conducive to cell adhesion, proliferation, and tissue regeneration. Cellulose itself, a linear polymer composed of β-1,4-linked D-glucopyranose units, forms nanofibers that offer substantial water retention capacity, low immunogenicity, and mechanical strength, making them ideal for maintaining a moist wound environment and protecting against microbial invasion. To enhance functional performance, cellulose nanofibers are often combined with bioactive agents such as antibiotics, growth factors, silver nanoparticles (AgNPs), or plant-derived extracts, facilitating antimicrobial action and accelerated healing.

Several studies have demonstrated the efficacy of cellulose-based electrospun nanofibers in wound management. For instance, carboxylated cellulose nanofibers incorporated with aminated AgNPs and gelatin formed hydrogel dressings that showed potent antibacterial activity against *S. aureus* and *Pseudomonas aeruginosa*, coupled with excellent in vivo wound closure rates and biocompatibility. Similarly, oxidized cellulose nanofiber-PVA hydrogels loaded with curcumin promoted granulation tissue formation and enhanced re-epithelialization in rat wound models. These materials provide controlled drug release and effective infection control, which are critical in managing both acute and chronic wounds. Additionally, cellulose nanofibers' inherent transparency allows for real-time wound monitoring without frequent dressing changes, improving patient comfort. Varied cellulose derivatives such as cellulose acetate (CA), CMC, and hydroxypropyl methylcellulose have also been electrospun into nanofibers with tailored properties suitable for different wound types, including diabetic ulcers and infected wounds. Overall, cellulose-based nanofibrous dressings represent a promising and versatile platform for next-generation wound care due to their biocompatibility, functionalization potential, and ability to closely mimic native tissue architecture [40].

Electrospun nanofibers continue to be at the forefront of advanced wound dressing development due to their biomimetic architecture, high porosity, and capability for controlled drug delivery. Ullah et al. [41] demonstrated the fabrication of CA nanofibrous mats incorporating Manuka honey (MH) via electrospinning. The addition of MH enhanced the antibacterial efficacy against common pathogens and improved antioxidant properties, while maintaining suitable mechanical strength and high porosity (85%–90%) for effective wound breathability. In vitro tests confirmed excellent cytocompatibility with NIH 3T3 fibroblast cells, supporting the use of CA-MH nanofibers as a promising antimicrobial wound dressing.

The incorporation of therapeutic agents into composite nanofibers has been further explored by Ullah et al. [42], who fabricated soy protein isolate (SPI) and hydroxyethyl cellulose (HEC) nanofibers loaded with DS and halloysite nanotubes

(HNTs) for sustained drug release and antibacterial activity. The electrospun mats displayed uniform morphology with an average diameter around 450 nm, and cross-linking enhanced their stability. Drug release studies revealed sustained delivery of DS over 14 days, while in vitro biocompatibility assays confirmed the non-cytotoxic nature of the mats. Antibacterial tests demonstrated effectiveness against *E. coli* and *Bacillus subtilis*, highlighting their applicability for infection control in wound care (Figure 7.2).

Similarly, Ullah et al. [43] incorporated *Blumea balsamifera* (Sambong) essential oil into CA nanofibers, showing enhanced antibacterial activity against *E. coli* and *S. aureus*. The electrospun mats exhibited adequate moisture vapor transmission rates (MVTR) and good cell viability (~92%), indicating their suitability as bioactive wound dressings. The study detailed the electrospinning parameters, polymer solution preparation, and characterization techniques, providing a comprehensive understanding of the formulation's properties and potential clinical applications.

Further advancing the functionalization of nanofibers, Haider et al. [44] synthesized AgNPs on PAN nanofibers using a green lignin-induced in situ reduction method. The resulting PAN/AgNP membranes showed enhanced antibacterial activity against both Gram-positive *S. aureus* and Gram-negative *E. coli*, with inhibition zones exceeding 18 mm. Characterization confirmed uniform AgNP distribution and significant improvement in hydrophilicity. The approach provided an environmentally friendly and cost-effective route for producing multifunctional antimicrobial wound dressings with potential for clinical translation.

Self-responsive electrospun nanofiber wound dressings represent a cutting-edge approach in wound care, designed to dynamically respond to the wound environment for optimized healing. These smart dressings are fabricated primarily through electrospinning techniques that incorporate stimuli-responsive polymers and bioactive agents capable of sensing and reacting to changes such as pH, temperature, bacterial presence, oxygen levels, or light exposure. Typically, the electrospinning setup produces nanofibrous mats that mimic the ECM structure, ensuring high porosity, breathability, and effective drug loading and release.

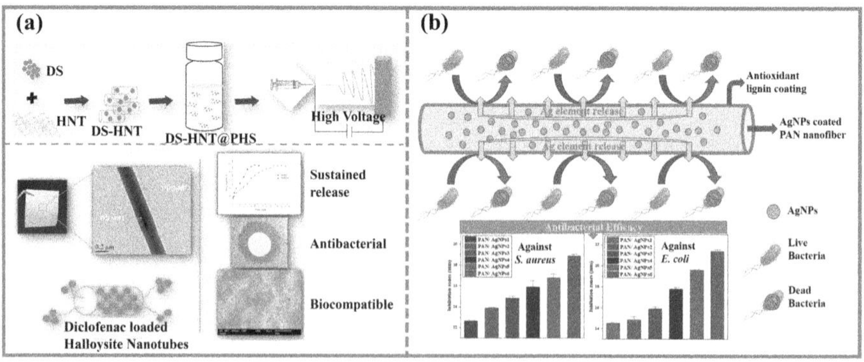

FIGURE 7.2 Schematic diagram of the fabrication and application of (a) PHSDH nanofibers [42] and (b) PAN/AgNPs [44].

A key advantage of self-responsive dressings is their ability to modulate therapeutic release in response to specific wound cues, such as elevated pH levels during infection or the presence of bacterial enzymes, thereby preventing unnecessary and constant drug elution that can lead to antimicrobial resistance or cytotoxicity. For instance, pH-responsive nanofibers incorporate halochromic dyes (e.g., bromothymol blue, bromocresol green, or natural anthocyanins) that change color as the wound pH shifts, enabling real-time visual monitoring of wound status without removing the dressing. Simultaneously, pH-sensitive polymers such as Eudragit L100-55 are used to control drug release, allowing antibiotics or anti-inflammatory agents to be released only at alkaline pH typical of infected wounds. This smart release mechanism enhances efficacy while minimizing side effects.

Temperature-responsive nanofibers leverage polymers like poly(N-isopropylacrylamide), which undergo phase transitions near physiological temperatures, enabling controlled drug delivery triggered by local temperature changes associated with inflammation. Bacteria-responsive nanofibers are designed with bacterial enzyme-sensitive polymers that degrade and release encapsulated antimicrobials in the presence of pathogenic bacteria. Additionally, oxygen-responsive nanofibers incorporating coordination polymers can detect reactive oxygen species (ROS) such as hydrogen peroxide, providing insights into wound oxidative stress and healing progression.

Light-responsive nanofibers utilize embedded photo-cleavable linkers or upconverting nanoparticles to achieve spatiotemporal control over drug release via external light stimuli, offering precise therapeutic dosing. Combining multiple responsive elements into dual or multi-stimuli systems further enhances functionality, enabling dressings to simultaneously monitor wound parameters and deliver drugs on demand.

Overall, self-responsive electrospun nanofibrous wound dressings offer an intelligent platform that integrates wound monitoring, infection detection, and controlled therapeutic delivery. These attributes reduce dressing change frequency, lower healthcare costs, and improve patient comfort and outcomes. Despite promising in vitro and some in vivo results, challenges remain in optimizing mechanical properties, biocompatibility, and scalability before widespread clinical adoption [45].

Collectively, these studies underscore the versatility of electrospun nanofibers as platforms for wound management. By optimizing polymer selection, electrospinning parameters, and functional agent incorporation, researchers have engineered wound dressings with tailored mechanical properties, controlled drug release, antimicrobial efficacy, and regenerative potential. The evidence supports their promising role in addressing challenges in both acute and chronic wound care, paving the way for multifunctional and smart wound dressings that improve healing outcomes and patient quality of life.

METAL-BASED NANOMATERIALS FOR WOUND DRESSING

Metal-based nanomaterials, including metallic nanoparticles and metal oxide nanoparticles, have gained significant attention in wound care due to their unique physicochemical properties, broad-spectrum antimicrobial activity, and ability to enhance the wound healing process. The nanoscale size and large surface area of these particles allow them to interact effectively with microbial cells, disrupting bacterial membranes and generating ROS that inhibit the growth of pathogenic organisms, including drug-resistant strains. Importantly, metal nanoparticles such as silver (AgNPs), gold (AuNPs), copper (CuNPs), zinc oxide (ZnO NPs), and titanium dioxide (TiO_2 NPs) have demonstrated potent antibacterial, anti-inflammatory, and pro-angiogenic effects that are critical for accelerating tissue regeneration and reducing infection-related complications [46–48].

These nanoparticles are often incorporated into biocompatible polymer matrices such as hydrogels, electrospun nanofibers, and composite membranes to form multifunctional wound dressings that not only provide physical protection and maintain a moist wound environment but also deliver therapeutic effects at the wound site. The incorporation of metal-based nanoparticles addresses key limitations of traditional dressings by enabling sustained antimicrobial activity, promoting cell proliferation, and modulating inflammatory responses. For instance, AgNPs have been widely used for their broad-spectrum bactericidal properties, while ZnO NPs contribute to angiogenesis and oxidative stress reduction. Advances in green synthesis and stabilization methods using polysaccharides or plant extracts have improved the biocompatibility and stability of metal nanoparticles in wound dressings, reducing cytotoxicity and enhancing therapeutic efficacy [47,48].

Despite promising preclinical and clinical outcomes, challenges remain regarding the optimal dosage, controlled release, and potential cytotoxic effects of metal nanomaterials. Continued research focuses on developing nanocomposites with tailored physicochemical characteristics that maximize healing benefits while minimizing adverse effects. Overall, metal-based nanomaterials represent a rapidly evolving class of wound dressing components with significant potential to transform chronic and acute wound management by combining antimicrobial protection with regenerative support [48].

AgNPs have emerged as a promising antimicrobial agent for wound dressings due to their broad-spectrum activity against bacteria, fungi, and viruses, including antibiotic-resistant strains. Their nanoscale size provides a high surface-area-to-volume ratio, enhancing interaction with microbial membranes and promoting efficient bacterial cell disruption through mechanisms such as ROS generation, membrane damage, and interference with microbial DNA replication. Incorporating AgNPs into wound dressings such as electrospun nanofibers, hydrogels, and composite membranes has been shown to accelerate wound closure by reducing microbial burden and modulating inflammation, thereby promoting tissue regeneration and minimizing infection-related complications. In vivo and in vitro studies have demonstrated that AgNP functionalized dressings inhibit pathogenic strains, including *S. aureus*, *E. coli*, and *P. aeruginosa*, and contribute to enhanced fibroblast proliferation and angiogenesis, which are key processes for effective healing [49].

However, despite these advantages, several downsides limit the clinical translation of AgNP wound dressings. One significant concern is cytotoxicity; high concentrations or uncontrolled release of silver ions can damage host cells, impede tissue repair, and cause delayed healing. Moreover, the potential for silver resistance development in bacteria, although currently less common than antibiotic resistance, raises concerns about long-term efficacy. The physicochemical properties of AgNPs, such as size, shape, surface charge, and coating, critically influence their antimicrobial potency and cytotoxicity, demanding precise synthesis and formulation control. Additionally, interactions with biological fluids and wound exudates can lead to nanoparticle aggregation or inactivation, reducing antimicrobial effectiveness. Challenges also exist in ensuring a sustained, controlled release of silver ions from dressings to maintain antimicrobial activity without adverse effects. Lastly, cost, scalability, and regulatory hurdles remain barriers to widespread adoption. Thus, optimizing AgNP concentration, surface functionalization, and integration into biocompatible matrices is essential to maximize therapeutic benefits while minimizing toxicity and resistance risks [49].

Building upon the established antimicrobial efficacy of AgNPs, other metal-based nanomaterials such as copper (Cu), gold (Au), zinc oxide (ZnO) nanoparticles, and their bimetallic combinations have garnered considerable attention for wound dressing applications due to their complementary and, in some cases, enhanced biological activities. Copper nanoparticles exert potent broad-spectrum antibacterial effects through the release of Cu^{2+} ions, generation of ROS, and disruption of bacterial membranes, while also offering photothermal properties under near-infrared (NIR) irradiation that enable synergistic antimicrobial therapy. Their ability to inhibit biofilm formation makes them especially valuable in treating chronic, infected wounds, sometimes demonstrating superior efficacy to AgNPs against resilient strains like *P. aeruginosa* [50].

AuNPs, renowned for their excellent biocompatibility, exert antibacterial activity by disrupting bacterial membranes and interfering with vital intracellular processes, including ATP synthesis and DNA transcription. The functionalization of AuNPs with bioactive molecules has further enhanced their antimicrobial and tissue regenerative properties, effectively targeting pathogens such as MRSA and promoting accelerated wound healing in vivo [50]. ZnO NPs contribute multifunctional benefits, combining antibacterial, anti-inflammatory, and pro-angiogenic effects essential for wound repair. ZnO NPs inhibit bacterial growth and biofilm formation through ROS generation and membrane disruption, and they have been successfully integrated into various biopolymer-based dressings to synergistically support tissue regeneration [50].

Moreover, bimetallic nanoparticles, such as Au–Ag and Ag–Cu hybrids, harness synergistic mechanisms to overcome bacterial resistance and enhance wound healing outcomes. These nanostructures disrupt multiple bacterial targets, including cell division proteins and membrane integrity, resulting in superior antimicrobial activity compared to monometallic counterparts. Experimental evidence demonstrates that bimetallic nanoparticle-containing dressings promote effective bacterial clearance and scar-free healing, offering promising alternatives or adjuncts to traditional antibiotics in wound management [50].

Collectively, these metal-based nanomaterials expand the armamentarium of antimicrobial agents available for advanced wound dressings, combining potent infection control with biological activities that facilitate tissue repair and regeneration.

Copper nanoparticles (CuNPs) have emerged as a promising nanomaterial in wound care due to their multifaceted role in promoting wound healing, antimicrobial activity, and tissue regeneration. CuNPs enhance wound repair by stimulating angiogenesis through upregulation of VEGF and hypoxia-inducible factor-1 alpha (HIF-1α), promoting ECM remodeling via increased collagen and elastin synthesis, and modulating inflammatory responses by inducing the secretion of anti-inflammatory cytokines such as IL-4 and IL-10. In vitro and in vivo studies demonstrate that CuNPs promote proliferation and migration of fibroblasts, keratinocytes, endothelial cells, and mesenchymal stem cells, which are critical for tissue regeneration. Furthermore, CuNPs exhibit potent broad-spectrum antimicrobial effects by releasing Cu^{2+} ions that disrupt bacterial membranes, generate ROS, and interfere with bacterial DNA and protein synthesis, thereby reducing infection risk in both acute and chronic wounds [51,52].

Despite these therapeutic advantages, CuNPs face several limitations and challenges. High concentrations or uncontrolled release of copper ions can lead to cytotoxicity, oxidative stress, and damage to host cells, as evidenced by reduced cell viability and induction of lipid peroxidation in cultured skin cells. Moreover, copper's propensity for rapid oxidation and nanoparticle aggregation can reduce bioavailability and antimicrobial efficacy. Balancing the beneficial pro-angiogenic and antimicrobial effects of CuNPs while minimizing toxicity requires careful control of nanoparticle size, concentration, surface modification, and incorporation into biocompatible polymeric matrices such as hydrogels and nanofibers. These composite systems can modulate copper ion release rates to achieve sustained therapeutic levels, improve nanoparticle stability, and enhance biocompatibility. Recent advances include copper sulfide nanoparticles combined with NIR photothermal therapy to synergistically eradicate bacteria while accelerating wound closure with minimal invasiveness. Nonetheless, further research is needed to optimize formulation parameters, fully elucidate long-term safety profiles, and translate CuNP-based dressings into clinical practice [51,52].

Following the promising role of copper-based nanomaterials in wound healing, ZnO NPs have also attracted considerable interest as effective antimicrobial and regenerative agents in wound care. Similar to copper, ZnO NPs exhibit broad-spectrum antibacterial activity primarily through the release of Zn^{2+} ions and generation of ROS, which disrupt bacterial membranes and metabolic functions. When incorporated into biopolymeric matrices such as cellulose, chitosan, and alginate, ZnO-based nanobiocomposites demonstrate enhanced antimicrobial efficacy against prevalent wound pathogens including *S. aureus* and *P. aeruginosa*, while also inhibiting biofilm formation, which is a critical factor in chronic wound infections. Additionally, ZnO NPs contribute to accelerated wound healing by promoting cellular proliferation, angiogenesis, and collagen synthesis, which is mediated through modulation of oxidative stress and inflammatory responses in the wound environment. These nanoparticles improve the mechanical properties, moisture retention, and biocompatibility of hydrogels, nanobiofilms, and electrospun dressings, creating conducive scaffolds for tissue regeneration and accelerated closure [53,54].

Despite their therapeutic benefits, the clinical application of ZnO NP-containing dressings faces challenges such as cytotoxicity at high concentrations due to excessive ROS, nanoparticle aggregation reducing bioavailability, and variability arising from diverse synthesis and formulation methods. Achieving controlled, sustained release of Zn^{2+} ions while maintaining biocompatibility remains essential.

Recent advances in green synthesis and surface modification have improved the safety of ZnO nanocomposites; however, comprehensive in vivo studies and long-term evaluations are still required to validate their efficacy and safety for clinical use. Thus, ZnO NPs complement copper-based nanomaterials as integral components of next-generation multifunctional wound dressings aimed at addressing infection control and tissue regeneration [53,54].

Apart from ZnO NPs, AuNPs have also been extensively explored for wound dressing applications due to their unique physicochemical properties and excellent biocompatibility. Several studies have reported the fabrication of AuNP-containing wound dressings using diverse matrices and preparation techniques to achieve effective antimicrobial activity, enhanced healing, and controlled drug release.

For example, Borges et al. [55] developed a novel wound dressing by incorporating metronidazole-loaded AuNPs into natural rubber latex (NRL). AuNPs were synthesized using the Turkevich–Frens method, yielding spherical particles (~35 nm). The NRL-based dressings exhibited appropriate mechanical properties for skin application, sustained drug release over 100 hours with a second-order exponential decay profile, excellent hemocompatibility, and fibroblast cell viability. This combination leveraged the antimicrobial properties of metronidazole and AuNPs to provide a synergistic effect in controlling infections and promoting wound healing, demonstrating promising potential for dermal applications.

In another study, Zepon et al. [56] fabricated polymer-based lyophilized wafers containing in situ–synthesized AuNPs within a matrix of κ-carrageenan, locust bean gum, and PVA. The AuNPs (~10–15 nm) were formed by the reduction of gold ions during gel preparation. These wafers exhibited porous morphology conducive to high exudate absorption and gaseous exchange, mechanical stability, and served effectively as a bacterial barrier against *S. aureus* and *P. aeruginosa*. Cytotoxicity assays confirmed the wafers' biocompatibility with NIH–3T3 fibroblasts, indicating their potential for chronic wound management where moisture balance and infection control are critical.

El-Naggar et al. [57] employed electrospinning to create PCL nanofibers blended with AuNPs and spearmint oil nanoemulsion, producing nanofibrous scaffolds with smooth morphology and improved mechanical properties. The composite nanofibers demonstrated significant antimicrobial activity against multiple pathogens including *E. coli*, *P. aeruginosa*, *S. aureus*, and *Candida albicans*. Additionally, the scaffolds exhibited good cell viability, highlighting their suitability as wound dressings that combine physical protection, antimicrobial function, and support for tissue regeneration.

Furthermore, Zhou et al. [58] developed a novel silk fabric wound dressing with in situ–synthesized AuNPs conjugated to the antibiotic gentamicin sulfate. This SF@Au/GM dressing showed enhanced antibacterial efficacy compared to gentamicin alone, allowing for reduced antibiotic dosages. In vivo animal experiments demonstrated accelerated epidermal growth and wound closure compared to commercial dressings. The facile, scalable method utilized the sericin component of silk as a reducing agent, representing a sustainable approach to manufacturing advanced biomedical textiles with improved therapeutic performance and minimized antibiotic resistance risk (Figure 7.3).

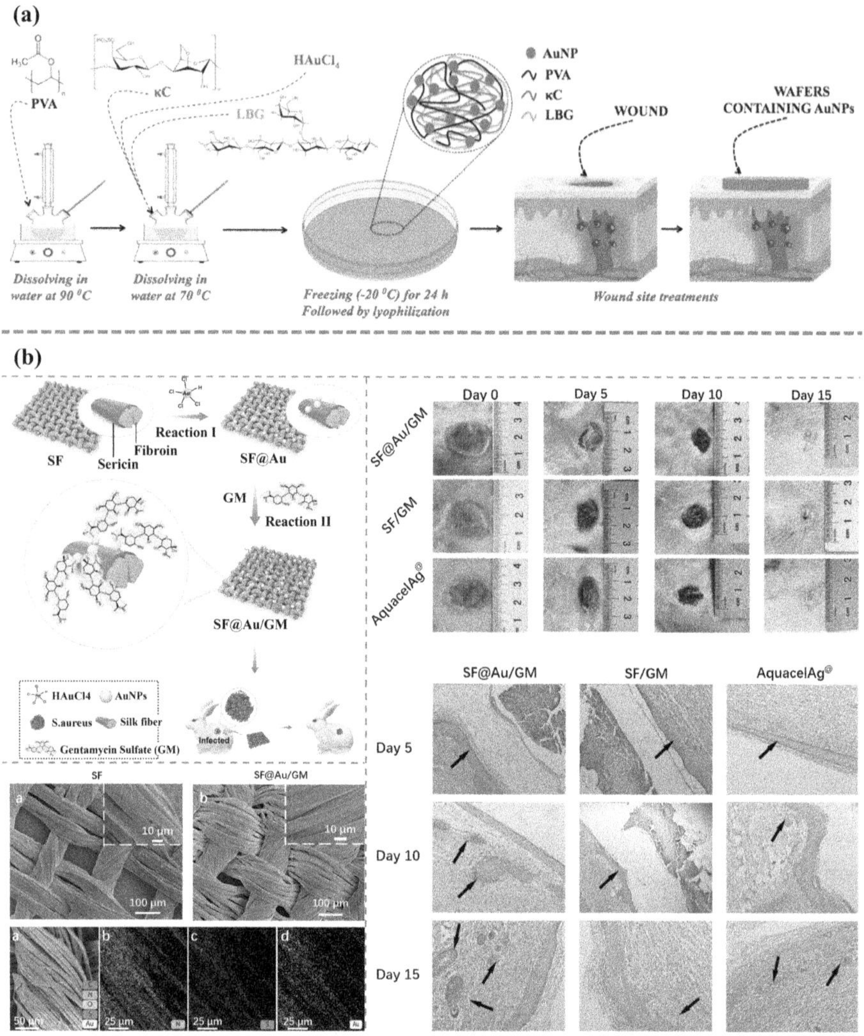

FIGURE 7.3 (a) Nanoparticle-based wound dressing: recent progress in the detection and therapy of bacterial infections [56]. (b) Minimizing antibiotic dosage through in situ formation of gold nanoparticles across antibacterial wound dressings: a facile approach using silk fabric as the base substrate [58].

Another class of metallic nanoparticles gaining attention in wound care is bimetallic nanoparticles, which combine two different metals to harness synergistic antimicrobial effects and enhanced wound healing properties compared to their monometallic counterparts. The unique physicochemical properties of BMNPs arise from their tunable composition, morphology (e.g., core–shell or alloy structures), and electronic interactions between the two metals, enabling improved antibacterial activity, reduced cytotoxicity, and multifunctional therapeutic effects compared to their monometallic counterparts.

One notable example involves silver-doped zinc oxide (Ag-ZnO) BMNPs synthesized via green methods using *Tridax procumbens* leaf extract, incorporated into ointment formulations. These Ag-ZnO BMNPs exhibited potent antimicrobial activity and significant wound healing acceleration in excision wound models, and this was attributed to the combined antibacterial action of Ag^+ ions and ZnO's pro-healing effects, alongside the antioxidant and anti-inflammatory phytochemicals from the plant extract. The ointment demonstrated suitable physicochemical properties, controlled-release behavior, and favorable biocompatibility, highlighting the promise of plant-mediated green synthesis for multifunctional wound dressings [59].

Similarly, silver-platinum (AgPt) BMNPs synthesized with citric acid and coated onto chitosan-fabricated cotton gauze showed superior antimicrobial and antioxidant activity against bacteria, yeast, and fungi compared to monometallic nanoparticles. The AgPt NP-coated gauze exhibited hydrophobic properties advantageous for wound protection, sustained pH-dependent release of silver and platinum ions, and improved in vitro fibroblast migration, accelerating wound closure. This multifunctional dressing addresses limitations of traditional gauze by combining antimicrobial efficacy with wound healing promotion [60].

Another advanced application involved bimetallic silver-magnesium oxide (Ag-MgO) nanoparticles loaded with Aloe vera extracts and xanthan gum to produce nanocomposites with synergistic antibacterial and wound healing properties. The nanocomposites effectively inhibited multidrug-resistant bacterial strains such as *E. coli* and *Bacillus cereus*, demonstrated low cytotoxicity, and accelerated wound closure in vitro, showcasing the therapeutic benefits of combining bimetallic nanoparticles with bioactive plant extracts and natural polymers for enhanced wound management [61] (Figure 7.4).

In addition, N,N,N-trimethyl chitosan-capped gold-silver (Au-Ag-TMC) BMNPs incorporated into PVA/chitosan nanofibers formed highly effective antimicrobial wound dressings against multidrug-resistant pathogens including *S. aureus*, *E. coli*, *P. aeruginosa*, and *C. albicans*. These nanofiber dressings exhibited potent antibacterial and antifungal activity, reduced microbial efflux pump expression, and promoted 99.34% wound closure in infected mice within 12 days. Advanced imaging confirmed enhanced re-epithelialization, angiogenesis, and oxygen saturation, demonstrating real-time wound healing progress and the potential of BMNP-nanofiber composites in clinical wound management [62].

Furthermore, copper-iron oxide ($Cu–Fe_3O_4$) bimetallic nanoclusters with multiple enzymatic activities (peroxidase, superoxide dismutase, and catalase-like) effectively scavenged free radicals and showed remarkable antibacterial activity against MRSA and *E. coli*. In vivo studies revealed that these nanozymes prevented MRSA infections and accelerated wound healing by interfering with bacterial metabolism and quorum sensing to inhibit biofilm formation. Their multifunctional catalytic behavior and excellent biosafety position $Cu–Fe_3O_4$ nanoclusters as a novel therapeutic agent for infection control and tissue regeneration in wound care [63].

Metal-based nanomaterials including monometallic nanoparticles such as silver, copper, gold, and zinc oxide, along with their bimetallic combinations offer a

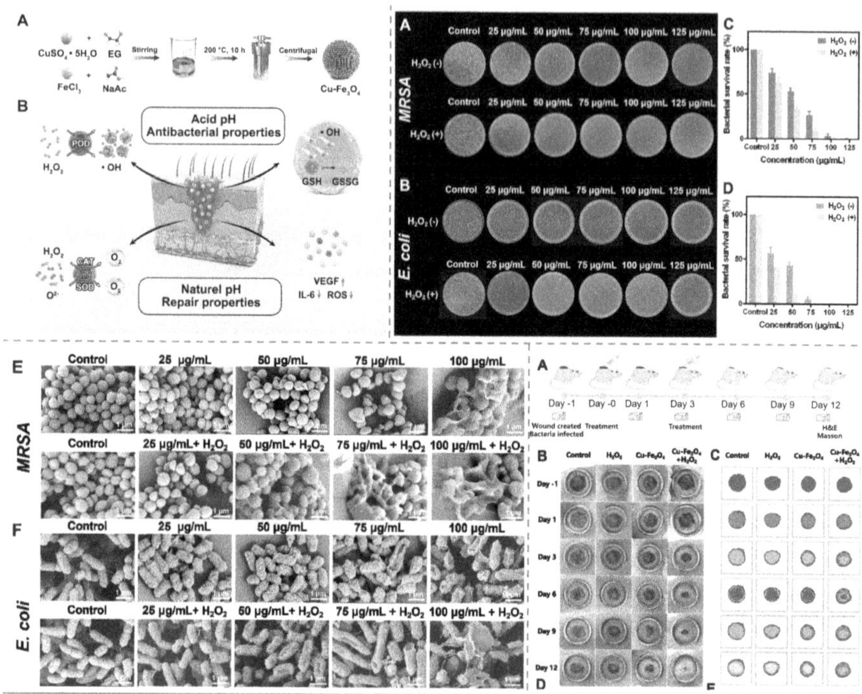

FIGURE 7.4 Bimetallic (Ag and MgO) nanoparticles, Aloe vera extracts loaded xanthan gum nanocomposite for enhanced antibacterial and in vitro wound healing activity (A) synthesis, (B) pH profile, (C) Bacterial survival rate for MRSA, (D) Bacterial Survival rate for E Coli, (E) Invitro activity for MRSA and (F) Invitro activity for E. Coli.

versatile and powerful approach to advancing wound dressing technologies. Their unique physicochemical characteristics enable strong antimicrobial effects, regulation of inflammation, and enhanced tissue regeneration, which are essential for effective wound repair. When integrated into biocompatible polymeric matrices and multifunctional platforms, these nanomaterials provide controlled therapeutic release, improved stability, and synergistic biological benefits. While challenges related to cytotoxicity, nanoparticle aggregation, and dosage optimization remain, ongoing innovations in synthesis, surface functionalization, and eco-friendly fabrication methods are addressing these issues. These advancements position metal-based nanomaterials as promising candidates for next-generation wound dressings that can effectively manage both acute and chronic wounds, ultimately improving patient care and reducing the burden on healthcare systems.

CBNs FOR WOUND DRESSING

CBNs have gained considerable attention in the development of advanced wound dressings due to their remarkable antibacterial properties, biocompatibility, and ability to promote tissue regeneration. Materials such as activated carbon, graphene and its derivatives, CNTs, and carbon quantum dots provide multifunctional platforms that can absorb toxins and exudates, inhibit microbial growth, and support cellular activities essential for wound healing. Liu et al. [64] highlights that micro/nano carbon materials exhibit broad-spectrum antibacterial effects through mechanisms involving physical disruption of bacterial membranes, oxidative stress induction, and interference with bacterial metabolism. These materials can be integrated into hydrogels, membranes, and composite dressings to enhance antimicrobial efficacy and maintain a moist wound environment conducive to healing.

Specifically, CNT-based hydrogels, as reviewed by Patil Tejal et al. [65], combine the exceptional mechanical strength and electrical conductivity of CNTs with the hydrophilic and biocompatible nature of hydrogels. These nanocomposite hydrogels exhibit significant bacterial eradication abilities while promoting cell proliferation and angiogenesis. Their multifunctionality enables not only infection control but also accelerated tissue repair, making them promising candidates for next-generation wound care. Despite their benefits, challenges such as potential cytotoxicity, aggregation, and long-term biocompatibility require further research focused on functionalization and hybrid material design to optimize clinical safety and efficacy. Together, these CBNs offer a versatile and potent approach for developing wound dressings that effectively address infection control and tissue regeneration.

CBNs have increasingly been incorporated into wound dressings due to their exceptional properties such as high surface area, mechanical strength, biocompatibility, and inherent antimicrobial activity. Among these, CNTs, carbon dots (CDs), and activated carbon have been extensively studied for their multifunctional roles in enhancing wound healing.

Shakiba et al. [66] developed a multifunctional nanofibrous composite by embedding a carboxylated multiwalled carbon nanotube-curcumin (CMWCNT-Cur) hybrid into a polyamide 6/poly(vinyl alcohol) nanofiber matrix via electrospinning. This composite demonstrated improved wettability, mechanical properties, and biodegradability. Importantly, the dressing exhibited significant antibacterial activity against *S. aureus* and *E. coli*, and controlled curcumin release was faster in mildly acidic conditions typical of wound sites. Cell viability assays indicated enhanced fibroblast proliferation, supporting tissue regeneration and highlighting its potential as an advanced chronic wound dressing (Figure 7.5).

Activated carbon has also been incorporated into PEG-based hydrogels to create dressings targeting malodorous wounds by adsorbing volatile compounds responsible for wound odor. Minsart et al. [67] synthesized hydrogel sheets and electrospun membranes combining acrylate-endcapped urethane-based polymers, methacrylated alginate, and activated carbon. These dressings showed tunable mechanical strength and swelling properties along with high adsorption capacity, surpassing commercial dressings in odor control. Their biocompatibility was confirmed, suggesting suitability for malodorous wound treatment, which improves patient quality of life.

CDs, a zero-dimensional carbon nanomaterial, have been incorporated into chitosan/PVA sponges to enhance hemostatic and antibacterial functions. Shakiba-Marani fabricated CS/PVA/CD sponges by freeze-drying, which exhibited high porosity, water absorption, flexibility, and excellent biocompatibility. The sponges promoted rapid hemostasis in vivo, demonstrating their promise as effective wound dressings that can manage bleeding and reduce infection risk [68].

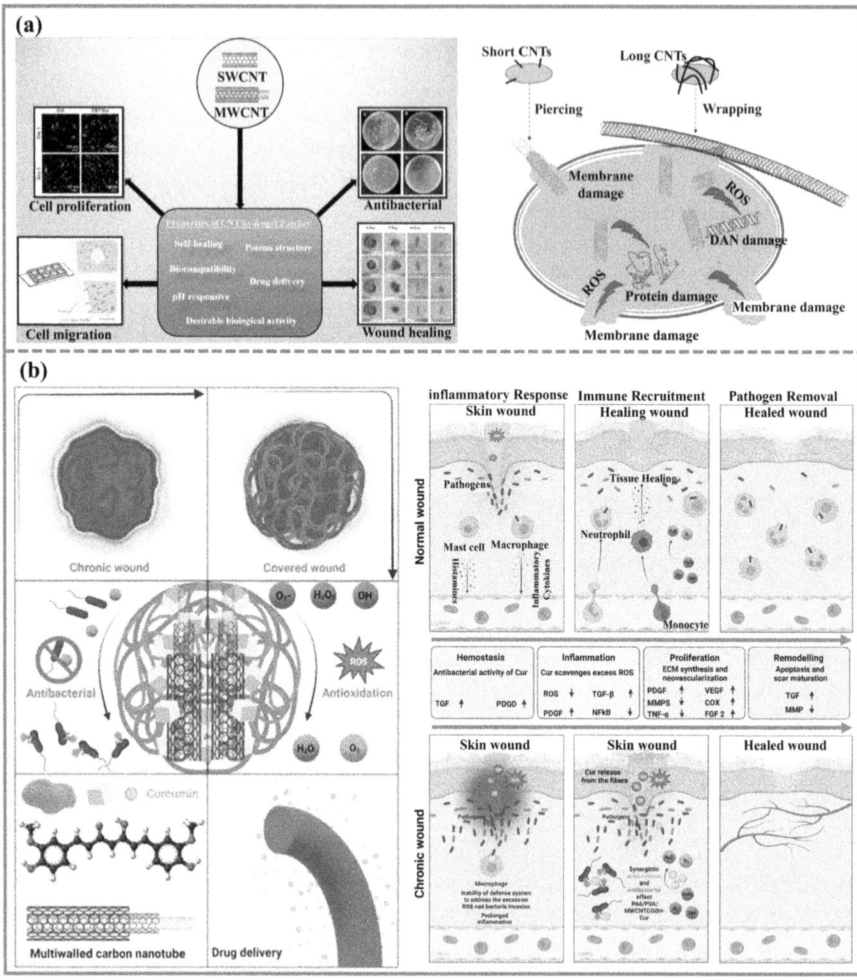

FIGURE 7.5 (a) Carbon nanotubes-based hydrogels for bacterial eradiation and wound-healing applications [65]. (b) Drug-loaded carbon nanotube incorporated into nanofibers: a multifunctional nanocomposite for smart chronic wound healing [66].

Similarly, Rezaei and Ehtesabi [69] prepared alginate/chitosan nanocomposite sponges incorporating green-synthesized CDs from Pyracantha plant precursors. The nanocomposites exhibited improved mechanical properties, increased porosity, enhanced water vapor transmission, and superior hemostatic potential. Cytocompatibility tests confirmed safety, and the enhanced blood-clotting ability indicated their potential for wound management applications.

Further, Faal et al. [70] utilized electrospinning to fabricate PLA nanofiber dressings loaded with curcumin and CNTs. The CNT incorporation enhanced mechanical strength, antibacterial activity (with nearly 79% inhibition against bacteria), and controlled curcumin release, while maintaining good cytocompatibility.

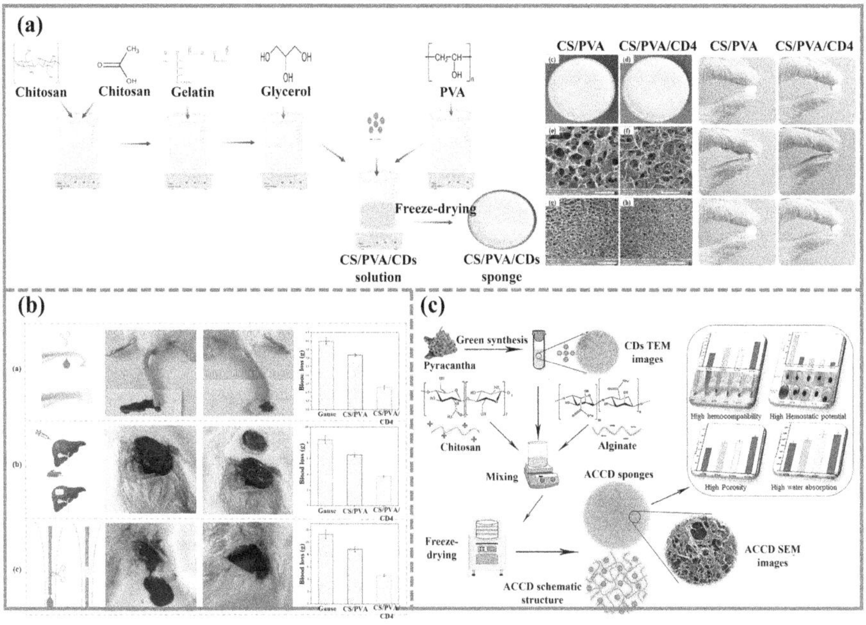

FIGURE 7.6 (a) and (b) A flexible and hemostatic chitosan, polyvinyl alcohol, carbon dot nanocomposite sponge for wound dressing application [68]. (c) Fabrication and evaluation of polylactic acid-curcumin containing carbon nanotubes (CNTs) wound dressing using electrospinning method with experimental and computational approaches [70].

These nanofibers showed promise as drug delivery platforms and physical wound barriers, improving both infection control and tissue regeneration (Figure 7.6).

Collectively, CBNs offer a multifaceted approach to wound management by combining antimicrobial activity, enhanced mechanical properties, and biofunctional support for tissue regeneration. The integration of activated carbon, CNTs, CDs, and their composites into diverse dressing platforms such as hydrogels, nanofibers, and sponges has demonstrated promising results in controlling infection, promoting hemostasis, and accelerating healing in both acute and chronic wounds. While challenges related to cytotoxicity, nanoparticle aggregation, and long-term biocompatibility persist, ongoing advances in material functionalization and hybridization continue to improve their safety and efficacy profiles. As research progresses, CBNs are poised to play a pivotal role in the development of next-generation wound dressings that offer targeted, effective, and patient-friendly therapeutic solutions.

FUTURE PERSPECTIVES AND CHALLENGES

The application of nanomaterials in wound dressings represents a transformative advance in wound care, offering multifunctional platforms that combine antimicrobial protection, inflammation modulation, and tissue regeneration. Despite promising preclinical and early clinical results, the translation of these innovations into widespread clinical use requires overcoming several critical challenges and capitalizing on emerging technological opportunities.

A key future direction involves the continued development of "smart" wound dressings that dynamically respond to the wound microenvironment. These self-responsive nanomaterials can detect changes in pH, temperature, bacterial load, or oxidative stress and subsequently modulate drug release or provide real-time wound status monitoring. Integration of biosensors with nanofibrous matrices holds potential for precision medicine approaches, allowing personalized treatment and reducing the frequency of dressing changes to minimize patient discomfort and healthcare costs. Further advances in multi-stimuli-responsive systems that combine pH-, enzyme-, and light-triggered mechanisms may optimize therapeutic delivery and efficacy in complex chronic wounds.

Material innovation is also essential for improving biocompatibility, biodegradability, and mechanical performance of nanomaterial-based dressings. Natural polymers like chitosan, gelatin, and cellulose derivatives show great promise due to their inherent bioactivity and environmental sustainability, yet challenges remain in achieving scalable fabrication with reproducible properties. Hybrid composites combining synthetic polymers with bioactive nanomaterials offer tunable degradation rates and enhanced mechanical strength, enabling dressings tailored for specific wound types. Additionally, progress in green synthesis methods for metallic and carbon-based nanoparticles enhances biocompatibility and reduces environmental impact, which is a crucial consideration for future clinical and commercial applications.

Another critical challenge concerns safety and regulatory approval. Nanomaterials exhibit complex interactions with biological systems that can vary depending on size, shape, surface chemistry, and dose. Cytotoxicity, inflammatory responses, and potential long-term accumulation require comprehensive in vitro and in vivo evaluation. Establishing standardized protocols for nanomaterial characterization, toxicity assessment, and clinical efficacy is imperative to streamline regulatory pathways and ensure patient safety. Collaborative efforts between academia, industry, and regulatory agencies are needed to develop consensus guidelines and quality control measures specific to nanoscale wound dressings.

Manufacturing scalability and cost-effectiveness remain practical barriers to commercialization. While electrospinning and centrifugal spinning techniques enable production of nanofibers with controlled architecture, translating lab-scale processes to industrial-scale manufacturing requires optimizing throughput, process stability, and reproducibility. Advances in needleless electrospinning and additive manufacturing may facilitate large-scale fabrication of multifunctional dressings with integrated sensors or controlled-release systems. Cost reduction strategies, including use of abundant natural polymers and sustainable nanoparticle synthesis, will be vital for broader adoption, especially in low-resource settings where chronic wounds impose substantial healthcare burdens.

Furthermore, clinical translation demands robust evidence from well-designed randomized controlled trials to validate safety and therapeutic superiority over existing dressings. Patient-centric outcomes such as pain reduction, scar quality, infection rates, and healing time must be prioritized alongside mechanistic biomarkers. Integration of digital health technologies to collect real-world data and monitor healing trajectories may accelerate clinical evaluation and personalized treatment adjustments.

In summary, the future of nanomaterial-enabled wound dressings lies in interdisciplinary innovation that combines materials science, bioengineering, clinical research, and regulatory science. Overcoming current challenges in safety, manufacturing, and clinical validation will unlock the full potential of these advanced therapies, improving outcomes for patients suffering from acute and chronic wounds worldwide. With ongoing research and technological progress, nanomaterial-based wound dressings are poised to become a mainstay of next-generation wound care, offering targeted, responsive, and efficacious solutions that address complex healing environments and reduce the global burden of non-healing wounds.

CONCLUSION

Nanomaterials have revolutionized the landscape of wound dressing development by providing multifunctional platforms that address critical challenges in wound healing, including infection control, inflammation modulation, and tissue regeneration. The unique physicochemical properties of metallic nanoparticles, CBNs, and polymeric nanofibers enable the design of advanced dressings with enhanced antimicrobial activity, controlled therapeutic delivery, and biomimetic architectures that support cellular functions essential for effective healing. While silver, copper, gold, zinc oxide, and bimetallic nanoparticles have demonstrated potent antibacterial and pro-healing effects, carbon-based materials and polymeric nanofibers contribute structural strength, biocompatibility, and versatile drug-loading capabilities.

Despite the promising outcomes reported in laboratory and animal studies, clinical translation remains a significant hurdle due to challenges related to safety, cytotoxicity, manufacturing scalability, and regulatory approval. Future efforts must focus on optimizing nanomaterial formulations to balance efficacy with biocompatibility, developing smart responsive systems for real-time wound monitoring and on-demand drug release, and establishing standardized testing protocols to ensure reproducibility and safety. Additionally, integration of sustainable and green synthesis methods will be critical for eco-friendly and cost-effective production.

In conclusion, the continued interdisciplinary collaboration across materials science, bioengineering, and clinical research is essential to fully harness the potential of nanomaterials in wound care. These advanced nanomaterial-based dressings hold great promise to transform the management of acute and chronic wounds, ultimately improving patient outcomes and reducing the global burden of non-healing wounds.

REFERENCES

1. Stoica AE, Chircov C, Grumezescu AM. Nanomaterials for wound dressings: an up-to-date overview. *Molecules*. 2020;25:2699.
2. Sangnim T, Puri V, Dheer D, Venkatesh DN, Huanbutta K, Sharma A. Nanomaterials in the wound healing process: new insights and advancements. *Pharmaceutics*. 2024;16(3):1–26.
3. Mihai MM, Dima MB, Dima B, Holban AM. Nanomaterials for wound healing and infection control. *Materials (Basel)*. 2019;12(13):1–16.

4. Nethi SK, Das S, Patra CR, Mukherjee S. Recent advances in inorganic nanomaterials for wound-healing applications. *Biomater Sci.* 2019;7(7):2652–74.
5. Chakrabarti S, Chattopadhyay P, Islam J, Ray S, Raju PS, Mazumder B. Aspects of nanomaterials in wound healing. *Curr Drug Deliv.* 2018;16(1):26–41.
6. Ling TZ, Nather A, Dennis HHW. Basic science of wound healing. *Diabet Foot.* 2012;15:89–96.
7. Irfan-Maqsood M. Classification of wounds: know before research and clinical practice. *J Genes Cells.* 2018;4:1.
8. Wang M, Huang X, Zheng H, Tang Y, Zeng K, Shao L, et al. Nanomaterials applied in wound healing: mechanisms, limitations and perspectives. *J Control Release.* 2021;337(May):236–47.
9. Akombaetwa N, Bwanga A, Makoni PA, Witika BA. Applications of electrospun drug-eluting nanofibers in wound healing: current and future perspectives. *Polymers (Basel).* 2022;14(14):1–26.
10. Liu X, Xu H, Zhang M, Yu DG. Electrospun medicated nanofibers for wound healing: *Review. Membranes (Basel).* 2021;11(10):770.
11. Gao C, Zhang L, Wang J, Jin M, Tang Q, Chen Z, et al. Electrospun nanofibers promote wound healing: theories, techniques, and perspectives. *J Mater Chem B.* 2021;9(14):3106–30.
12. Parham S, Kharazi AZ, Bakhsheshi-Rad HR, Kharaziha M, Ismail AF, Sharif S, et al. Antimicrobial synthetic and natural polymeric nanofibers as wound dressing: a review. *Adv Eng Mater.* 2022;24(6):1–22.
13. Pormohammad A, Monych NK, Ghosh S, Turner DL, Turner RJ. Nanomaterials in wound healing and infection control. *Antibiotics.* 2021;10(5):473.
14. Mendes C, Thirupathi A, Corrêa MEAB, Gu Y, Silveira PCL. The use of metallic nanoparticles in wound healing: new perspectives. *Int J Mol Sci.* 2022;23(23):15376.
15. Faghani G, Azarniya A. Emerging nanomaterials for novel wound dressings: from metallic nanoparticles and MXene nanosheets to metal-organic frameworks. *Heliyon.* 2024;10(21):e39611. https://doi.org/10.1016/j.heliyon.2024.e39611.
16. Wang Y, Zhang M, Yan Z, Ji S, Xiao S, Gao J. Metal nanoparticle hybrid hydrogels: the state-of-the-art of combining hard and soft materials to promote wound healing. *Theranostics.* 2024;14(4):1534–60.
17. Chauhan N, Saxena K, Jain U. Carbon-based nanomaterials in wound care management: a new and pristine strategy. *Biomed Mater Devices.* 2023;1(1):108–21. https://doi.org/10.1007/s44174-022-00030-3.
18. Islam M, Lantada AD, Mager D, Korvink JG. Carbon-based materials for articular tissue engineering: from innovative scaffolding materials toward engineered living carbon. *Adv Healthc Mater.* 2022;11(1):1–25.
19. Dalla Colletta A, Pelin M, Sosa S, Fusco L, Prato M, Tubaro A. Carbon-based nanomaterials and SKIN: an overview. *Carbon.* 2022;196(April):683–98. https://doi.org/10.1016/j.carbon.2022.05.036.
20. Balasubramanian P, Mari Selvam S. Valorization of biomass to activated carbon for wound dressing applications: recent trends and future challenges. *Bioresour Technol Reports.* 2023;23(July):101562. https://doi.org/10.1016/j.biteb.2023.101562.
21. Chen K, Hu H, Zeng Y, Pan H, Wang S, Zhang Y, et al. Recent advances in electrospun nanofibers for wound dressing. *Eur Polym J.* 2022;178(July):111490. https://doi.org/10.1016/j.eurpolymj.2022.111490.
22. Rajchal B, Thapa YN, Karki D, Prajapati P, Adhikari R. Insights into electrospun polymeric nanofiber mats: an innovative dressing for wound healing applications. *Polym Int.* 2025;74(5):391–404.
23. Zhang X, Wang Y, Gao Z, Mao X, Cheng J, Huang L, et al. Advances in wound dressing based on electrospinning nanofibers. *J Appl Polym Sci.* 2024;141(1):1–28.

24. Gavande V, Nagappan S, Seo B, Lee WK. A systematic review on green and natural polymeric nanofibers for biomedical applications. *Int J Biol Macromol.* 2024;262(P2):130135. https://doi.org/10.1016/j.ijbiomac.2024.130135.
25. Alturki AM. Rationally design of electrospun polysaccharides polymeric nanofiber webs by various tools for biomedical applications: a review. *Int J Biol Macromol.* 2021;184(February):648–65. https://doi.org/10.1016/j.ijbiomac.2021.06.021.
26. Alavi M, Nokhodchi A. Antimicrobial and wound healing activities of electrospun nanofibers based on functionalized carbohydrates and proteins. *Cellulose.* 2022;29(3):1331–47. https://doi.org/10.1007/s10570-021-04412-6.
27. Anusiya G, Jaiganesh R. A review on fabrication methods of nanofibers and a special focus on application of cellulose nanofibers. *Carbohydr Polym Technol Appl.* 2022;4(November):100262. https://doi.org/10.1016/j.carpta.2022.100262.
28. Xu H, Yagi S, Ashour S, Du L, Hoque ME, Tan L. A review on current nanofiber technologies: electrospinning, centrifugal spinning, and electro-centrifugal spinning. *Macromol Mater Eng.* 2023;308(3):1–13.
29. Hiwrale A, Bharati S, Pingale P, Rajput A. Nanofibers: a current era in drug delivery system. *Heliyon.* 2023;9(9):e18917. https://doi.org/10.1016/j.heliyon.2023.e18917.
30. Satish S, Priya R. A mini review on centrifugal spinning technique for production of nanofibers and its applications in drug delivery. *J Med Pharm Allied Sci.* 2022;11(1):4349–52.
31. Kazeminava F, Javanbakht S, Nouri M, Adibkia K, Ganbarov K, Yousefi M, et al. Electrospun nanofibers based on carboxymethyl cellulose/polyvinyl alcohol as a potential antimicrobial wound dressing. *Int J Biol Macromol.* 2022;214(January):111–9. https://doi.org/10.1016/j.ijbiomac.2022.05.175.
32. Nezhad-Mokhtari P, Kazeminava F, Abdollahi B, Gholizadeh P, Heydari A, Elmi F, et al. Matricaria chamomilla essential oil-loaded hybrid electrospun nanofibers based on polycaprolactone/sulfonated chitosan/ZIF-8 nanoparticles for wound healing acceleration. *Int J Biol Macromol.* 2023;247(July):125718. https://doi.org/10.1016/j.ijbiomac.2023.125718.
33. Wang B, Lu G, Song K, Chen A, Xing H, Wu J, et al. PLGA-based electrospun nanofibers loaded with dual bioactive agent loaded scaffold as a potential wound dressing material. *Colloids Surfaces B Biointerfaces.* 2023;231(September):113570. https://doi.org/10.1016/j.colsurfb.2023.113570.
34. Zhang X, Lv R, Chen L, Sun R, Zhang Y, Sheng R, et al. A multifunctional janus electrospun nanofiber dressing with biofluid draining, monitoring, and antibacterial properties for wound healing. *ACS Appl Mater Interfaces.* 2022;14(11):12984–3000.
35. Ren Y, Huang L, Wang Y, Mei L, Fan R, He M, et al. Stereocomplexed electrospun nanofibers containing poly (lactic acid) modified quaternized chitosan for wound healing. *Carbohydr Polym.* 2020;247(March):116754. https://doi.org/10.1016/j.carbpol.2020.116754.
36. Hwang PA, Chen HY, Chang JS, Hsu FY. Electrospun nanofiber composite mat based on ulvan for wound dressing applications. *Int J Biol Macromol.* 2023;253(P1):126646. https://doi.org/10.1016/j.ijbiomac.2023.126646.
37. Amani M, Rakhshani A, Maghsoudian S, Rasoulzadehzali M, Yoosefi S, Keihankhadiv S, et al. pH-sensitive bilayer electrospun nanofibers based on ethyl cellulose and Eudragit S-100 as a dual delivery system for treatment of the burn wounds; preparation, characterizations, and in-vitro/in-vivo assessment. *Int J Biol Macromol.* 2023;249(September):126705. https://doi.org/10.1016/j.ijbiomac.2023.126705.
38. Li T, Sun M, Wu S. State-of-the-art review of electrospun gelatin-based nanofiber dressings for wound healing applications. *Nanomaterials.* 2022;12(5):784. https://doi.org/10.3390/nano12050784.
39. Huang C, Xu X, Fu J, Yu DG, Liu Y. Recent progress in electrospun polyacrylonitrile nanofiber-based wound dressing. *Polymers (Basel).* 2022;14(16):1–33.
40. Datta D, Bandi SP, Colaco V, Dhas N, Saha SS, Hussain SZ, et al. Cellulose-based nanofibers infused with biotherapeutics for enhanced wound-healing applications. *ACS Polym Au.* 2025;5(2):80–104.

41. Ullah A, Ullah S, Khan MQ, Hashmi M, Nam PD, Kato Y, et al. Manuka honey incorporated cellulose acetate nanofibrous mats: fabrication and in vitro evaluation as a potential wound dressing. *Int J Biol Macromol.* 2020;155:479–89. https://doi.org/10.1016/j.ijbiomac.2020.03.237.
42. Ullah A, Sarwar MN, Wang F, Kharaghani D, Sun L, Zhu C, et al. In vitro biocompatibility, antibacterial activity, and release behavior of halloysite nanotubes loaded with diclofenac sodium salt incorporated in electrospun soy protein isolate/hydroxyethyl cellulose nanofibers. *Curr Res Biotechnol.* 2022;4(May):445–58. https://doi.org/10.1016/j.crbiot.2022.09.008.
43. Ullah A, Saito Y, Ullah S, Haider MK, Nawaz H, Duy-Nam P, et al. Bioactive Sambong oil-loaded electrospun cellulose acetate nanofibers: preparation, characterization, and in-vitro biocompatibility. *Int J Biol Macromol.* 2021;166:1009–21. https://doi.org/10.1016/j.ijbiomac.2020.10.257.
44. Haider MK, Ullah A, Sarwar MN, Yamaguchi T, Wang Q, Ullah S, et al. Fabricating antibacterial and antioxidant electrospun hydrophilic polyacrylonitrile nanofibers loaded with AgNPs by lignin-induced in-situ method. *Polymers (Basel).* 2021;13(5):1–20.
45. Adamu BF, Gao J, Gebeyehu EK, Beyene KA, Tadesse MG, Liyew EZ. Self-responsive electrospun nanofibers wound dressings: the future of wound care. *Adv Mater Sci Eng.* 2022;2022. https://doi.org/10.1155/2022/2025170.
46. Aminzai MT, Patan A. Recent applications and evaluation of metal nanoparticle-polymer hybrids as chronic wound dressings. *J Nanomater.* 2024;2024. https://doi.org/10.1155/2024/3280349.
47. Yudaev P, Mezhuev Y, Chistyakov E. Nanoparticle-containing wound dressing: antimicrobial and healing effects. *Gels.* 2022;8(6):329.
48. Kwiatkowska A, Drabik M, Lipko A, Grzeczkowicz A, Stachowiak R, Marszalik A, et al. Composite membrane dressings system with metallic nanoparticles as an antibacterial factor in wound healing. *Membranes (Basel).* 2022;12(2):215. https://www.mdpi.com/2077-0375/12/2/215.
49. Kalantari K, Mostafavi E, Afifi AM, Izadiyan Z, Jahangirian H, Rafiee-Moghaddam R, et al. Wound dressings functionalized with silver nanoparticles: promises and pitfalls. *Nanoscale.* 2020;12(4):2268–91.
50. Xu C, Akakuru OU, Ma X, Zheng J, Zheng J, Wu A. Nanoparticle-based wound dressing: recent progress in the detection and therapy of bacterial infections. *Bioconjug Chem.* 2020;31(7):1708–23.
51. Diao W, Li P, Jiang X, Zhou J, Yang S. Progress in copper-based materials for wound healing. *Wound Repair Regen.* 2024;32(3):314–22.
52. Sandoval C, Ríos G, Sepúlveda N, Salvo J, Souza-Mello V, Farías J. Effectiveness of copper nanoparticles in wound healing process using in vivo and in vitro studies: a systematic review. *Pharmaceutics.* 2022;14(9):1838.
53. Pino P, Bosco F, Mollea C, Onida B. Antimicrobial nano-zinc oxide biocomposites for wound healing applications: a review. *Pharmaceutics.* 2023;15(3):970.
54. Alavi M, Nokhodchi A. An overview on antimicrobial and wound healing properties of ZnO nanobiofilms, hydrogels, and bionanocomposites based on cellulose, chitosan, and alginate polymers. *Carbohydr Polym.* 2020;227(September 2019):115349. https://doi.org/10.1016/j.carbpol.2019.115349.
55. Borges FA, de Camargo Drago B, Baggio LO, de Barros NR, Sant'Ana Pegorin Brasil G, Scontri M, et al. Metronidazole-loaded gold nanoparticles in natural rubber latex as a potential wound dressing. *Int J Biol Macromol.* 2022;211(February):568–79.
56. Zepon KM, Marques MS, Hansen AW, Pucci CAF, Morisso FDP, Ziulkoski AL, et al. Polymer-based wafers containing in situ synthesized gold nanoparticles as a potential wound-dressing material. *Mater Sci Eng C.* 2020;109(August 2019):1–8.

57. El-Naggar ME, Shalaby ES, Abd-Al-Aleem AH, Abu-Saied MA, Youssef AM. Synthesis of environmentally benign antimicrobial dressing nanofibers based on polycaprolactone blended with gold nanoparticles and spearmint oil nanoemulsion. *J Mater Res Technol.* 2021;15:3447–60. https://doi.org/10.1016/j.jmrt.2021.09.136.
58. Zhou L, Yu K, Lu F, Lan G, Dai F, Shang S, et al. Minimizing antibiotic dosage through in situ formation of gold nanoparticles across antibacterial wound dressings: a facile approach using silk fabric as the base substrate. *J Clean Prod.* 2020;243:118604. https://doi.org/10.1016/j.jclepro.2019.118604.
59. Raju SK, Sekar P, Sankarganesh M, Bhat AR, Ahmed M, Ahmed S, et al. Synthesis, characterization, formulation and wound healing activity of silver doped zinc oxide bimetallic nanoparticles using Tridax procumbens leaf extract. *J Mol Struct.* 2025;1344(May):142813. https://doi.org/10.1016/j.molstruc.2025.142813.
60. Sathiyaseelan A, Saravanakumar K, Wang MH. Bimetallic silver-platinum (AgPt) nanoparticles and chitosan fabricated cotton gauze for enhanced antimicrobial and wound healing applications. *Int J Biol Macromol.* 2022;220(May):1556–69. https://doi.org/10.1016/j.ijbiomac.2022.09.045.
61. Saravanakumar K, Sathiyaseelan A, Zhang X, Choi M, Wang MH. Bimetallic (Ag and MgO) nanoparticles, Aloe vera extracts loaded xanthan gum nanocomposite for enhanced antibacterial and in-vitro wound healing activity. *Int J Biol Macromol.* 2023;242(P2):124813. https://doi.org/10.1016/j.ijbiomac.2023.124813.
62. Malik AK, Singh C, Mehata AK, Vikas, Setia A, Muthu MS, et al. Corrigendum to "Nanofibers of N,N,N-trimethyl chitosan capped bimetallic nanoparticles: preparation, characterization, wound dressing and in vivo treatment of MDR microbial infection and tracking by optical and photoacoustic imaging". Int. J. Biol. Macromol. 263 (2024) 130327](S0141813024009577)(10.1016/j.ijbiomac.2024.130154). *Int J Biol Macromol.* 2024;277(February). https://doi.org/10.1016/j.ijbiomac.2024.133036.
63. Jin X, Shan J, Zhao J, Wang T, Zhang W, Yang S, et al. Bimetallic oxide Cu–Fe_3O_4 nanoclusters with multiple enzymatic activities for wound infection treatment and wound healing. *Acta Biomater.* 2024;173:403–19.
64. Liu Y, Li QQ, Zhang H, Yu SP, Zhang L, Yang YZ. Research progress on the use of micro/nano carbon materials for antibacterial dressings. *New Carbon Mater.* 2020;35(4):323–35. https://doi.org/10.1016/S1872-5805(20)60492-9.
65. Patil T V., Patel DK, Dutta SD, Ganguly K, Randhawa A, Lim KT. Carbon nanotubes-based hydrogels for bacterial eradiation and wound-healing applications. *Appl Sci.* 2021;11(20):9550.
66. Shakiba M, Jahangiri P, Rahmani E, Hosseini SM, Bigham A, Foroozandeh A, et al. Drug-loaded carbon nanotube incorporated in nanofibers: a multifunctional nanocomposite for smart chronic wound healing. *ACS Appl Polym Mater.* 2023;5(7):5662–75.
67. Minsart M, Mignon A, Arslan A, Allan IU, Van Vlierberghe S, Dubruel P. Activated carbon containing PEG-based hydrogels as novel candidate dressings for the treatment of malodorous wounds. *Macromol Mater Eng.* 2021;306(1):1–12.
68. Shakiba-Marani R, Ehtesabi H. A flexible and hemostatic chitosan, polyvinyl alcohol, carbon dot nanocomposite sponge for wound dressing application. *Int J Biol Macromol.* 2023;224(July 2022):831–9. https://doi.org/10.1016/j.ijbiomac.2022.10.169.
69. Rezaei A, Ehtesabi H. Fabrication of alginate/chitosan nanocomposite sponges using green synthesized carbon dots as potential wound dressing. *Mater Today Chem.* 2022;24:100910. https://doi.org/10.1016/j.mtchem.2022.100910.
70. Faal M, Faal M, Ahmadi T, Dehgan F. Fabrication and evaluation of polylactic acid-curcumin containing carbon nanotubes (CNTs) wound dressing using electrospinning method with experimental and computational approaches. *Sci Rep.* 2025;15(1):1–17.

8 Technologies in Advanced Wound Dressings Development

Gul I. Zahra, Maham Raza, and Rashid Masood

INTRODUCTION

Wound healing is a complex and dynamic biological process that involves coordinated events of acellular and cellular mechanisms; after injury, it helps to restore the affected tissue. This process depends on factors like type of wound and overall health of the patient. As traditional processes often come up short, advanced technologies such as nano-based dressings have been formed to improve the process of healing. There are different phases of wound healing that include hemostasis, inflammation, proliferation, and remodeling or maturation. The process starts with hemostasis, which occurs right after injury. In this process, the blood vessels contract to reduce loss of blood, and platelets combined to form a clot at the wound site through fibrin mesh, and they also release signaling molecules such as platelet-derived growth factor (PDGF) and transforming growth factor-beta (TGF-β), which trigger other cells to come and start the process of healing [1–3].

Following hemostasis, the next stage is an inflammatory phase that lasts up to 72 hours or a few days. This stage includes the placement of immune cells to remove germs and cellular debris. Neutrophils arrive first, executing phagocytosis and releasing reactive oxygen species and proteolytic enzymes. Macrophages go to the wound area and remove dead cells and repair the tissue by releasing cytokines and growth factors. Lymphocytes also help to control the immune response. This phase is characterized by redness, pain, swelling, and functional disturbance.

Next is the proliferative phase, in which the body starts to regenerate tissue structure. Fibroblasts travel toward the wound site and initiate producing components such as collagen, glycosaminoglycans, and other extracellular matrix (ECM) components that form granulation tissue. Simultaneously, angiogenesis arises, and new blood vessels are formed to restore the delivery of nutrients and oxygen. Keratinocytes migrate across the wound bed; this process is known as re-epithelialization. This stage depends on a suitable supply of nutrients and oxygen and is influenced by various growth factors.

The last stage is the remodeling or maturation phase, which lasts from weeks to some months or even years. In this phase, type III collagen that is produced in the proliferation stage is exchanged by other stronger type I collagen, which leads to increased tensile strength of the healed tissue. Particularly, contractile fibroblasts,

DOI: 10.1201/9781003616726-10

Myofibroblasts, contribute to the contraction of the wound, which results in reducing the size of the wound. Unsystematic and excessive ECM components are degenerated by matrix metalloproteinases (MMPs), controlled by tissue inhibitors of metalloproteinases (TIMPs), which helps to restore the structure of normal tissue. As unnecessary new vessels regress, the vascular thickness also proceeds to baseline. Many factors also affect the healing like poor nutrition, low oxygen, diabetes, infection, age, stress, and so on. Understanding how wound healing cells and molecules work not only provides insight into normal tissue repair but also informs strategies for managing chronic or excessive wound healing conditions such as ulcers or keloids [4–7].

Types of Wounds

Wounds are disturbances in the skin's integrity, many factors cause wounds and characteristically classified on the basis of their depth, origin, time, and potential of healing. Some types of wounds are acute, chronic, diabetic ulcer, pressure ulcers, burn wounds, surgical wounds, and so on.

Acute wounds are injuries that heal within 8–12 weeks, and these types of injuries are majorly caused by the minor incidents like cuts, abrasion, minor burns, and surgical slits. These wounds heal by normal healing phases that are hemostasis, inflammation, proliferation, and remodeling. If treated properly, wounds heal in a short term. If wounds don't heal and complications start, then the wounds may transition into chronic wounds, which lasts about months or years. These are caused mainly by diabetes, infections, vascular diseases, or repeated injury. These wounds show inflammation, poor regeneration of cells, and ECM degradation. These wounds need advanced care approaches [8,9].

Surgical wounds are usually caused during operations, and they heal naturally within a short time just like acute wounds. But if these wounds get complicated because of any infection or poor postoperative care, it can also become chronic. Precautionary hygiene and sterilized techniques are essential for healing. Pressure ulcers progress because of the long pressure on the skin, mainly on the bony areas. These wounds are staged from stage I to IV based on how severe the wound is. These types of ulcers can be painful, heal slowly, and cause infections. They are very common in old people and bedbound patients [10]. The main cause of diabetic ulcer is because of diabetic-related issues such as poor circulation of blood and neuropathy. Diabetic ulcers are classified into numerous types such as neuropathic ulcers, which occur due to the loss of protective sensation, ischemic ulcers occur due to arterial blockage, and neurochemical ulcers both above types and hard to manage, and the last is diabetic ulcers due to trauma, caused when the external force like sharp things, any burns, and frictional forces applies to foot, which leads towards ulceration. Proper foot care is needed for diabetic patients. Burn wounds caused by chemical, thermal, or electrical injuries also vary from one to four stages. First-degree burns usually harm the surface of the skin only; if the burn is deeper, then it can also destroy the tissues. Severe burning increases the danger of having infection and loss of fluid [11–14].

Factors Affecting Wound Healing

Wound healing is a physiological process that is influenced by several local and systemic factors. Local factors are considered as those that directly affect the wound environment. As oxygen is important for cellular metabolism, synthesis of collagen, microbial killing, and angiogenesis, oxygenation is considered as the important mechanism. If insufficient oxygen is supplied, it delays the process of healing. Infection plays a critical role in the healing process by prolonging the stage of inflammation by releasing enzymes and cytokines. Poor circulation of blood also delays healing, promoting inflammation and damaging regeneration of tissue [2–4,15].

Systematic factors include the biological conditions of the individual that affect the healing of wounds. Age is considered as a prominent factor; in elders, delay in the process of healing is seen due to the weakened immune responses, slower migration of cells, and reduced angiogenesis. Hormonal effects play a role in healing; estrogen helps in promoting healing and reducing inflammation, while androgens delay the process of healing and promote a chronic inflammatory phase. Emotional stress can also affect healing by disrupting the immune system and hormonal functions. Mainly, high cortisol and less cytokine activity reduce the inflammatory response that is important for the early phase of healing. Obesity has an influence on the healing process of wounds by increasing the chances of having infection and decreasing the perfusion of tissue, resulting in mechanical stress. Alcohol, smoking, and medicines also interfere with the process of repairing wounds, affecting the immune system and reducing the delivery of oxygen to tissues and delay synthesis of collagen [16–19].

PRINCIPLES OF WOUND ASSESSMENT

Wound assessment includes assessing the wound size, shape, wound bed, and condition of adjacent tissue, which involves checking infections, pain, and other factors that affect the healing. This detailed evaluation of wounds guides treatment decisions and monitor's progress [20].

Wound Classification Systems

Wound classification systems play an important role in evaluating wounds and guiding suitable treatment approaches. Each component shows different properties such as T removal and identification of non-viable tissues. 'I' shows the inflammation or any infection in the wound, which can be examined by seeing signs like swelling, redness, and so on. 'M' focuses on the balancing of moisture; selection of dressing must support optimal hydration. 'E' stands for the importance of healthy wound edges; if any rolled edge is seen, then there is a need for further treatment for healing. National pressure ulcer advisory panels are another classification system. This system's main focus is on pressure ulcers, and it has four stages. In Stage 1, the skin appears red when pressure is applied and it did not turn white; the skin surface is unbreakable. Stage 2 shows that some layers of skin are damaged. In Stage 3, the whole skin is damaged. Stage 4 is the deeper wounds that show bones, tendons, and muscles [20,21].

TABLE 8.1
These Classification Systems Help to Examine Wound Assessment and Management

System	Best For	Focus Area	Key Use
TIME	Chronic wounds	Tissue, infection, moisture, edges	Wound bed preparation
NPUAP	Pressure ulcers	Stages 1–4, deep tissue	Documentation and treatment plan
Wanger	Diabetic foot ulcers	Depth, infections	Surgical, clinical intervention planning

The Wagner system is used to check the depth of the wound and the presence of any infection in the diabetic foot ulcers wound. It ranges from grade 0 to grade 4. At grade 0, the skin is undamaged but at risk. Grade 5 involves high infection of the foot. Grade 1 involves superficial ulcers, whereas grade 2 shows wounds that are deep and reaching tendons or ligaments. Grade 3 reflects deep infections, whereas grade 4 contains infection of the forefoot. These steps are helpful for planning and predicting outcomes of healing in diabetic patients [22] (Table 8.1).

Documentation and Measurement of Wounds

Nurses are responsible for maintaining comprehensive and accurate records of wounds. This meticulous documentation is crucial for monitoring the wound's progress and guiding the selection of appropriate treatments to facilitate healing. A key aspect of wound management is regular and thorough assessment, which should be performed initially and at consistent intervals. To ensure the reliability of these assessments, they must be conducted using a standardized method, with the patient in the same position each time. Changes in the dimensions of a wound, including its length, width, and depth, serve as significant indicators of the healing process. To streamline this process and enhance both the continuity of care and the consistency of documentation, the use of a wound assessment chart is highly recommended. These charts, whether in paper or electronic format, provide a structured framework for recording relevant wound parameters.

i. **Wound Size**

   Regularly measuring wound size is of paramount importance in evaluating the effectiveness of the treatment being administered. Accurate monitoring of wound size necessitates the use of consistent measurement methods. This ensures that any changes in the wound's dimensions are reliably tracked over time, providing valuable insights into whether the wound is healing as expected.

ii. **Wound Depth**

   In addition to length and width, wound depth is another critical parameter that should be measured and documented as part of a comprehensive wound assessment. Accurate measurement of wound depth helps healthcare professionals to fully understand the extent of tissue damage and to tailor treatment plans accordingly.

iii. **Exudate**

Wound exudate, often referred to as wound fluid or drainage, is a natural component of the healing process. However, it is essential to maintain a delicate balance. Excessive amounts of exudate, exudate in an inappropriate location, or exudate with an abnormal composition can all impede the healing process. Therefore, a thorough assessment of wound exudate should be an integral part of a structured and holistic wound assessment. This assessment should not only focus on the exudate itself but also consider the patient's overall health, the specific wound management strategies in place, and any other pertinent factors that may influence wound healing. Key aspects of exudate assessment include quantifying the amount of exudate, characterizing its type (appearance), and evaluating its consistency. While measuring exudate can provide valuable data, it is not always feasible in clinical settings. When measurement is possible, methods such as weighing dressings or utilizing negative pressure wound therapy (NPWT) canisters can be employed. Normal exudate plays a crucial role in supporting healing by maintaining a moist wound environment, facilitating the diffusion of immune mediators and growth factors, acting as a medium for cell migration, supplying essential nutrients for cell metabolism, and promoting autolysis (the separation of dead or damaged tissue). The inflammatory process, a natural response to injury, increases fluid production, which in turn contributes to the formation of exudate. Wound exudate is derived from blood and contains a complex mixture of components, including proteins, growth factors, and enzymes. In addition to these beneficial substances, exudate may also contain metabolic waste products, microorganisms, and tissue debris, highlighting the importance of proper management to prevent complications.

iv. **Wound Edges**

The condition of the wound edges is a significant factor in the overall assessment of a wound. A healthy wound edge is indicative of active healing, while unhealthy or deteriorating edges may signal underlying problems. Assessment of the wound edge is a key component of the Triangle of Wound Assessment, a framework used by clinicians to evaluate various aspects of the wound. Additionally, the TIME(S) framework, a widely used tool for wound bed preparation, also emphasizes the importance of assessing the edge of the wound. TIME(S) is an acronym that stands for Tissue, Inflammation/Infection, Moisture balance, Edge of wound, and social factors [23] (Figure 8.1).

Identifying Infection and Biofilm Presence

Identifying infection and biofilm presence in wounds is critical for guiding effective treatment and improving patient outcomes. Clinically, wound infections are typically recognized through signs such as redness, swelling, warmth, delayed healing, excess

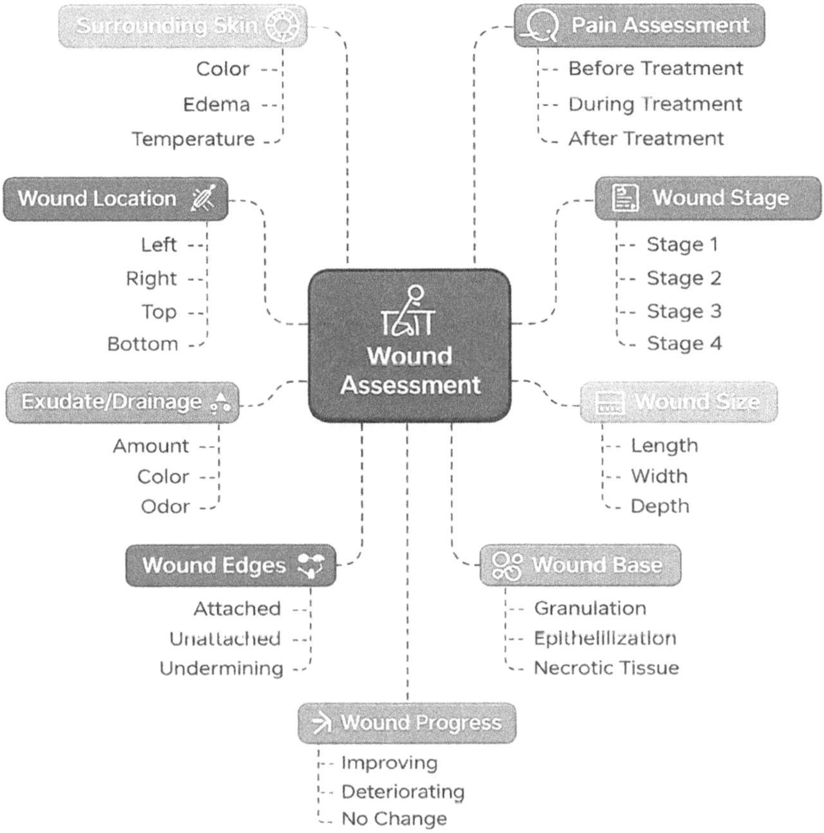

FIGURE 8.1 Documentation and measurement of wound.

exudate, foul odor, friable granulation tissue, and increased pain. In chronic wounds, the signs can be subtler, including hyper-granulation, epithelial bridging, pocketing, and wound breakdown, which may be misinterpreted or masked by underlying conditions like diabetes or vascular disease. Diagnostic tools commonly used include wound swab cultures particularly the Levine method, which collects bacteria from tissue fluid rather than just the surface, deep tissue biopsies (considered the gold standard but invasive), and needle aspiration for localized infections. Laboratory markers such as C-reactive protein (CRP), procalcitonin (PCT), and bacterial protease activity can also help differentiate infection from mere inflammation [8,24,25].

Biofilms are enclosed in an ECM, which protects immune responses and is resistant to antibiotics. Finding the biofilm in wounds adds complexity. Usually, the sessile bacteria sometimes are unable to detect by standard laboratory cultures, contributing to chronic and non-healing wounds. Methods to detect biofilms are PCR, which detect biofilms that are related to genes, and several forms of microscopy like scanning electron microscopy, transmission electron microscopy, and confocal laser scanning microscopy are used to detect the structure of biofilm. Although emerging techniques like MALDI-TOF mass spectrometry and omics-based analyses show promise for rapid and specific biofilm detection, they remain limited in routine clinical use due to cost, technical demands, and the need for specialized equipment. Therefore, current best practices rely on integrating careful clinical assessment, targeted laboratory investigations, and molecular diagnostics, when available, to accurately identify both infection and biofilm presence in wounds and to guide effective, tailored treatment strategies [26,27].

Pain Assessment and Management

Pain assessment is a crucial part of wound management, as it affects patient comfort, treatment adherence, and healing outcomes. Because pain is subjective, clinicians must rely on the patient's report using tools like the Visual Analog Scale (VAS), Numeric Rating Scale (NRS), or Faces Pain Scale-Revised (FPS-R). Evaluating only the intensity of pain is not enough; so, also check the location, type, time, and triggers of pain. When dressing, special care is needed so it doesn't cause discomfort and use non-adherent materials. Complete approach is needed because biological factors such as fear can also increase pain. Doing daily assessments and documentation guarantees pain management plans to remain patient positioned and effective [28,29].

TRADITIONAL VS. ADVANCED DRESSINGS

Traditional dressings such as bandages and gauze are cost-effective, but they stick to tissue that causes pain while advanced dressings like films, alginates, and hydrocolloids help protect from bacteria and maintain a humid environment. Comparing both, advanced dressings are much more convenient as they reduce pain during changing and less wound disturbance. For antimicrobial activity, growth factor, and regulation of moisture, they include bioactive components. Modern methods in chronic wound management focus on biodegradability, biocompatibility, and comfort of patients. It also shows an important improvement in wound care that promotes good healing and better outcomes [30–33].

INNOVATIVE TECHNIQUES AND TECHNOLOGIES

Smart Wound Dressings

Traditional wound dressings mainly act as a protective shield, but advanced methods have been directed toward the smart dressings, which actively interact with wound environment and play an important role in wound care management. Smart dressings integrate biosensors that monitor the condition of wounds all the time. The sensors also shows the pH, temperature, and exudate levels, as well as changes in the wound environment. Several biosensors are studied to use in wound dressings that include electrochemical sensors that measure the pH and glucose levels, optical sensors that display saturation of oxygen, and Aptamer-based sensors that are helpful for detecting bacteria that are harmful. Materials that are used for making these types of biosensors include synthetic and natural polymers that biodegrade easily and are biocompatible such as polyurethane and polyethylene glycol (PEG), alginate, silk fibroin, and chitosan [34–36].

Key Parameters Monitored by Smart Dressings

Smart dressings are designed to monitor several key parameters within the wound microenvironment (Figure 8.2).

Change in pH shows infection and other difficulties. High temperature suggests inflammation; examples of this include nanodiamond-silk fibroin membranes with temperature-sensing abilities. Extreme and inadequate exudate can delay the process of healing. Mainly, monitoring glucose levels is important in diabetic wounds, where decrease in glucose metabolism can result in healing wounds. Oxygen plays a very important part in the process of healing, and some other smart dressings are manufactured for detecting specific bacteria that includes antibiotic-resistant strains. Examples of Innovative Smart Dressings include Nanodiamond-Silk Fibroin Membranes. As mentioned, these membranes have temperature-sensing capabilities, aiding in early infection detection. Development of Chitosan-Alginate Polyelectrolyte: These materials are used for creating films with good water vapor permeability and good mechanical properties. Thyme Oil Nanoemulsions: The use of thyme oil nanoemulsions in dressings provides antimicrobial activity. Electroactive Dressing materials like polyurethane/siloxane can be engineered to be electroactive, antibacterial, and antioxidant, promoting wound healing [35,37].

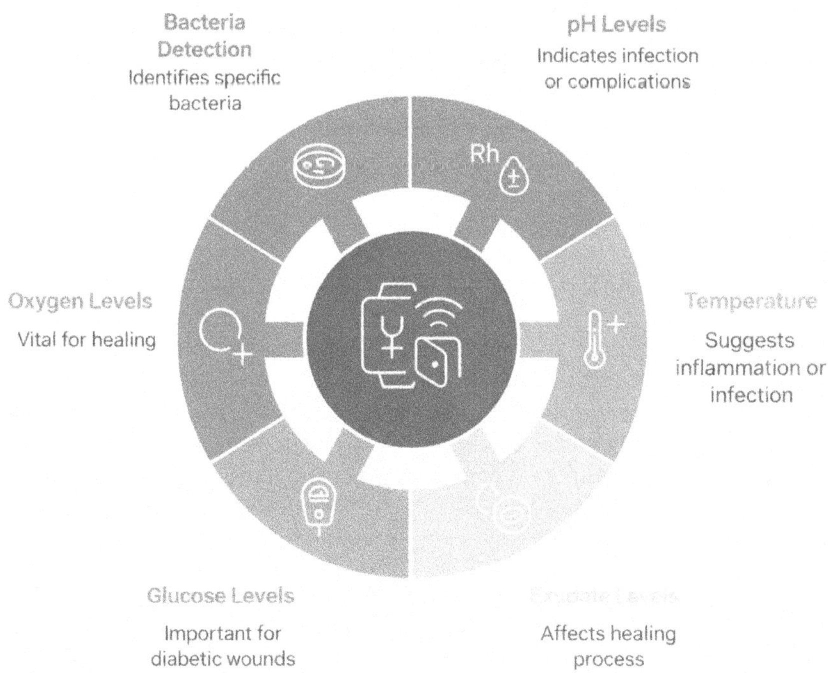

FIGURE 8.2 Several key parameters within the wound microenvironment.

Advantages of Smart Dressings

Smart dressing offers numerous advantages over traditional dressings as follows. Real-time Monitoring: Continuous monitoring of wound conditions allows for timely intervention. Early Detection of Complications: Smart dressings can detect infections and other problems early on, preventing further complications. Individualized Treatment: With the help of the data acquired by smart dressings, we can adapt the treatment according to the wound. Better Healing Results: Depending on the wound, smart dressings can heal the wounds faster and effectively. Less Need for Changing: Due to its ability to stay in place for a long time, there will be less need to change dresses frequently. Delivery of Drug: Smart dressings can also provide drugs in a controlled manner directly to the wound. Antimicrobial Properties: Many smart dressings have antibacterial properties to prevent any sort of infection. Biocompatibility: Smart dressings are usually made from biocompatible substances to decrease harmful activity. Cost-Effectiveness: It can lead to cost cutting eventually due to all its properties, whereas it can be expensive in the beginning [34,35,38].

Challenges and Future Directions

Despite all the advantages smart dressing can provide, it has some significant challenges as follows. Cost: The high cost can be a hurdle for its adoption globally. Measurability: Making these smart dresses at a large level can be challenging. Integration of Multiple Sensing Element: Using multiple sensing elements into a dressing can be difficult to keep it biocompatible and functionable. Data Management: Managing and interpreting the large amounts of data generated by smart dressings requires sophisticated systems. Supply of Power: Always having a power source to wireless dressing can be difficult. Researchers are working on alternate options like battery operated or bio-resourceful options. Long-Term Stability: Ensuring the long-term stability and functionality of the sensors and other components within the dressing is essential.

Addressing these challenges and finding their solutions is the focus of future research, which includes developing more cost-effective and scalable manufacturing methods; integrating a wider range of sensors to monitor additional parameters; developing closed-loop systems that can automatically adjust treatment based on sensor data; exploring new materials with enhanced properties; improving the wireless capabilities and power efficiency of smart dressings; and creating more user-friendly interfaces for data management and interpretation. Smart dressings represent an important advancement in wound care technology. By using biosensors and other advanced options, these dressings can transform the wound handling ways, resulting in better healing and comfort to patients. With all the continuing research, smart dressing will play a very important role in skin medicine in the near future.

Drug-Delivery Wound Dressings

There has been significant progress in the field of drug-delivery wound dressings. While in traditional ways, the sole purpose of dressing was to protect it from physical interaction, now in modern ways, dressings will also provide with the necessary drug required to heal the wound. The core purpose is to use the dressings to heal the wound more effectively. Drug-delivery wound dressing's main purpose is to release the drug directly to the wound to help it heal. It will keep the drug locked in, which will help with the faster healing of the wound as dressings will not require frequent changes. These dressings take part in the healing process actively, address the required need for healing, and promote a wound friendly environment. Examples of drug-delivery wound dressings include cotton gauze bandages coated with chitosan and zinc oxide nanoparticles (NPs), combined with electrospun nanofibers loaded with diclofenac sodium (for anti-inflammatory and antibacterial effects), chitosan-alginate PEC films loaded with thyme oil nanoemulsions (for antibacterial activity), Carbopol hydrogels embedded with oxygen nanobubbles (ONBs), and collagenase [39,40].

Classification of Drug-Delivery Wound Dressings

Drug-delivery wound dressings can be categorized based on various factors, including composition, mechanisms, and types of therapy substances they include. Dressings can be made of a variety of materials, each of which has its own properties. These dressings are often made of biocompatible polymers such as polyurethane, silicone, or hydrogels. They can be configured to be occlusive or semi-occlusive, rendering a barrier to allow some moisture vapor to transmit. These are three-dimensional schemes of hydrophilic polymers that can absorb large sums of biological fluids and water. They make the environment damp, which is important for cell motion and proliferation. Hydrogels are peculiarly well-suited to deliver drugs that are water soluble. These dressings have gel-forming agents, such as sodium carboxymethylcellulose, and adhesives. They can form a gel when they interact with wound exudation, create a damp environment, and provide some level of autolytic debridement. It is obtained from seaweed. They have high absorbent properties and get into a gel form after having an interaction with sodium ions. They are useful for heavy wounds and can be useful in delivering drugs to wounds. These dressings have NPs that carry drugs. Nanoparticles can be useful in drug solubility, are more bioavailable, and deliver the drug targeted to specific tissues or cells in the body. Composite materials combining hydrogels or electrospun constructs with NPs offer a wide range of applications. Electrospinning is the way to produce fine fibers that can be converted into non-woven mats. Due to its high surface, these mats are ideal for loading the drug and controlled release [41–43].

Drug Release Mechanism

The way the drug is released is the critical factor in the efficiency of the drug-delivery wound dressings. Diffusion-Controlled Release: The drug is discharged from the dressing by the process of diffusion, which is derived by the concentration gradient between the dressing and the wound. Swelling-Controlled Release: When the wound fluids are absorbed, it causes the swelling of the dressing, resulting in the release of drug. Degradation-Controlled Release: The drug is also released when the material of the dressing degrades. Triggered Release: pH changes, enzymes, or temperature can also cause the release of drug [6].

Therapeutic Agents

A variety of therapeutic factors can be merged into wound dressings, depending on the particular needs of the wound. Antimicrobials were used to prevent or treat infection (e.g., antibiotics, silver, chlorhexidine). Growth factors were used to stimulate cell proliferation and tissue regeneration (e.g., epidermal growth factor, PDGF). Anti-inflammatory agents were used to reduce the inflammation and pain (e.g., corticosteroids, nonsteroidal anti-inflammatory drugs). Analgesics were used to alleviate pain. Angiogenic factors were used to promote new blood vessel formation [35,44].

Advantages of Drug-Delivery Wound Dressings

Drug-delivery wound dressings provide many benefits than traditional dressings, including better and fast healing and patient comfort. Targeted Drug Delivery: Drugs are directly delivered to the wound, which maximize the therapeutic effect and minimize possible side effects. Controlled Release: Dressings can be fashioned to release drugs at a planned rate, guaranteeing an uninterrupted healing effect and also reduce the frequency of dressing changes. Improved Patient Compliance: Application of single dressing can help the patient in having the treatment with no delays as wounds take time, patients usually stop coming, and let it heal on its own, which is a dangerous practice. Enhanced Wound Healing: The delivery of drugs and not so frequent changing can fasten up the healing process and better tissue build-up after that. Reduced Risk of Infection: Antimicrobial dressings can prevent infections caused by wounds, which are a major reason that delays the healing process. Figure 8.3 represents how a drug is released from the dressing. The fluid coming out of the wound has a critical role to play in the whole process, as it interacts with the material of the dressing. The drug is then released through different mechanisms. For example, the fluid may dissolve the drug, which will help it diffuse into the wound. In the case of hydrogel dressings, the dressing can swell, which can lead to the release of the drug. As an alternative, the fluid may contain enzymes that degrade

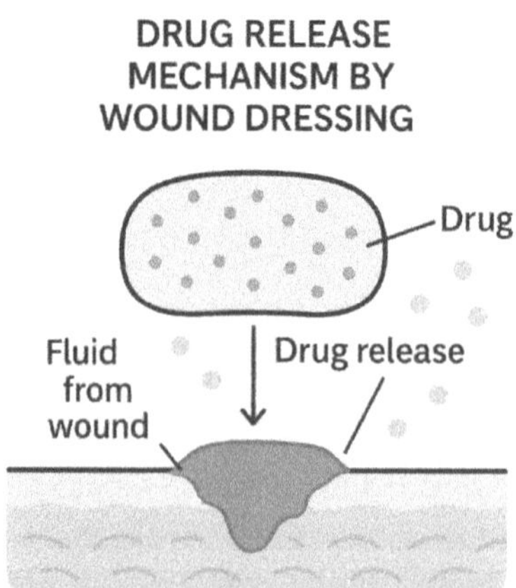

FIGURE 8.3 Drug release mechanism.

the material of dressing, resulting in drug release. Therefore, the characteristics of the wound fluid, such as its composition and volume, can significantly influence the rate and extent of drug release [39–42,45].

Mechanisms of Drug Release from Wound Dressings

The image also presents the drug release process. The mechanisms involved can be different depending on the type of dressing and the drug that is being delivered. Here are some of the key mechanisms. Diffusion: This is the easiest mechanism, driven by the concentration gradient between the dressing and the wound. Drug molecules move from an area of high concentration (the dressing) to an area of low concentration (the wound). Swelling-Controlled Release: In this mechanism, the dressing, often a hydrogel, swells by absorbing the fluid coming out of the wounds. As the dressing expands, the drug molecules are released from the polymer network. Degradation-Controlled Release: Some dressings are made of biodegradable materials. Enzymes or other components in wound fluid can break down these materials, leading to the release of the drug. Environmentally Responsive Release: Some dressings are designed to release drugs in response to specific stimuli in the wound environment, such as changes in pH, temperature, or the presence of specific enzymes [40,41].

Conclusion and Future Directions

In conclusion, the drug-delivery wound dressings play an important role in the care of wounds. It not only offers protection but also heals the process. These dressings with its characteristics can promote healing and can enhance patient care. Moreover, further research has been going on to overcome the challenges and obstacles we are facing at the moment including the delivery system, the use of more biodegradable options, advancement in carrying of drugs, and individualized approaches to the wounds. The future of wound dressings is likely to be focused on these challenges.

Stem Cell-Infused Dressings

The dressings that are stem cell-infused present a unique approach toward healing of wounds, leveraging the productive potential of stem cells to speed up tissue repair and regeneration. There are many innovative techniques and technologies working on this method, with a particular focus on how these dressings increase tissue regeneration by delivering progenitor cells straight to the wound, which promotes angiogenesis and alleviates ECM formation. The main concept behind these stem cell-infused wound dressings is to give a contributing microenvironment for cellular activity of the wound. Traditional dressings mainly offer protection, but stem cell–infused dressings also provide Delivering Progenitor Cells; these dressings act as a vehicle for stem cells, typically mesenchymal stem cells (MSCs) or other relevant cell types, directly to the wound. To promote angiogenesis, stem cells have factors, which help in faster regrowth of new blood vessels, which are very crucial for the supply of nutrients. Also, it removes the waste of the healing process. To assist ECM formation, stem cells synthesize and organize the ECM, which is the functional structure that assists growth of cells and repairing of tissues [46].

Key Innovative Techniques and Technologies

Many techniques are used to create useful stem cell-infused wound dressing. Some are as follows:

Biomaterial Scaffolds:

i. **Biocompatible**: They are non-toxic and well tolerated by the body.
ii. **Biodegradable**: They are able to degrade over time, allowing for tissue integration.
iii. **Porous**: They provide space for cell growth, migration, and nutrient diffusion.
iv. **Mechanically stable**: During the application and healing, structural integrity is maintained.

Biomaterials that are common include:

i. **Collagen**: A natural protein that is found in skin that provides excellent biocompatibility and cell adherence.
ii. **Hyaluronic acid (HA)**: A glycosaminoglycan that boosts cell proliferation and migration.
iii. **Alginate**: A polysaccharide taken from algae that forms a gel-like matrix that can encapsulate cells.
iv. **Synthetic polymers**: Synthetic polymers such as poly lactic-co-glycolic acid (PLGA) that offers controlled mechanical properties and degradation rates.

Hydrogels are used as a matrix to load and deliver therapeutic agents. For example, Carbopol hydrogels can be used to deliver ONBs and drugs like collagenase. This approach can enhance oxygen supply to the wound, which is crucial for the healing process [47,48].

Cell Source and Preparation

The efficiency of dressing is impacted by the condition and type of stem cells. The common sources of cells include Mesenchymal Stem Cells (MSCs). These multipotent cells can differentiate into various cell types involved in tissue repair, such as fibroblasts, endothelial cells, and keratinocytes. MSCs can be acquired from several tissues, including bone marrow, adipose tissue, and the umbilical cord. Adipose-Derived Stromal Cells (ASCs): Similar to MSCs, ASCs are readily available and have demonstrated effectiveness in promoting skin regeneration. Induced Pluripotent Stem Cells (iPSCs): These cells are derived from adult cells that have been reprogrammed to an embryonic stem cell-like state [39]. The preparation of cells involves the following. Isolation and Expansion: To increase the number of stem cells, they are obtained from source tissues and later cluttered. Characterization:

To make sure that the stem cells have all the required properties and are valid. Delivery: The cells are preserved to maintain their validity and are loaded onto the biomaterial scaffold to keep them functioning [40,42,43].

Growth Factor and Cytokine Incorporation

To enhance the tissue's regrowth, the stem cell–infused dressings can be made according to growth factors and have signaling molecules that can regulate the cells like cytokines. Some examples are Vascular Endothelial Growth Factor (VEGF), which stimulates angiogenesis; PDGF, which promotes cell proliferation and migration; and Transforming Growth Factor-beta (TGF-β), which regulates ECM synthesis and remodeling. These factors can be directly incorporated into the biomaterial scaffold. These are released from stem cells, which naturally secrete a variety of growth factors, and delivered via NPs for controlled and sustained release [49,46].

Advanced Fabrication Techniques

Advanced composition methods are important to create dressings that have optimal properties as follows. Electrospinning: In this technique, nanofibers are created from polymer solution by using an electric field. It forms a scaffold that has a high surface-area-to-volume ratio [50]. 3D Bioprinting: This technology allows for the precise deposition of cells and biomaterials layer by layer, creating complex three-dimensional structures tailored to the wound defect [47]. Microfluidics: Fluid flow at the microscale can be controlled by this technology. It facilitates the creation of microengineered scaffolds [51].

Mechanisms of Action

Wound healing with the help of stem cell-infused dressings is promoted through various ways. The first type is Cellular Differentiation and Replacement, where stem cells that are delivered can be categorized into special cells, such as keratinocytes and fibroblast. They will replace the damaged tissues and restore the integrity of the skin. The second type is Paracrine Signaling, where stem cells have a variety of growth factors like cytokines and other signaling molecules that induce surrounding cells to take part in the healing process. This paracrine is important for boosting angiogenesis. It also reduces inflammation and stimulates ECM. The third one is Immunomodulation, where stem cells can also affect the response of the immune system, reduce the inflammation, and promote a more pleasing healing environment. The last one is ECM Remodeling, where the process of the synthesis and organization of the ECM is contributed by stem cells, which provides support and also promotes the process of regeneration of tissues [49,52,53].

Clinical application of stem cell–infused dressings embrace huge potential for treating a wide range of wounds that include chronic wounds like diabetic foot ulcers, venous leg ulcers, and pressure ulcers that are difficult to heal, as well as acute wounds like surgical wounds, burns, and injuries to quicken healing. Future directions include finding cost-effective types of stem cells and developing methods to improve their therapeutic potential, create dressings that respond to changes in the environment of the wound, and improve the time delivery methods of stem cells at the wound site [46].

Customization and Architectural Control

An individualized dressing can be made according to the needs of the patient through 3D printing, considering the points like size, depth, and geometry of the patient's wound. Using data from medical imaging (e.g., 3D scanning), customized designs can be generated. Computer-Aided Design (CAD) systems, such as the Computer-Aided System for Tissue Scaffolds (CASTS), facilitate the design of scaffolds with controlled architectures, including precise pore sizes, interconnectivity, and overall porosity. Mimicking the ECM, scaffolds are designed to emulate the natural ECM, providing structural support and a conducive environment for cell attachment, migration, proliferation, and differentiation. Precise control over pore size (ideally 100–400 μm for skin regeneration) and interconnectivity is crucial for nutrient diffusion, waste removal, and vascularization. Functionally Graded Scaffolds are natural tissues like bone that exhibit property gradients. 3D printing allows the fabrication of functionally graded scaffolds where properties like porosity and mechanical stiffness vary spatially within the structure, better matching the host tissue and improving integration [51,54].

Biomaterials for 3D-Printed Dressings and Scaffolds

The choice of material is critical for the success of 3D-printed wound care products. Materials must be biocompatible, often biodegradable, and possess appropriate mechanical and biological properties. Natural Polymers are often favored for their inherent biocompatibility and bioactivity. Chitosan, derived from chitin, is biodegradable, biocompatible, inherently antimicrobial, and hemostatic [55]. It promotes cell proliferation and tissue regeneration, making it highly suitable for wound dressings. Its positive charge interacts favorably with negatively charged biological surfaces. Collagen and gelatin, as major components of the natural ECM, provide excellent cell adhesion sites and support tissue formation [48]. Gelatin is also thermosensitive, which can be utilized in some printing and application processes. Alginate, extracted from seaweed, forms hydrogels in the presence of divalent cations (like Ca^{2+}). It is biocompatible, absorbent, and widely used in bioinks, where it is often blended with other polymers to improve cell adhesion. Hyaluronic acid (HA), a key glycosaminoglycan in the ECM, plays roles in hydration, cell signaling, and inflammation modulation. Silk fibroin, derived from silk, offers good mechanical strength and biocompatibility. Cellulose is abundant and biocompatible, and it is often used in modified forms (like carboxymethyl cellulose, CMC) or as bacterial cellulose for hydrogels and scaffolds. Synthetic polymers offer tunable mechanical properties, controlled degradation rates, and processability. PCL and PLA/PLGA, biodegradable polyester is commonly used for scaffold fabrication via FDM or SLS due to their thermoplastic nature and mechanical strength. PCL degrades slowly, making it suitable for long-term support, while PLA/PLGA offer tunable degradation rates. PEG and polyvinyl alcohol (PVA) are hydrophilic polymers that are often used to form hydrogels. PEG is biocompatible and reduces non-specific protein adsorption. PVA hydrogels can be formed via physical methods like freeze-thawing, avoiding chemical crosslinkers. Composite materials and hydrogels blend natural and synthetic polymers to enhance mechanical properties while retaining bioactivity. Hydrogels are particularly important as they form 3D networks capable of holding large amounts of water, creating a moist environment ideal for wound healing. Thermosensitive hydrogels (e.g., using Pluronic F-127) that transition from liquid to gel at body temperature are advantageous for extrusion printing and maintaining structural integrity post-printing [47,48,56].

Functionalization: Incorporating Bioactive Components

3D printing allows for the integration of various bioactive agents directly into the dressing or scaffold structure to enhance healing. Cells (Bioprinting): Techniques like inkjet and micro-extrusion printing that enable the deposition of living cells (fibroblasts, keratinocytes, stem cells) within hydrogel bioinks to create acellularized constructs or skin substitutes. This promotes faster tissue integration and regeneration. Growth Factors: Incorporating growth factors (e.g., VEGF for angiogenesis, EGF for epithelialization, and FGF for fibroblast proliferation) provides localized biochemical cues to stimulate specific stages of the healing process. Controlled release mechanisms ensure sustained activity. Antimicrobial Agents: To combat infection, a major complication in chronic wounds, antimicrobial agents like antibiotics (e.g., gentamicin, levofloxacin), silver NPs, or inherently antimicrobial polymers like chitosan can be loaded into the scaffold. Stimuli-responsive systems can release these agents on demand (e.g., in response to pH changes indicative of infection) [57,58].

Creating a Conducive Healing Environment

3D printed dressings and scaffolds facilitate wound healing by optimizing the local environment by Moisture Balance; hydrogel-based dressings maintain a moist wound environment, which is crucial for cell migration, preventing scab formation, and promoting epithelialization. The porosity can be tuned to manage exudate levels effectively. The next is Gas Exchange, in which the porous structure allows for adequate oxygen supply to the wound bed, which is essential for cellular metabolism and tissue viability, while also permitting the escape of carbon dioxide. The third one is Protection, in which the dressing acts as a physical barrier against external contaminants and bacterial invasion. The last one is Controlled Release, in which functionalized scaffolds provide sustained, localized delivery of therapeutic agents, improving efficacy and reducing systemic side effects [1,49].

Challenges and Future Directions

Despite significant progress, challenges remain. Achieving adequate and rapid vascularization within thick 3D-printed constructs is crucial for their survival and integration. The long-term biocompatibility and degradation profiles of novel materials require thorough investigation. Production at large scale, cost hurdles, and having approvals at every step are noticeable hurdles for more advancement. In future, innovations in the field of wound dressing will include the use of sensors and monitoring devices to monitor the healing of wounds. The emergence of 4D printing will help with the change in function or shape of dressing according to the wound, which offers possibilities that the dressing will be according to the wound to its least extent. We can also optimize better dressings by using 3D printing with both machine learning and artificial intelligence. It can help in predicting the healing outcomes.

To conclude, we can say that 3D printing is a powerful tool to make advance dressings for wounds. By customizing dressings, the use of bioactive components, and drug delivery by dressings, these can beat the many limitations of the traditional ways of dressings, especially the healing process for chronic wounds. Still, continuing the research and finding out new ways hold a promise for best healing processes.

NANOTECHNOLOGY-BASED WOUND DRESSINGS

Nanotechnology develops materials at the nanoscale, i.e., 1–100 nm, offers advanced solutions in wound management, and enhances properties such as drug delivery, antimicrobial activity, and regeneration of tissue while promoting healing. To improve the functionality of wound dressings, nanomaterials like nanofibers and NPs are incorporated into it. These materials prevent infections and promote cell proliferation [59]. Nanotechnology improves healing in many ways such as enhanced tissue regeneration that consists of nanofibers like ultra-fine fibers made by electrospinning technique, which encourages skin cells to grow, migrate, attach, and form new tissue and blood vessels more efficiently; next, it fights with bacterial infection with the rise of antibiotic-resistant strains. Antimicrobial NPs like silver, zinc oxide, gold, and copper integrate in nanodressings. These NPs play an important role in killing bacteria via several mechanisms that include disrupting the cell walls, interfering with important DNA and proteins, and creating harmful reactive oxygen species that makes it difficult for bacteria to develop resistance. Combination of NPs with other materials like chitosan or inserting them in hydrogels helps in controlling their release and decreasing toxicity [59].

The controlled drug delivery consists of nanomaterials such as polymeric NPs like chitosan, nanofibers, hydrogels, and so on; these include anti-inflammatory drugs, antibiotics, essential oils, plants extract, and growth factors that stimulate healing phases and stem cells. These nanomaterials permit them to be released gradually over time in response to specific wound conditions such as pH and bacterial enzymes. Another one is optimal healing environment, where nanodressing keeps a moist wound environment that is vital for healing, allows for necessary gas exchange, absorbs excess fluid, and offers protective walls against external impurities [60].

Nanomaterial-Based Wound Dressings

Manufacturing nanomaterial-based wound dressings, as illustrated in Figure 8.4, starts with synthesis and functionalization of NPs such as zinc oxide. To form nanocomposite mixture, these are then spread into a solution of polymer. By using methods like electrospinning, the mixture is fabricated into a scaffold, a nanofiber mat. Post-processing steps like crosslinking and freeze-drying improve stability and porosity. Lastly, the whole dressing undergoes sterilization and sterile packaging for clinical application [10,35].

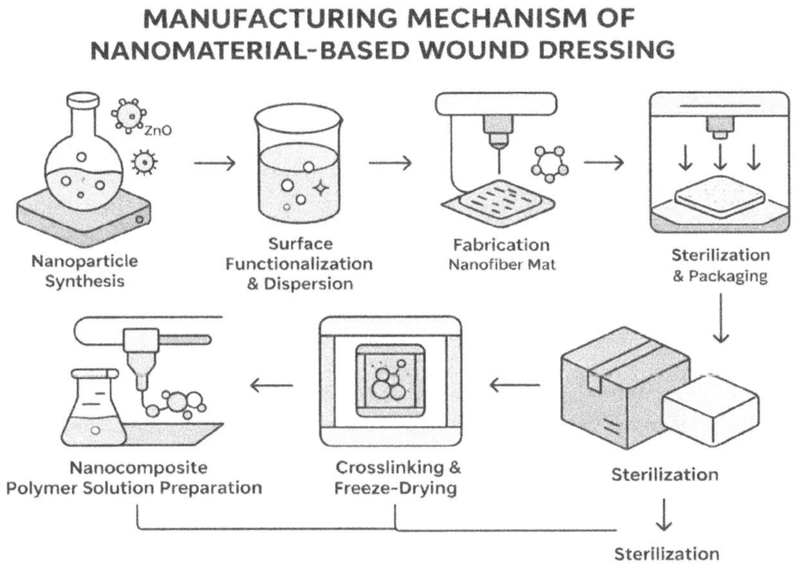

FIGURE 8.4 Nanomaterial-based wound dressings.

Types of Nanotechnology Dressings

Nanotechnology-based wound dressings come in several forms frequently using natural polymers, synthetic polymers, and both. Nanofiber mats mimic the ECM that promotes cell incorporation.

Hydrogels deliver drugs and keep the wound moist. Films protect and control permeability. Sponges have porous structures that are good for absorbing large amounts of exudate. Nanomaterials such as hydrogels or nanofibers are combined to attain numerous functions [43,61]. Smart dressings have nanosensors integrated in the dressings. These sensors help to monitor the condition of wounds such as temperature, pH, and level of oxygen, trigger drug release when needed, and create customized patient-specific scaffolds; technologies like 3D printing are also explored. Some challenges remain, such as long-term safety, biocompatibility and toxicity of some NPs, scaling up production cost-effectively, and navigating regulatory approval [31,38].

Electrospinning Techniques for Nanofiber Mats

Electrospinning method is used to produce nanofibers with diameters that range from nanometer to micrometer. Working mechanisms include electrical forces that stretch a liquid, such as a polymer solution or melt, into a jet that solidifies into fiber. Because of its unique properties and versatility of the resulting nanofiber mats, such as porosity and high surface area, this technique is used broadly [62,63]. The setup consists of high voltage source, collector plate, and spinneret. So, the liquid is driven via the spinneret, then high voltage is applied and an electrically charged jet is ejected toward the collector. The jet solidifies into a fiber when the solvent evaporates and cools down, then the jet endures twisting viability, which thins it down and forms nanofibers [64].

Some main factors influence the process and the outcome; adjusting these factors allows control over fiber diameter; these consist of properties of liquid such as conductivity, viscosity, surface tension and processing parameters like voltage, flow, distance, and the ambient conditions such as humidity and temperature. There are several electrospinning techniques like multi-needle setups for higher production, coaxial electrospinning for core sheath fibers, and melt electrospinning. Materials vary from several polymers to composites and also small molecules. Collector design and other manipulations of the electric field alignment and mat structure can be attained [65].

Electrospinning-Based Manufacturing Process for Nanocomposite Wound Dressings

The process of manufacturing nanocomposite wound dressings starts with two sources of polymer solution, one categorized as polymer solution and the other is Polycaprolactone/Polyethylene glycol (PCL/PEG + therapeutics). Then, these solutions are fed into the apparatus of electrospinning, polymer solution is emitted with spinneret, and nanofibers are assembled at a rotating drum; the process of electrospinning is categorized by a lightning bolt symbol that indicates the application of high voltage. After being electrospun and collected on the rotary drum as a nanofiber mat, the mat passes via crosslinking or curing oven. Then, it goes through UV sterilization, and the sterilized nanofiber mat is then cut and processed as a separate wound dressing unit. Lastly, the final wound dressings should be UV sterilized before they are used or packaged [50,66]. Figure 8.5 shows the process from start to the final product of wound dressing.

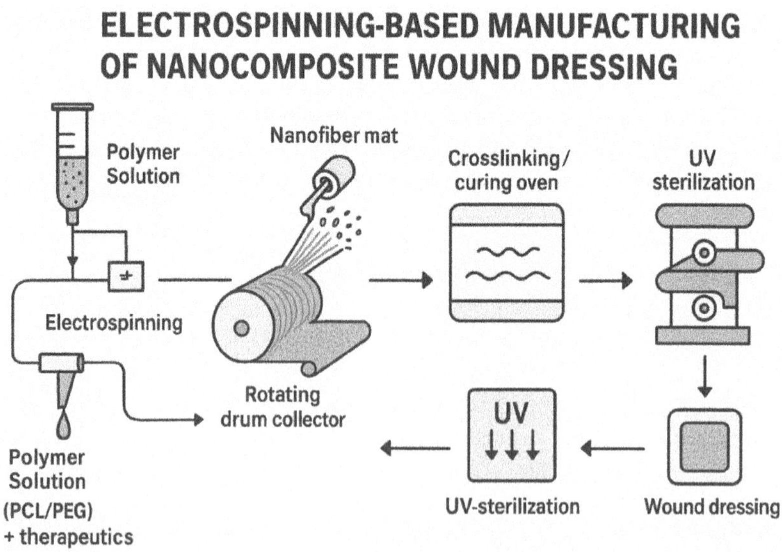

FIGURE 8.5 Electrospinning techniques for nanofiber mats.

Layer-by-Layer (L-b-L) Self-Assembly

This technique is used for creating complex ultra-thin films and multilayer films with detailed control over their nanoscale structure on a various range of substrates. In this method, the surface is dipped into a solution containing positively and negatively charged materials, such as polyanions and polycations, which stick together mostly via electrostatic attraction. Layer-by-Layer (L-b-L) also uses hydrogen bonding, charge transfer, and hydrophobic interactions, which expand the range of usable materials. In every step of dipping, rinsing is done to remove the excess resources and avoid infection. During assembly, the final thickness of film is controlled by adjusting material concentrations, number of layers, pH, salt content, and temperature during assembly [67] (Figure 8.6).

Other materials used in L-b-L consist of NPs, micelles, proteins, DNA, larger colloidal particles, and nanogels. To start the process of layering, the main condition is that the surface has an initial charge. This works on both surfaces' flat materials, such as glass, metals, silicon, and complex materials such as fibers, membranes, and NPs. This technique has shown substrates like cotton fabrics, polyester, glass, quartz, silicon, mica, metal electrodes, and carbon-based materials. Also, the integration of nanomaterials like clay NPs, carbon nanotube, silver NPs, and titanium dioxide NPs into films is used to improve specific functional properties [68].

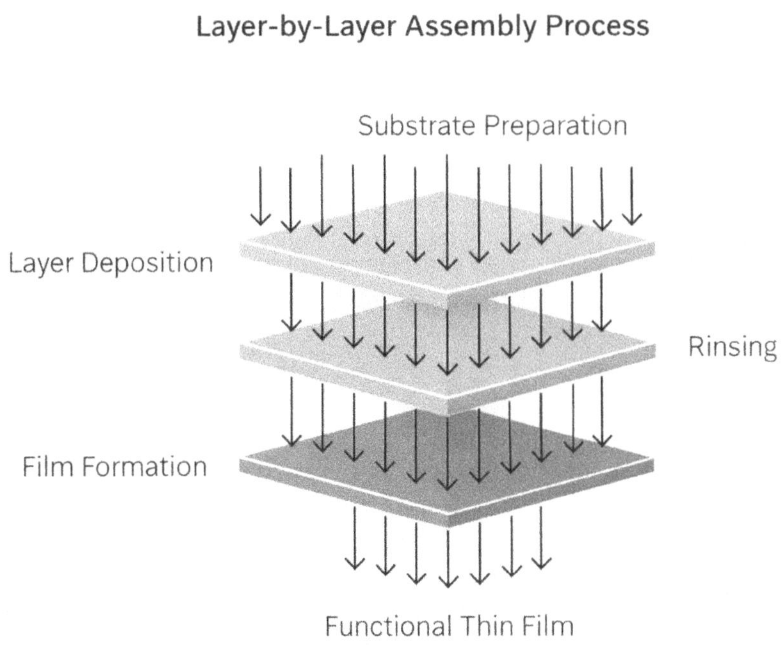

FIGURE 8.6 Layer-by-layer (L-b-L) self-assembly.

Diverse Applications of L-b-L Self-Assembly

Because of its ability to create coatings with custom-designed properties, L-b-L self-assembly is used widely across many fields. In the biomedical and healthcare sectors, it finds important efficacy in advanced drug delivery systems, tissue scaffolds, and wound healing, which recover implant surfaces and release medicines in a controlled way that contributes to improved patient outcomes. For textile materials, this method imparts multifunctionality including flame retardancy, antibacterial effects, improved resistance to UV radiation, water repellency, and electromagnetic shielding. It also plays an important part in developing sensitive sensors for detecting hydrogen and gases and in creating parts for nanoelectronics. Moreover, it also contributes to energy-related technologies, including solar energy conversion systems and components for fuel cells. Some key benefits of using L-b-L are that it is a low-cost and easy to implement method that doesn't need complex machines and can also be used in many research areas. It offers precise control over both the film thickness and internal structure, allowing fine tuning of material performance. This works with an exceptionally wide range of materials, making it adaptable for different purposes; it also enables the fabrication of films at any surface regardless of the size or shape. Additionally, this process is conducted under mild conditions such as room temperature and solution that are water-based, which is mainly beneficial for conserving the biological activity of delicate biomolecules that are incorporated into the films. It is an economical and highly effective method for creating advanced functional coating [68–72].

Surface Functionalization

Surface functionalization is a process in nanotechnology that includes adjusting the outermost layer of a material and its chemical, biological, and physical properties. To enhance the characteristics of materials such as nanofibers, this modification can transform an inert material like pristine graphene into a multi-purpose and reactive stage. These modifications can be purposely intended to get detailed functionalities for applications that range from drug delivery to biosensing, and they can also contact biological fluids that lead toward the formation of a bimolecular corona that influences the behavior of material. Monitoring nanomaterial surfaces is important for their safety and use [73,74]. The flow process is illustrated in Figure 8.7.

Methods of Surface Functionalization

Surface functionalization utilizes numerous simple methods like physical and chemical methods. Physical methods, such as physical vapor deposition, ion beam, and plasma treatment, play a role in changing the surface by using energy but don't create a strong chemical bond. Chemical methods include cross-linking, grafting, chelation, and wet chemical treatments that form strong covalent bonds between functional molecules and nanomaterial surfaces [73]. Nanotechnology-based techniques, including sol-gel methods, electroless deposition, atomic deposition, L-b-L assembly, and molecular imprinting, use nanoscale control to coat and functionalize pattern onto surfaces. Bio-inspired functionalization utilizes molecules such as dopamine

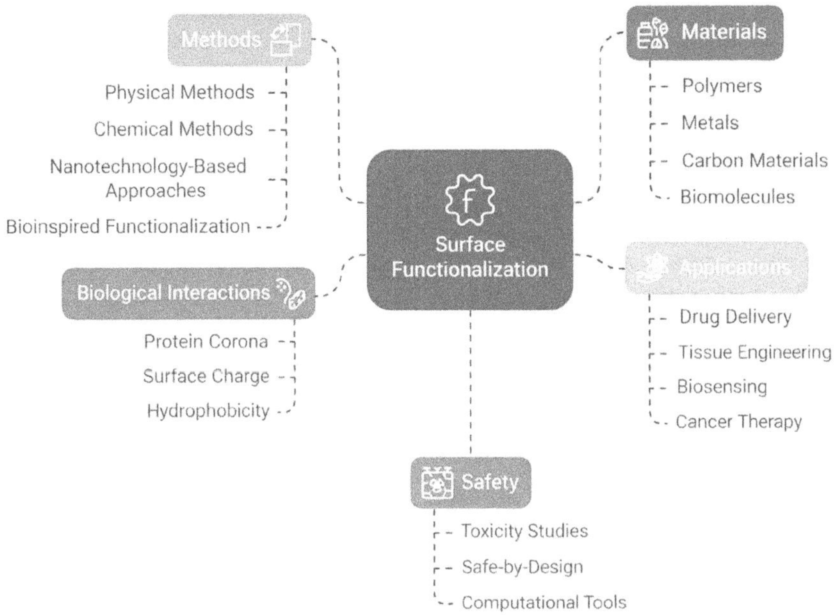

FIGURE 8.7 Surface functionalization process.

that mimic natural adhesion abilities, resulting in a multi-purpose coating strategy. Moreover, covalent functionalization directly attaches molecules such as polymers, DNA, and proteins, while non-covalent methods depend on weaker forces such as π–π stacking, electrostatic interactions, or hydrogen bonding, which help to preserve material's original properties. To modify their surface chemistry, plasma hydrogenation is applied to graphene-based materials [69].

Material Used for Surface Functionalization

To change the surface of nanomaterials, different materials are used depending on what they are needed for. Biocompatibility and solubility are improved by polymers such as PEG, dextran, chitosan, and polycaprolactone, while metals like silver, copper, gold, and nickel NPs offer conductive and antibacterial properties. Carbon materials such as graphene oxide proposed built-in functional groups for attachment. Some chemical groups such as –COOH, $-NH_2$, –OH, and halogens regulate surface charge and reactivity. For the attachment of cells, biomolecules like proteins and peptides help with biological interactions. Zinc oxide and nanohydroxyapatite offer special functional properties. Zwitterionic compounds help to prevent unwanted protein binding on surfaces [74].

Applications for Surface Functionalization

Surface functionalization plays a role in many applications, especially in medicine. In drug delivery, this helps in carrying more drug, control release, target specific area, and also increasing effectiveness. For repairing of tissue, these functionalized materials support the growth of cells and also mimic natural tissue. They also provide antibacterial properties and regenerate tissue during wound healing. Also, they help in detecting and visualizing specific biological markers in biosensing and imaging, as well as in the treatment of cancer, disease diagnosis, removing heavy metals, and improving conditions of cell culture. Nanomaterials via their surface interact with the body, where they attract biomolecules and form proteins that affect how the body reacts to them. Because of the stronger interactions with cell membranes, the positively charged surfaces are more harmful and the negatively charged surfaces are safer. Adding biocompatible coatings such as PEG helps in reducing toxicity, but small chemical groups can have mixed effects. The shape, size, and surface features of nanomaterials determine how cells take in these materials and where they end up in the body. Computational tools, such as molecular simulations and machine learning, combined with continued research, play a vital role in designing nanomaterials that perform effectively while remaining safe and sustainable over the long term [74–76].

Spray Coating and 3D Printing Nanotechnology

The merging of spray coating, 3D printing, and nanotechnology offers exciting paths for creating advanced materials and devices. To improve functionality by integrating nanomaterials, 3D printing allows for the precise fabrication of complex three-dimensional structures. Spray coating offers a multi-purpose method for spreading thin layers of materials, consisting of those incorporated with nanotechnology, onto numerous surfaces with 3D-printed objects [4,6].

3D Printing and Nanomaterials

3D printing, also called additive manufacturing, is a transformative technology that builds objects layer by layer on the basis of digital models. It helps in making detailed complex shapes that are useful in the healthcare sectors. It includes different methods such as light, extrusion, inkjet, or lasers. Nanotechnology works with super tiny materials ranging from 1 to 100 nm, having special properties. When nanomaterials are added to 3D printing, it's known as nano printing; this enhances strength, antibacterial effects, and conductivity, while also controlling drug release. For example, silver NPs are used in 3D printing that helps to prevent wounds and infections [32,33].

Spray Coating Techniques and Applications

Spray coating is a technique, which is used to spray fine tiny droplets of material onto a surface to create a coating. This method can be used on several different surface shapes and materials. With advancements in nanotechnology, spray coating is used to apply ultra-thin nanolayers with enhanced features such as water repellency, stain resistance, and antimicrobial properties. Ultrasonic spray technology uses the waves of sound that break clumps and then produce fine and even droplets. This makes sure that the nanosuspensions spread smoothly and evenly on the surface. So, the coatings are uniform and provide improved performance. Generally, it's used to enhance the properties of surfaces by using nanomaterials [77].

Combining Spray Coating and 3D Printing Nanotechnology

Combining 3D printing and spray coating with nanotechnology offers many benefits; spray coating plays a role in adding advanced features by special nanolayers onto 3D-printed parts, including water-repellency, antimicrobial properties, and stain resistance. It can also apply materials like conductive inks or electroluminescent layers to create interactive or glowing designs on complex shapes. Another technique that builds 3D structure by spraying powder at high speed shows how spray-based techniques can create both shapes and apply coating; this technique is known as cold additive manufacturing. Using smart materials that can sense or respond according to the environment, an advanced robotic spray system is developed to coat 3D-printed parts. With this, we can design multifunctional products and devices. This mix is opening new possibilities in many fields such as medicine, electronics, and advanced manufacturing [78–80].

Nano Silver Dressing Acticoat

Acticoat is a kind of wound dressing that uses nanocrystalline silver; it consists of very small particles of silver, created by using a special technology called nanotechnology. These tiny silver crystals are designed to manage wounds because they are highly reactive. Acticoat dressings typically contain layers of core material sandwiched between layers of mesh coated with this nanocrystalline silver. Also, an absorbent version is made with alginate. When the Acticoat dressing is moisturized with sterile water, it starts to release the nanocrystalline silver onto the wound surface, and this release lasts for several days such as 3–7 days, which means there is no need to change dressing daily like some older silver treatments such as silver sulfadiazine cream. Released silver attacks harmful microbes such as fungi and bacteria, damaging their cell walls and interfering with their important functions that include replicating their DNA and breathing, ultimately killing them [81].

Acticoat has strong and broad-spectrum antimicrobial action, which means that it is very effective against a wide variety of common wound bacteria and also consists of difficult ones such as Methicillin-Resistant *Staphylococcus aureus* (MRSA) and *Pseudomonas aeruginosa* and fungi. This helps in reducing overall bacterial load in wounds by killing these microbes. Other than fighting infection, Acticoat also supports the healing process, helps in reducing inflammation, and promotes the growth of new tissue; it also enhances the organization of collagen that leads to less damage. This is used on several types of wounds like burns, surgical wounds, chronic ulcers, and donor sites [82].

The main advantage of Acticoat is that it doesn't need to change frequently as compared to traditional silver creams or solutions, and this makes it easier and less painful for patients and reduces the cost of treatment. There is less pain while changing the dressings, so it's important to use Acticoat properly. This needs moisture to work efficiently. Silver-containing dressings need moisture to work but also harm healing cells at certain levels and can slightly delay skin closure, so they should be used cautiously and not combined with irritant products like povidone-iodine [83] (Figure 8.8).

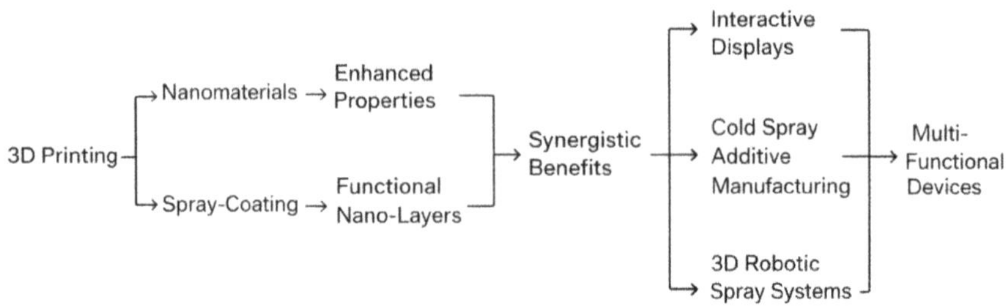

FIGURE 8.8 Spray coating and 3D printing nanotechnology.

Chitosan-Silver Nanocomposites

When we combine chitosan, a natural biopolymer, with silver NPs, we get an advanced material known as Chitosan-silver nanocomposites. Chitin is the source of the second most widely available natural polymer chitosan after cellulose. It is found in fungi, insects, and crustaceans [84]. Chitosan is well known for its beneficial biological properties, including biocompatibility, biodegradability, non-toxicity, and antimicrobial activity. Due to these properties, chitosan is suitable for different applications like dressings for wounds and drug delivery systems [85].

Synthesis Methods

The synthesis method of Chitosan-silver nanocomposites often includes combining AgNPs into a chitosan polymer matrix. Different methods like chemical reduction and reducing agents like sodium citrate or hydrazine hydrate reducing silver ions are used in the presence of chitosan. Green synthesis, which uses chitosan not only as a matrix but also as the stabilizing and reducing agent, is also a popular approach [83]. The amino and hydroxyl groups within the chitosan structure can lessen silver ions to metallic silver (Ag^0) and then cap the NPs, which prevents them from clumping together and ensures stability. Synthesis conditions like temperature (often elevated, e.g., 70°C–90°C) and pH (often alkaline, using NaOH) can affect the reaction rate and formation of NPs. The formation of AgNPs is usually shown by a change of color in the solution, often to brown or yellow. The amount of chitosan used can affect the size of the resulting AgNPs, with higher chitosan amounts sometimes leading to smaller NPs [54,86].

Properties and Characterization

ChAgNPs have unique properties derived from both chitosan and AgNPs. Techniques of characterization confirm their successful formation and structure. UV–Visible spectroscopy typically shows a surface plasmon resonance (SPR) peak characteristic of AgNPs, often in the 400–450 nm range. Techniques like Transmission Electron Microscopy (TEM) and Scanning Electron Microscopy (SEM) disclose the morphology and size of the NPs, which are often spherical and typically range from a few nanometers to around 50 nm that are dispersed within the chitosan matrix [55]. X-ray Diffraction (XRD) confirms the crystalline nature of the embedded AgNPs and can show changes in chitosan's crystallinity upon nanocomposite formation. Fourier Transform Infrared Spectroscopy (FTIR) identifies functional groups and interactions, often showing shifts in chitosan's characteristic peaks (like those for –OH and $-NH_2$ groups) due to bonding with AgNPs. Zeta potential measurements indicate the surface charge and stability of the nanocomposites in dispersion; positive values (e.g., +19 mV to +56 mV) suggest good stability due to electrostatic repulsion. Thermogravimetric analysis (TGA) and Differential Scanning Calorimetry (DSC) can assess thermal stability, which sometimes shows enhanced stability compared to pure chitosan [87].

Antibacterial Activity and Applications

A key characteristic of ChAgNPs is its enhanced antibacterial property compared to chitosan alone. This is very effective against a broad range of bacteria, including both Gram-positive (like *S. aureus*) and Gram-negative (like *Escherichia coli* and *P. aeruginosa*) strains, and even some fungi [88]. The process involves the synergistic effects of chitosan, which disrupts bacterial membranes via its positive charge and AgNPs release silver ions, which generate reactive oxygen species, interact with thiol groups in proteins, and damage DNA. Smaller AgNPs normally show higher activity. Due to these properties, ChAgNPs are explored to use in various forms, mainly as antibacterial agents for wound dressings, food packaging, antibacterial coatings (e.g., for mobile phones), and antifungal agents in agriculture. They also show antioxidant and wound healing properties, which makes them multifunctional. Studies often show that ChAgNPs induced wound closure, reduced inflammation, and enhanced tissue regeneration [81,89] (Figure 8.9).

Characteristic	Chitosan	Silver Nanoparticles	Chitosan-Silver Nanocomposites
Source	Derived from chitin, abundant natural polymer	Metallic element, often from silver nitrate	Combination of chitosan and silver nanoparticles
Properties	Biocompatible, biodegradable, non-toxic, antimicrobial	Antibacterial properties, surface plasmon resonance	Enhanced antibacterial activity, antioxidant, wound-healing
Synthesis	Matrix for nanoparticle incorporation	Incorporated into chitosan matrix	Chemical reduction, green synthesis methods
Characterization	Functional groups, interactions	Surface plasmon resonance peak	UV-Vis, TEM, SEM, XRD, FTIR, Zeta potental, TGA, DSC
Characterization	Functional groups, interactions	Surface plasmon resonance peak	UV-Vis, TEM, SEM, XRD, FTIR, Zeta potental, TGA, DSC
Applications	Wound dressings, drug delivery systems	Antibacterial agent	Antibacterial materials, wound dressings, food packaging, coatings

FIGURE 8.9 Comparison of Chitosan silver nanocomposites.

Hydrogel Dressings with Embedded Nanoparticles

Hydrogel dressings are advanced dressings that are used to cover wounds. They maintain a moist environment around the wound because they resemble soft, water-rich gels, which are recognized to speed up the process of healing [45]. These dressings are beneficial because they absorb excess fluid and allow the skin to breathe, and these dressings are soft and gentle on the skin. Tiny particles are integrated into the hydrogel structure to improve their healing characteristics and the ability to kill harmful microbes [90,91].

NPs that are derived from metals like silver, copper, gold, and zinc are incorporated into hydrogels to enhance wound management; the main function of these NPs is to provide antimicrobial properties, prevent from having infections that can delay the healing process, or lead to any complications [92]. NPs accomplish this via several mechanisms, including disrupting cell walls of bacteria and interfering with their essential processes. Besides fighting infection, various NPs also possess anti-inflammatory properties, which can cause the skin tissue regeneration and form new blood vessels, that is, angiogenesis. Among several types that are utilized, silver NPs are used frequently because of their broad-spectrum efficiency against bacteria, fungi, viruses, which also reduces inflammation and enhances better regeneration of tissue [93,94]. Gold NPs are appreciated for their antioxidant and anti-inflammatory effects that help to protect healing tissue from oxidative stress and also support angiogenesis through their antimicrobial strength that might be less effective than silver unless combined with other activated external stimuli like light. Zinc oxide and copper oxide also play an important role in rebuilding the skin's ECM. Often, combinations of different NPs are used synergistically within a single hydrogel dressing to maximize therapeutic benefits by leveraging the unique advantages of each nanoparticle type. The integration of NPs into hydrogel dressings has many advantages for wound care. It controls infections, reduces reliance on traditional antibiotics, and helps to combat the growing issue of antibiotic resistance. These dressings improve the quality of tissue repair and healing [33,95].

Nano-Enhanced Foams and Films

Nano-enhanced foams include integrating tiny particles, known as NPs, into foam structures to advance their properties, particularly stability. These foams contain gas bubbles dispersed within a continuous liquid phase, often stabilized by substances like surfactants. NPs, characteristically ranging from 1 to 100 nm in size, are added to improve this stability, especially under challenging conditions like high temperatures and pressures often found in industrial applications. Similarly, nano-enhanced films can be formed, sometimes in layered structures with foams, to attain specific properties like electromagnetic interference (EMI) shielding [96].

Stabilization Mechanisms

The main role of NPs in foams is stabilization. Foams are naturally unstable and tend to break down through processes like drainage liquid flowing out, coarsening smaller bubbles merging into larger ones, and coalescence bubbles rupturing and combining. NPs help to counter these processes. They can adsorb irreversibly onto the gas–liquid interfaces on the surface of the bubbles due to high adsorption energy [48].

This makes a protective layer or network. This layer delays liquid drainage from the thin films that are lamellae, separating bubbles, increases the film's elasticity and viscosity, and acts as a barrier preventing bubbles from merging or gas from diffusing between them. The effectiveness frequently depends on the nanoparticle's properties, such as size and wettability, and how well they interact with the liquid. Particles with intermediate hydrophobicity are often most effective [76].

Several NPs are used, with silicon dioxide being common due to its abundance, cost-effectiveness, and favorable surface chemistry. Other NPs like aluminum oxide, calcium carbonate, titanium dioxide, iron oxides, carbon dots, and MXene, which is a type of 2D material, have also been explored. Often, NPs need surface modification to achieve optimality, especially in harsh conditions like high salinity or temperature, where they might otherwise aggregate. Modification techniques include altering surface groups like adjusting hydrophobicity by controlling Si-OH groups on SiO_2, adding surfactants, or grafting functional groups or long-chain molecules onto the nanoparticle surface. For instance, treating SiO_2 NPs to achieve moderate hydrophobic contact angles around 90 degrees can significantly enhance foam stability. Combining NPs with surfactants often shows synergistic effects, enhancing stability further [92,96].

Nano-enhanced foams have significant applications in Enhanced Oil Recovery. In this, the foams help control the mobility of injected gases such as CO_2, N_2, or methane, preventing them from bypassing oil zones through high-permeability channels or due to gravity override, thus improving oil sweep efficiency. NPs enhance foam stability under harsh reservoir conditions like high temperature, salinity, and the presence of oil, making this process more effective. Studies show that nanoparticle-stabilized foams can increase oil recovery significantly. Foams, including nano-enhanced ones, are also used for CO_2 sequestration, improving storage capacity by trapping CO_2 more effectively in subsurface formations. Other applications include foamed concrete, where NPs like nano-Al_2O_3 improve foam stability, leading to a uniform pore structure and enhanced mechanical strength. Layered foam/film polymer nanocomposites using materials like MXene and Si-C nanowires show promise for lightweight, efficient EMI shielding with low reflection [96,97] (Figure 8.10).

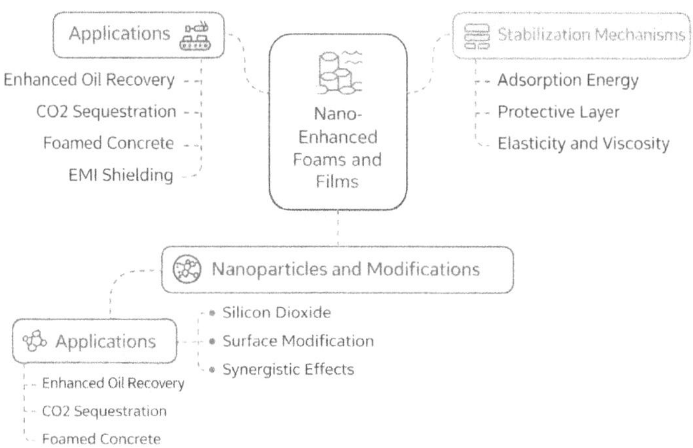

FIGURE 8.10 Properties, mechanisms, and applications of nano-enhanced foams and films.

REFERENCES

1. F. Mahyudin, M. Edward, M. H. Basuki, Y. Basrewan, and A. Rahman, "Modern and Classic Wound Dressing Comparison in Wound Healing, Comfort and Cost," *Jurnal Ners*, vol. 15, no. 1, pp. 31–36, Apr. 2020. doi:10.20473/jn.v15i1.16597.
2. V. Kotteeswaran, M. Saravanakumar, R. M. Alexander, R. S. Nair, and K. M. Ramnath, "Advancement of Nanofibers in Wound Healing: A Review," 2024. doi:10.13005/bpj/2953.
3. M. Rybka, Ł. Mazurek, and M. Konop, "Beneficial Effect of Wound Dressings Containing Silver and Silver Nanoparticles in Wound Healing—From Experimental Studies to Clinical Practice," 2023. doi:10.3390/life13010069.
4. K. Anderson and R. L. Hamm, "Factors that Impair Wound Healing," 2012. doi:10.1016/j.jccw.2014.03.001.
5. S. Guo and L. A. DiPietro, "Critical Review in Oral Biology & Medicine: Factors Affecting Wound Healing," *J Dent Res*, vol. 89, no. 3, pp. 219–229, 2010. doi:10.1177/0022034509359125.
6. F. Rosyid, "Wounds: Physiological Mechanisms and Factors Affecting Healing," *Int J Res Med Sci*, vol. 10, no. 4, p. 1001, 2022. doi:10.18203/2320-6012.ijrms20221000.
7. Fda, "Guidance for Industry Chronic Cutaneous Ulcer and Burn Wounds—Developing Products for Treatment," 2006. https://www.fda.gov/cdrh/ggpmain.html
8. R. Wolcott, K. Cutting, S. Dowd, and S. Percival, "Types of Wounds and Infections," In: S. Percival, K. Cutting, and B. Lipsky (Eds.), *Microbiology of Wounds*, CRC Press, 2010, pp. 219–232. https://doi.org/10.1201/9781420079944-7.
9. S. Jais, "Various Types of Wounds That Diabetic Patients Can Develop: A Narrative Review," 2023. doi:10.1177/2632010X231205366.
10. F. Abaszadeh, M. H. Ashoub, G. Khajouie, and M. Amiri, "Nanotechnology Development in Surgical Applications: Recent Trends and Developments," 2023. doi:10.1186/s40001-023-01429-4.
11. C. Münter, D. Doughty, J. L. Lázaro Martínez, and P. Scnct, *Advances in Wound Care: The Triangle of Wound Assessment* [Position document]. World Union of Wound Healing Societies, 2016. www.wuwhs.net.
12. M. Pollini, R. Striani, F. Paladini, A. Kiani, M. R. Acocella, and C. Esposito Corcione, "Nanotechnological Antibacterial and Conductive Wound Dressings for Pressure Ulcer Prevention," *Nanomaterials*, vol. 14, no. 15, 2024. doi:10.3390/nano14151309.
13. L. E. Edsberg, J. M. Black, M. Goldberg, L. McNichol, L. Moore, and M. Sieggreen, "Revised National Pressure Ulcer Advisory Panel Pressure Injury Staging System," *J Wound Ostomy Contin Nursing*, vol. 43, no. 6, pp. 585–597, 2016. doi:10.1097/WON.0000000000000281.
14. D. Stang and M. Young, "Selection and Application of a Diabetic Foot Ulcer Classification System in Scotland: Part 2," 2018.
15. P. H. Wang, B. S. Huang, H. C. Horng, C. C. Yeh, and Y. J. Chen, "Wound Healing," *J Chin Med Assoc*, 2018. doi:10.1016/j.jcma.2017.11.002.
16. S. Mani, "Wound Healing and It's Importance: A Review," *MCMed J*, 2012. www.mcmed.us/journal/dps
17. S. Mani, "Wound Healing and It's Importance-A Review," www.mcmed.us/journal/dps.
18. X. Zhou et al., "3D Printing-based Hydrogel Dressings for Wound Healing," *Adv Sci*, 2024. doi:10.1002/advs.202404580.
19. T. Sangnim, V. Puri, D. Dheer, D. N. Venkatesh, K. Huanbutta, and A. Sharma, "Nanomaterials in the Wound Healing Process: New Insights and Advancements," *Pharmaceutics*, 2024. doi:10.3390/pharmaceutics16030300.
20. A. Brown, "The Principles of Holistic Wound Assessment," *Nursing Times*. www.nursingtimes.net
21. K. Zulkowski, *Wound Classification*. Montana State University.

22. C. Dowsett and H. Newton, "Wound Bed Preparation: TIME in Practice," *Wounds UK*, vol. 1, 2005, pp. 58–70.
23. L. Van Rijswijk and M. Eisenberg, "Wound Assessment and Documentation," *Ostomy Wound Management*. https://www.o-wm.com/article/association-
24. S. Li, P. Renick, J. Senkowsky, A. Nair, and L. Tang, "Diagnostics for Wound Infections," *Wound Repair Reg*, 2021. doi:10.1089/wound.2019.1103.
25. N. B. S. Silva, L. A. Marques, and D. D. B. Röder, "Diagnosis of Biofilm Infections: Current Methods Used, Challenges and Perspectives for the Future," *J Appl Microbiol*. 2021. doi:10.1111/jam.15049.
26. E. Haesler, T. Swanson, K. Ousey, and K. Carville, "Clinical Indicators of Wound Infection and Biofilm: Reaching International Consensus," *J Wound Care*, vol. 28, no. Sup3b, pp. S4–S12, 2019. doi:10.12968/jowc.2019.28.sup3b.s4.
27. R. Alipoor, M. Ayan, M. R. Hamblin, R. Ranjbar, and S. Rashki, "Hyaluronic Acid-Based Nanomaterials as a New Approach to the Treatment and Prevention of Bacterial Infections," *Front Bioeng Biotechnol,* 2022, doi:10.3389/fbioe.2022.913912.
28. A. Brown, "The Assessment and Treatment of Wound Pain," *Nursing Times*, 2015. www.nursingtimes.net.
29. R. White, "A multinational Survey of the Assessment of Pain When Removing Dressings," *Wounds UK*, vol. 4, pp. 14–22, 2008.
30. H. M. Nguyen, T. T. Ngoc Le, A. T. Nguyen, H. N. Thien Le, and T. T. Pham, "Biomedical Materials for Wound Dressing: Recent Advances and Applications," *RSC Adv*, 2023. doi:10.1039/d2ra07673j.
31. N. Rani Raju, E. Silina, V. Stupin, N. Manturova, S. B. Chidambaram, and R. R. Achar, "Multifunctional and Smart Wound Dressings—A Review on Recent Research Advancements in Skin Regenerative Medicine," 2022, *Pharmaceutics*. doi:10.3390/pharmaceutics14081574.
32. A. E. Stoica, C. Chircov, and A. M. Grumezescu, "Nanomaterials for Wound Dressings: An Up-to-Date Overview," *Molecules*. 2020. doi:10.3390/molecules25112699.
33. Q. Pang, Z. Jiang, K. Wu, R. Hou, and Y. Zhu, "Nanomaterials-based Wound Dressing for Advanced Management of Infected Wound," *Antibiotics*, 2023. doi:10.3390/antibiotics12020351.
34. "Introduction to Smart Textile-Passive Smart Textile, Active Smart Textile," In: In: P. Kumar (Ed.), *Smart Textiles and Wearable Technologies*, Springer, 2022, pp. 1–18.
35. S. Nasra, S. Pramanik, V. Oza, K. Kansara, and A. Kumar, "Advancements in Wound Management: Integrating Nanotechnology and Smart Materials for Enhanced Therapeutic Interventions," *Nanosc Res Lett*, 2024. doi:10.1186/s11671-024-04116-3.
36. B. Ellouze and M. Damak, "The Use of Smart Textiles in the Healthcare Space: Towards an Improvement of the User-Patient Experience," *J Textile Sci Technol*, vol. 10, no. 02, pp. 41–50, 2024. doi:10.4236/jtst.2024.102003.
37. V. R. Ragnaboina, T. M. Jang, S. Han, and S. W. Hwang, "Recent Advancements in Smart Bandages for Wound Healing," *J Sensor Sci Technol*, vol. 32, no. 6, pp. 357–369, 2023. doi:10.46670/JSST.2023.32.6.357.
38. M. Naser, M. M. Nasr, and L. H. Shehata, "Smart Wound Dressings Integrating Biosensors for Real-Time Monitoring of Wound Conditions," *Int J Progre Sci Technol*, vol. 48, no. 2, pp. 456–488, 2025. https://ijpsat.org/
39. S. Saghazadeh et al., "Drug Delivery Systems and Materials for Wound Healing Applications," *Adv Drug Deliv Rev*, 2018. doi:10.1016/j.addr.2018.04.008.
40. J. S. Boateng, K. H. Matthews, H. N. E. Stevens, and G. M. Eccleston, "Wound Healing Dressings and Drug Delivery Systems: A Review," *J Pharm Sci*, 2008. doi:10.1002/jps.21210.
41. S. Hassan, M. N. Ali, M. Mir, A. Ahmed, and M. Arshad, "Development and Evaluation of Drug Delivery Patch for Topical Wound Healing Application," *SN Appl Sci*, vol. 3, no. 10, 2021. doi:10.1007/s42452-021-04809-9.

42. W. Ren, M. Sands, X. Han, M. Tsipursky, and J. Irudayaraj, "Hydrogel-Based Oxygen and Drug Delivery Dressing for Improved Wound Healing," *ACS Omega*, vol. 9, no. 22, pp. 24095–24104, 2024. doi:10.1021/acsomega.4c03324.
43. R. Abdulhussain, A. Adebisi, B. R. Conway, and K. Asare-Addo, "Electrospun Nanofibers: Exploring Process Parameters, Polymer Selection, and Recent Applications in Pharmaceuticals and Drug Delivery," *J Drug Deliv Sci Technol*, vol. 90, 2023. doi:10.1016/j.jddst.2023.105156.
44. S. M. Galvis Escobar, J. D. Molina Sierra, J. P. Ruíz Soto, M. A. Rego Londoño, and C. Pineda Molina, "Skin Wound Classification and Therapeutic Techniques for Skin Repair," *CES Enfermería*, vol. 4, no. 2, pp. 26–41, 2023. doi:10.21615/cesenferm.7262.
45. Y. Wang, M. Zhang, Z. Yan, S. Ji, S. Xiao, and J. Gao, "Metal Nanoparticle Hybrid Hydrogels: The State-of-the-Art of Combining Hard and Soft Materials to Promote Wound Healing," 2024. doi:10.7150/thno.91829.
46. A. El-Badawy and N. El-Badri, "Clinical Efficacy of Stem Cell Therapy for Diabetes Mellitus: A Meta-Analysis," *PLoS One*, vol. 11, no. 4, 2016. doi:10.1371/journal.pone.0151938.
47. Y. Jadhav, O. Bhingoli, A. Mali, V. Pawar, and V. Shinde, "Leveraging 3D Printing for Advanced Wound Dressing Technologies by Using Polymeric Materials and Polymeric Biomaterials," 2025. doi:10.1016/j.hybadv.2024.100364.
48. A. C. Bîrcă et al., "Nanoparticle-Enhanced Collagen Hydrogels for Chronic Wound Management," *J Funct Biomater*, vol. 16, no. 3, 2025. doi:10.3390/jfb16030091.
49. B. Farabi, K. Roster, R. Hirani, K. Tepper, M. F. Atak, and B. Safai, "The Efficacy of Stem Cells in Wound Healing: A Systematic Review," 2024. doi:10.3390/ijms25053006.
50. J. Xue, T. Wu, Y. Dai, and Y. Xia, "Electrospinning and Electrospun Nanofibers: Methods, Materials, and Applications," 2019. *Am Chem Soc*. doi:10.1021/acs.chemrev.8b00593.
51. S. M. Naghib, S. N. Hosseini, and A. Beigi, "3D 4D Printing of Chitosan-based Scaffolds for Wound Dressing Applications," 2024. doi:10.1016/j.carpta.2024.100594.
52. S. Wu, S. Sun, W. Fu, Z. Yang, H. Yao, and Z. Zhang, "The Role and Prospects of Mesenchymal Stem Cells in Skin Repair and Regeneration," 2024. doi:10.3390/biomedicines12040743.
53. X. Chen et al., "The Role of Gel Wound Dressings Loaded with Stem Cells in the Treatment of Diabetic Foot Ulcers," 2021. www.ajtr.org
54. S. Alven and B. A. Aderibigbe, "Chitosan-Based Scaffolds Incorporated with Silver Nanoparticles for the Treatment of Infected Wounds," 2024. doi:10.3390/pharmaceutics16030327.
55. H. L. Loo, B. H. Goh, L. H. Lee, and L. H. Chuah, "Application of Chitosan-based Nanoparticles in Skin Wound Healing," 2022. doi:10.1016/j.ajps.2022.04.001.
56. K. Las Heras, M. Igartua, E. Santos-Vizcaino, and R. M. Hernandez, "Cell-based Dressings: A Journey through Chronic Wound Management," 2022. doi:10.1016/j.bioadv.2022.212738.
57. A. A. El-Kheir and L. K. El-Gabry, "Potential Applications of Nanotechnology in Functionalization of Synthetic Fibres (A Review)," *Egypt J Chem*, vol. 65, no. 9, pp. 67–85, 2022. doi:10.21608/EJCHEM.2022.106369.4891.
58. J. Domínguez-Robles et al., "Poly(Caprolactone)/Lignin-based 3D-Printed Dressings Loaded with a Novel Combination of Bioactive Agents for Wound-Healing Applications," *Sustain Mater Technol*, vol. 35, 2023. doi:10.1016/j.susmat.2023.e00581.
59. J. A. Ataide et al., "Nanotechnology-Based Dressings for Wound Management," 2022.
60. A. Tahir et al., "Nanotechnology-based Approaches for Efficient Wound Monitoring and Healing," *Pakist BioMed J*, pp. 10–18, 2023. doi:10.54393/pbmj.v6i12.974.
61. Q. Bai et al., "Potential Applications of Nanomaterials and Technology for Diabetic Wound Healing," 2020. doi:10.2147/IJN.S276001.

62. A. Nadaf et al., "Recent Update on Electrospinning and Electrospun Nanofibers: Current Trends and their Applications," 2022. doi:10.1039/d2ra02864f.
63. P. Ramesh Kumar, N. Khan, S. Vivekanandhan, N. Satyanarayana, A. K. Mohanty, and M. Misra, "Nanofibers: Effective Generation by Electrospinning and their Applications," *J Nanosci Nanotechnol*, 2012, pp. 1–25. doi:10.1166/jnn.2012.5111.
64. A. Haider, S. Haider, and I. K. Kang, "A Comprehensive Review Summarizing the Effect of Electrospinning Parameters and Potential Applications of Nanofibers in Biomedical and Biotechnology," 2018. doi:10.1016/j.arabjc.2015.11.015.
65. A. Ahmadian, A. Shafiee, N. Aliahmad, and M. Agarwal, "Overview of Nano-Fiber Mats Fabrication via Electrospinning and Morphology Analysis," 2021. doi:10.3390/textiles1020010.
66. M. S. Islam, B. C. Ang, A. Andriyana, and A. M. Afifi, "A Review on Fabrication of Nanofibers Via Electrospinning and their Applications," 2019. doi:10.1007/s42452-019-1288-4.
67. C. Gallo et al., "Synergistic Nanocoating with Layer-by-Layer Functionalized PCL Membranes Enhanced by Manuka Honey and Essential Oils for Advanced Wound Healing," *Sci Rep*, vol. 14, no. 1, 2024. doi:10.1038/s41598-024-71466-4.
68. L. Wågberg and J. Erlandsson, "The Use of Layer-by-Layer Self-Assembly and Nanocellulose to Prepare Advanced Functional Materials," 2021. doi:10.1002/adma.202001474.
69. M. J. McShane and Y. M. Lvov, "Electrostatic Self-Assembly: Layer-by-Layer," In: J. A. Schwarz, S. E. Lyshevski, & C. I. Contescu (Eds.), *Dekker Encyclopedia of Nanoscience and Nanotechnology, Third Edition*, Taylor & Francis, 2014, pp. 1342–1358. doi:10.1081/e-enn3-120013616.
70. W. Tian, A. VahidMohammadi, Z. Wang, L. Ouyang, M. Beidaghi, and M. M. Hamedi, "Layer-by-layer self-assembly of pillared two-dimensional multilayers," *Nat Commun*, vol. 10, no. 1, 2019. doi:10.1038/s41467-019-10631-0.
71. D. Rawtani and Y. K. Agrawal, "ARTICLE Nanobiomedicine Emerging Strategies and Applications of Layer-by-layer Self-Assembly," *Nanobiomedicine*, vol. 1, pp. 1–8, 2014.
72. D. Dey, M. N. Islam, S. A. Hussain, and D. Bhattacharjee, "Layer by Layer (LbL) Technique for Fabrication of Electrostatic Self Assembled Ultrathin Films," 2008. https://www.ripublication.com/ijpap.htm
73. D. Kulkarni et al., "Surface Functionalization of Nanofibers: The Multifaceted Approach for Advanced Biomedical Applications," 2022. doi:10.3390/nano12213899.
74. Z. Guo et al., "Surface Functionalization of Graphene-Based Materials: Biological Behavior, Toxicology, and Safe-By-Design Aspects," 2021. doi:10.1002/adbi.202100637.
75. M. Afshar et al., "Nanomaterial Strategies in Wound Healing: A Comprehensive Review of Nanoparticles, Nanofibres and Nanosheets," 2024. doi:10.1111/iwj.14953.
76. K. Jangir, U. Kumar, N. K. Suniya, N. Singh, and K. Parihar, "Enhancing the Aqueous foam Stability Using Nanoparticles: A Review," 2022. doi:10.12691/wjce-10-2-5.
77. Y. Pan et al., "Layer-by-Layer Self-Assembly Coating for Multi-Functionalized Fabrics: A Scientometric Analysis in CiteSpace (2005–2021)," 2022. doi:10.3390/molecules27196767.
78. M. E. Astaneh and N. Fereydouni, "Silver Nanoparticles in 3D Printing: A New Frontier in Wound Healing," *Am Chem Soc,* 2024. doi:10.1021/acsomega.4c04961.
79. X. Zhou et al., "3D Printing-Based Hydrogel Dressings for Wound Healing," 2024. doi:10.1002/advs.202404580.
80. A. G. Tabriz and D. Douroumis, "Recent advances in 3D printing for wound healing: A systematic review," 2022. doi:10.1016/j.jddst.2022.103564.
81. R. Thakur, G. Jambheshwar, A. Chaudhury, P. Kaur, and A. Choudhary, "Synthesis of Chitosan-Silver Nanocomposites and their Antibacterial Activity," *Int J Sci Eng Res*, vol. 4, no. 4, 2013. https://www.ijser.org

82. D. Chicea, A. Nicolae-Maranciuc, and L. M. Chicea, "Silver Nanoparticles-Chitosan Nanocomposites: A Comparative Study Regarding Different Chemical Syntheses Procedures and their Antibacterial Effect," *Materials*, vol. 17, no. 5, 2024. doi:10.3390/ma17051113.
83. V. N. Okafor, B. A. Abimbola, A. D. Iwe, and O. F. Mbume, "Comparative Studies of Chitosan-Silver Nanocomposites from Commercial and Biowaste Sources," *Nanochem Res*, vol. 8, no. 1, pp. 78–86, 2023. doi:10.22036/ncr.2023.01.008.
84. G. Vanti et al., "Synthesis and Characterization of Multifunctional Chitosan–Silver Nanoparticles: An In-Vitro Approach for Biomedical Applications," *Pharmaceuticals*, vol. 17, no. 9, 2024. doi:10.3390/ph17091229.
85. G. J. C. Canama, M. C. L. Delco, R. A. Talandron, and N. P. Tan, "Synthesis of Chitosan-Silver Nanocomposite and Its Evaluation as an Antibacterial Coating for Mobile Phone Glass Protectors," *ACS Omega*, vol. 8, no. 20, pp. 17699–17711, 2023. doi:10.1021/acsomega.3c00191.
86. G. Ramachandran et al., "Chitosan/Silver Nanocomposites Enhanced the Biofilm Eradication in Biofilm Forming Gram Positive *S. aureus*," *J King Saud Univ Sci*, vol. 35, no. 4, 2023. doi:10.1016/j.jksus.2023.102597.
87. S. Gowda and S. Sriram, "Green Synthesis of Chitosan Silver Nanocomposites and Their Antifungal Activity against Colletotrichum Truncatum Causing Anthracnose in Chillies," *Plant Nano Biology*, vol. 5, 2023. doi:10.1016/j.plana.2023.100041.
88. A. Regiel, "Chitosan-Silver Nanocomposites-Modern Antibacterial Materials," https://www.ecdc.europa.eu/en/publications/Publications/0909_TER_
89. S. O. Ogungbesan et al., "Synthesis and Characterization of Chitosan–Silver Nanocomposite Film: Antibacterial and Cytotoxicity Study," *ChemistrySelect*, vol. 9, no. 42, 2024. doi:10.1002/slct.202404909.
90. F. M. Aldakheel et al., "Green Silver Nanoparticle-Embedded Chitosan-Alginate Hydrogel: A Novel Antibacterial Approach for Potential Wound Healing," *Polym Compos*, vol. 33, 2025. doi:10.1177/09673911251320463.
91. Y. Liu, S. Song, S. Liu, X. Zhu, and P. Wang, "Application of Nanomaterial in Hydrogels Related to Wound Healing," 2022. doi:10.1155/2022/4656037.
92. C. Liang et al., "Advances in the Application of Mxene Nanoparticles in Wound Healing," 2023. doi:10.1186/s13036-023-00355-7.
93. Y. Yang, P. Wang, G. Zhang, S. He, and B. Xu, "Inorganic-Nanomaterial-Composited Hydrogel Dressings for Wound Healing," 2024. doi:10.3390/jcs8020046.
94. S. Sheikh-Oleslami et al., "A Review of Metal Nanoparticles Embedded in Hydrogel Scaffolds for Wound Healing In Vivo," 2023. doi:10.3390/gels9070591.
95. R. Zhao, C. Zhao, Y. Wan, M. Majid, S. Q. Abbas, and Y. Wang, "In Vitro and In Vivo Evaluation of Alginate Hydrogel-based Wound Dressing Loaded with Green Chemistry Cerium Oxide Nanoparticles," *Front Chem*, vol. 11, 2023. doi:10.3389/fchem.2023.1298808.
96. Z. Xu et al., "Investigation of the Effect of Nanoparticle-Stabilized Foam on EOR: Nitrogen Foam and Methane Foam," *ACS Omega*, vol. 5, no. 30, pp. 19092–19103, 2020. doi:10.1021/acsomega.0c02434.
97. H. Zhang, Z. Wang, T. Zhang, and Z. Li, "Foam Stabilization Process for Nano-Al2O3 and Its Effect on Mechanical Properties of Foamed Concrete," *Nanomaterials*, vol. 14, no. 18, 2024. doi:10.3390/nano14181516.

9 Clinical Applications of Advanced Wound Dressings

Maham Raza and Muhammad Tauseef Khawar

INTRODUCTION

Skin is the outermost layer of the body that protects it and helps in healing the wound naturally or by some other methods. There are four main processes that occur to repair the damage like burn, cuts, etc. These include clotting, inflammation, new tissue growth, and final healing. Different kinds of medications and treatments are required for the nature of the wound like acute wound and chronic wound. Some wounds follow the normal healing process, and some are chronic, meaning they don't heal properly or take long time to heal. It is mostly stuck in the inflammation phase. There are many pressure risk areas that produce serious wounds and affect the quality of life. Some conditions like diabetes, poor circulation, any kind of infections, and old ages can all contribute to chronic wounds [1]. In such cases, the body's immune system works more actively, and instead of healing the wound, it may cause further damage. Neutrophils and macrophages may continue to flood the wound site, but maybe they produce too many enzymes and reactive oxygen species (ROS), which break down the tissue instead of repairing it [2]

Figure 9.1 shows various pressure sores in the human body. Wounds often have poor blood flow, which means that cells involved in healing don't get enough oxygen or nutrients to do that job. Additionally, the immune system's response can cause the destruction of the important growth factors and proteins like collagen and fibronectin, which are needed to rebuild the tissue [3]. This cycle prevents the wound from healing and can even lead to infection, making the situation worse. Chronic wounds are common in people, which have some health issues like venous leg ulcers, pressure ulcers, and diabetic foot ulcers (DFUs) [4]. Managing chronic wounds is a challenge, and researchers are looking for new ways to help them heal. One promising area is the use of natural plant compounds that have antimicrobial, anti-inflammatory, and antioxidant properties. These compounds can potentially help in reduction of the excessive inflammation in chronic wounds and promote the growth of new tissue [5].

The increasing aging population has increased the number of long-term bedridden patients, which create a burden and challenge to socioeconomic and public healthcare organizations. Bedsores are the common cause of prolonged stay in bed [6], and chronic diseases take 8 weeks or more and need a proper care. This kind of serious condition needs proper care and treatment. Bed sore is mainly caused by tissue

DOI: 10.1201/9781003616726-11

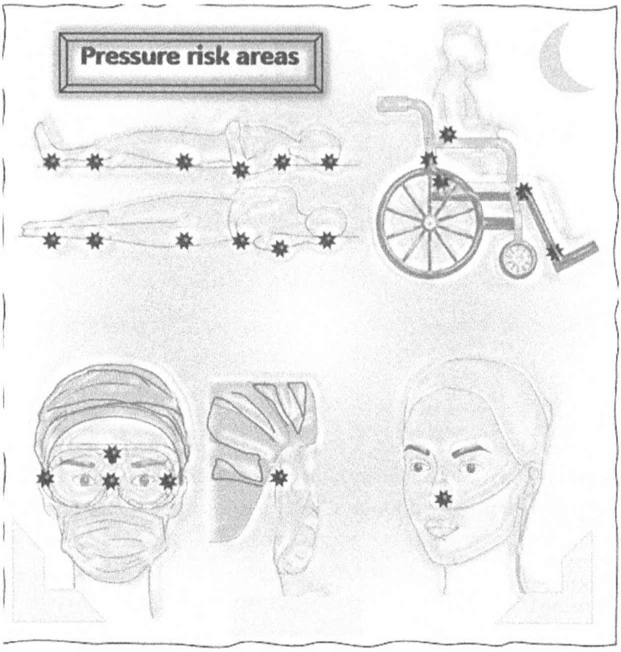

FIGURE 9.1 Pressure risk areas.

nutrition disorder. The area where the body is connected to the hard mattress causes interruption in blood flow [7].

This kind of diseases can be prevented by changing position or by continuously monitoring the humidity in that area [8] because humidity is the main cause of healing. Bedsores reduce the quality of a patient's life. Researchers thought that some bedsores can be avoidable by initial care and monitoring, as well as the use of smart technology, which has many benefits in treatment. Temperature can make the wound worse [9]. Mostly, when the temperature is high in any part of the body, especially in the case of bedridden patients, that area can be affected and damaged by wound-causing bacteria. Mostly for bedridden patients, bedsore occurs in the lower back area because more pressure occurs at that point because of weight [10].

MECHANISMS OF ACTION IN WOUND HEALING

Skin is the body's outer protective layer and the most exposed organ of the body. This gets damaged by different factors like cuts, burns, or many kinds of chemicals [11]. When any kind of damage occurs, the human body starts a complex procedure to repair the skin, which happens in four major stages: clotting, inflammation, new tissue growth, and final healing (remodeling) [12]. The wound healing process is pretty complicated. These four processes describe how the human body's immune system helps to get the wound healing process faster [13]. Figure 9.2 shows the complete process of the wound healing.

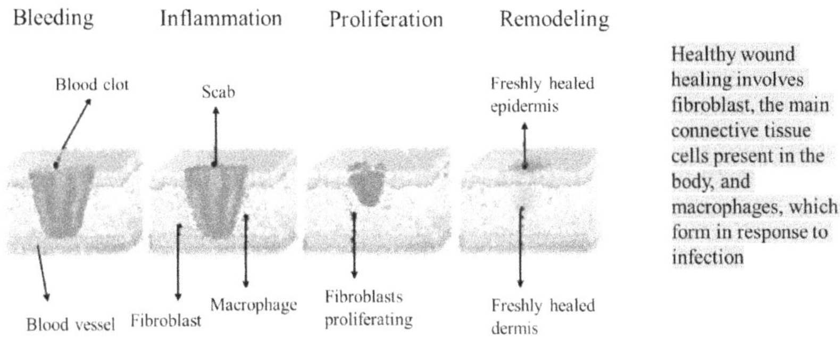

FIGURE 9.2 Mechanisms of action in wound healing.

Clotting

Clotting is the body's quick response to any damage to the skin and the underlying tissues. The major priority is to stop bleeding, so as to control the significant blood loss that could compromise the body's stability. When any kind of skin damage occurs, the blood vessels constrict, reducing blood flow. Simultaneously, platelets, which are very small cells in the blood, quickly run to the site of injury. These platelets stick to the wound surface, forming a clot and clumping the edges together. This action creates the foundation of what will become a clot, sealing off the wound to help in the prevention of blood loss [14].

As the platelets stick together, they release the chemicals that signal for more platelets to come and help in the clotting process. These chemicals also trigger the protein release like fibrin, which weave through the platelets and form a mesh-like structure that stabilizes the clot. This clot works as a temporary bandage, holding the wound together when the deeper healing processes are set in motion. Additionally, growth factors such as platelet-derived growth factor (PDGF) are emitted during this phase, which starts the recruitment of other cells involved in the healing process. These are the important growth factors that play a key role in setting the stage for inflammation and tissue regeneration.

The clotting process is crucial not only to stop bleeding but also to make the environment for the subsequent healing phases. If the clot does not occur, bacteria and other risky substance could easily enter the bloodstream, which cause infections [15]. Moreover, the clot acts as a temporary protective layer, which allows the time for the body's immune response to mobilize. It's important to keep in mind that this phase begins almost immediately, within a minute of injury, and happens quickly, as time is of the essence to stabilize the wound and prevent complications.

Inflammation

Once the clotting procedure is successfully controlled and the bleeding is stopped, the next phase is where the inflammation begins. This phase is sometimes distinguished by visible signs like redness, swelling, heat, and pain around the site of the wound. Inflammation is like the body's defense mechanism that is prompted to remove any harmful bacteria, dirt, or dead cells from the wound. The immune system sends specialized white blood cells, mainly neutrophils and macrophages, which help to clean the area of the injury site. Neutrophils respond first. They arrive within hours of the injury damage to fight against any potential infection by covering and digesting harmful bacteria and debris [16].

As neutrophils eliminate bacteria and dead cells, they also emit pro-inflammatory cytokines like interleukins and tumor necrosis factor. These are the cytokines that help to enhance the immune system, which ensure that more immune cells are recruited to the site of injury. After neutrophils have completed their initial cleanup, macrophages take over. Macrophages are versatile immune cells that not only continue the cleaning but also enhance the tissue repair by releasing growth factors that prepare the wound for the next level of healing. These cells are critical because they help to transition the wound from inflammation to the proliferation phase by recruiting fibroblasts and other cells necessary for tissue regeneration [3].

So, while inflammation is an important part in the wound healing process, too much inflammation can also be harmful. In cases where the inflammatory excessively or prolonged respond, it can lead to more tissue damage. Chronic wounds often remain stuck in that phase, with the immune system overreacting and releasing too many destructive enzymes and reactive oxygen species (ROS). This prolonged inflammation helps in the prevention of the wound in proper healing process, which is why controlling inflammation is often a target in the treatment of wound [17].

Building New Tissues

This phase is where the actual recreation of the damaged tissue begins. This phase usually starts a few days after the injury occurs and lasts for weeks, majorly depending on the size and depth of the wound. During this phase, the body focuses on creating new tissue that replaces the damaged one. Fibroblasts, a type of connective tissue cells, are the major key players in this stage. They transfer to the wound site and start producing collagen, the protein that gives the skinks its strength and structure. Initially, the body produces type III collagen, which is more flexible and forms the basis for new tissues [11].

Along with collagen production, the body also works on developing granulation tissue. This tissue consists of the newly formed blood vessels, extracellular matrix, and fibroblasts. Granulation tissue fills the wound that provides a scaffold that supports further healing. This time, new blood vessels are critical because they supply oxygen and nutrients to cells that are repaired actively. This process is called angiogenesis, and it is caused by growth factors like vascular endothelial growth factor (VEGF). If the new blood vessels do not occur, the wound will not receive enough oxygen to heal it properly [18].

Another major part of the proliferation phase is re-epithelialization, where new skin cells known as keratinocytes come across the wound to form a fresh layer of skin. These cells work from the inward edges of wound, slowly covering the exposed area. At the same time, myofibroblasts, which are a special type of fibroblast, help to contract the wound by pulling the corners of the wound closer together and reducing the size of the wound. At the end of the phase, the wound is mostly filled with new tissues, but it is not as strong as the original skin. The wound is still vulnerable and can easily reopen if disturbed [19].

FINAL HEALING FORMATION

The last and final phase is the remodeling, which can take months or maybe years to complete the procedure. In this phase, the newly formed tissue is reorganized and may strengthen to become more like the original skin. The type III collagen [20] that lays down during the proliferation phase is replaced by the stronger type I collagen. This switch is important because type I collagen provides high tensile strength, making the skin less likely to break or tear. Even now, the wound is closed and functional, so the new skin will never be as strong as the original. The maximum strength in the skin can regain, which is about 80% of what it was before the injury.

When the collagen fiber is reorganized, scar tissue becomes less vascular and more compact. The number of new blood vessels is now decreasing, and the scar that was once red and swollen begins to fade. After some time, the wound site becomes flatter and smoother. It causes scars because the skin repairs itself immediately and not exactly as it was before. The systematic structure of the original tissue is replaced by a more chaotic arrangement of the collagen fibers, which is why the scar looks different from the normal skin. In some cases, scars can become raised or spread beyond the wound boundary, depending on how the body heals [21]. This final wound healing formation process phase involves cellular turnover, where excess cells that are no longer needed for the healing process are removed by apoptosis, which is a programmed cell death. This helps to refine the tissue and remove any kind of unnecessary cells or structures. While the wound may seem fully healed at this level, it is important to note that the newly formed skin is still somewhat fragile. Some external factors like UV exposure or mechanical stress can affect the final appearance of the scar and the overall quality of the skin. Figure 9.3 represents the graphical flow of the wound healing process from clotting to final healing.

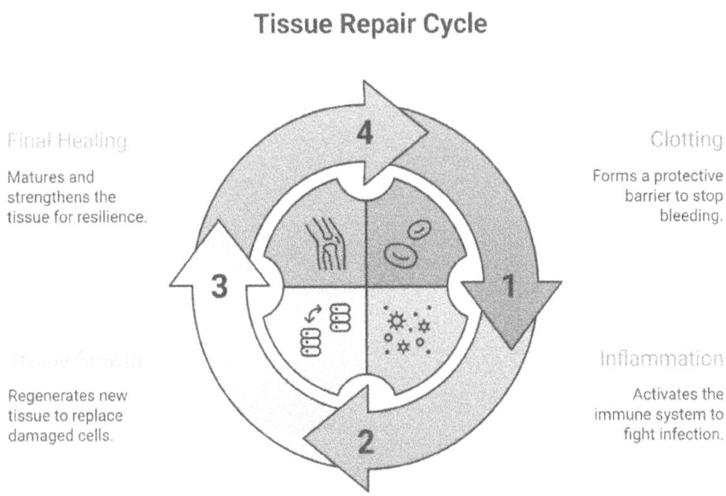

FIGURE 9.3 Mechanism of wound healing.

ROLE OF HYDROCOLLOID DRESSING

Hydrocolloid dressing is a very important innovation in wound care that is designed to promote healing by creating a moist environment. This type of dressing is designed to create a barrier that protects from the germs. This kind of dressing consists of hydrophilic materials like gelatin and pectin, which absorb wound exudate and swell into a gel-like substance. This gel not just keeps the wound moist but also helps in natural healing processes, such as autolytic debridement, where the body self-cleanses the wound of dead or necrotic tissue. By maintaining a consistent moisture level, hydrocolloid dressings help to enhance the healing process, reducing the likelihood of scab formation and promoting quicker recovery. One of the important key benefits of hydrocolloid dressing is their ability to provide a barrier against bacteria and external contaminants. The outer layer that is waterproof prevents the moisture loss and keeps the harmful pathogens out, which is complex in minimizing the risk of infection [22]. This makes the hydrocolloid dressings particularly suitable for moderate exuding wounds, pressure ulcers, and minor burns. Their semi-occlusive nature allows for the exchange of gas, which protects the wound from external irritants, thus creating the optimal environment for healing [23].

Figure 9.4 represents the benefits of the hydrocolloid dressing. The other major advantage of hydrocolloid dressings is comfort. Their flexible and soft nature of texture allows them to conform the body, which makes it ideal for use on high-friction areas like the heels and sacrum. Hydrocolloid dressings can be placed on the wound for several days. It can reduce the fatigue of the daily changes and the discomfort during the removal process. Mean hydrocolloid materials react with wound fluids,

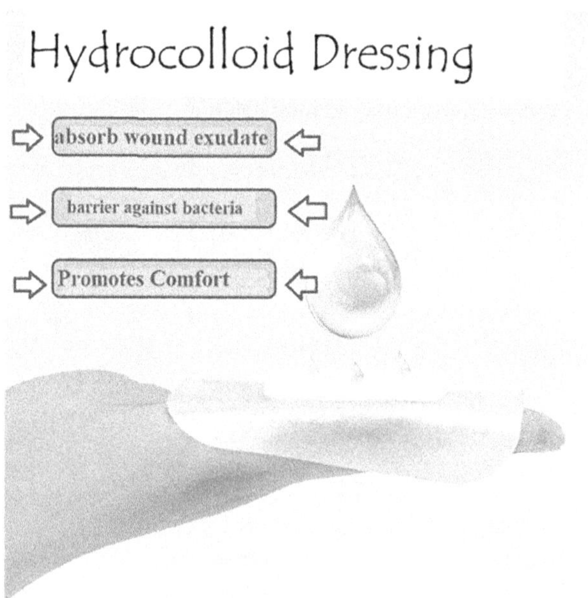

FIGURE 9.4 Hydrocolloid dressing and benefits.

forming a gel. When we removed the dressing, it would not damage the newly formed skin that can avoid the interference of the healing process [24]. This not only enhances the comfort of the patient but also helps in maintaining the integrity of the healing tissue beneath the dressing. However, it is essential to use hydrocolloid dressing carefully. It is not used on infected wounds, heavily exuding wounds, or wounds with deep spaces, as their sealed nature can make these conditions worse. Mostly, the wound may smell or look larger because of the gel formation, but it's a part of the healing process. Hydrocolloid dressing should be larger than the wound size (e.g., 2 cm) so that it covers the wound fully and avoid leakage. It is important to evaluate the wound and choose the correct type of dressing to ensure the best results in healing [25].

Effectiveness in Preventing Facial Pressure Ulcers

Hydrocolloid dressings are particularly useful for patients, which undergo non-invasive ventilation, as the masks exert significant pressure on the skin, causing pressure ulcers. These kinds of dressings significantly reduce the incidence of facial pressure ulcers by providing a moist and protective barrier on the skin. The dressings maintain necessary moisture balance, which help in preventing the skin breakdown and facilitating faster healing of any minor wounds or skin irritation caused by the mask [26]. This reduces the risk of infection and promotes patient comfort, which is crucial in most critical care settings where NIV (non-invasive ventilation) is commonly used [22].

Role in Postoperative Wound Healing

In maxillofacial surgery, hydrocolloid dressings have been shown to help in wound healing and reduce scarring. Since the face has complex structure and is very visible, taking care of wounds properly is important for both healing and appearance. These kinds of dressings keep the wound moist, which helps new tissues grow and speed up the recovery. They also protect the wound from germs and other harmful things, lowering the chance of infection. Patients who used hydrocolloid dressings had less scarring than those who didn't, highlighting how effective these dressings are for healing after the surgery [27].

BENEFITS OF ALGINATE DRESSING

Alginates are a special type of dressing that is formed from seaweed, and they are mostly known for their fluid absorbency ability. These seaweed fibers are rich in alginic acid. It is mostly beneficial for the wounds that produce a lot of the exudate. This wound dressing is very flexible and can be used to fill the deep wounds or the uneven one. Alginate dressing also provides hemostasis, which means they stop the bleeding; if the bleeding is not controlled, then it is used. This dressing helps in preventing the wound from drying out. These wounds are used for low to heavy exudate, including chronic ulcers, pressure sore, and surgical wound [28]. This dressing prevents softening and breakdown of the skin around the wound. Alginate dressing

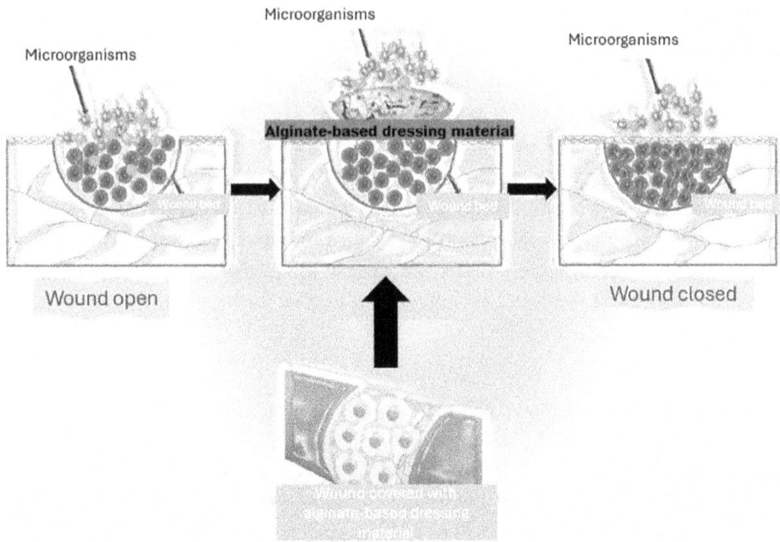

FIGURE 9.5 Alginate dressing and its working mechanism.

traps the grams produced by the exudate, reducing the risk of infection. Those are more suitable for those wounds that have more chance of being affected. It is easy to use, and it should minimize the pain and the trauma while dressing changes. Overall, the natural ability of alginate dressing in faster healing and promoting healthier skin makes it a powerful tool [29]. Figure 9.5 represents how the alginate-based dressing helps in the wound recovery process and how the material is used in wound covering.

Different Types of Alginate Dressings

There are different types of alginate dressings. Primarily, the hydrogel dressing is water or glycerin-based materials that prevent the wound from drying and provide moisture. They are mostly effective in wounds that need debridement, which involves removing dead and necrotic tissues. The content of water in the hydrogel dressing softens the dead tissue, making it easier for the healthcare professionals to remove that. This promotes the growth of healthy new tissues. Hydrogels provide the cooling and soothing effect that helps to reduce the pain, making them suitable for burns and sores that are caused by the pressure, as well as wounds that are painful and sensitive. Wound inflammation is also reduced by the cooling effect of the dressing [30].

When it combines with alginate, hydrogel dressing is more effective to manage the moisture and fluid. If the hydrogel gives moisture to the dry wound, then the alginate once can absorb excess fluid of the wound that prevents the wound from becoming too wet. So, this balance makes the alginate-hydrogel wound dressing more versatile for different wound types. This gel also formed an antibacterial barrier, which protects from infection. This provides extra protection for the wound. This wound dressing is like transparent one, which allows the healthcare professionals to carefully monitor the wound healing without the frequent removal of the wound dressing [23].

Film dressing is a thin, transparent sheet that provides the wound with a protective barrier and allows them to exchange the oxygen and moisture vapor. These dressings are mostly used for minor wounds like abrasions, cuts, or surgical minor mounds. This wound dressing transparency allows for easy wound monitoring without any need to remove the dressing, reducing the chances of disturbing the healing process of the wound. Film dressings prevent the bacteria and other contaminants from entering the wound, making them suitable for the wound with low risk of infection [31].

So, in alginate dressings, film can also complement alginate's ability to absorb the fluid. For the wounds with minimum exudate, the film protects not only the wound for maintaining the moist environment but also if that would be used with an alginate layer beneath. It helps them in the moisture balancing that is at risk of drying out or that requires protection from external factors. This film dressing also provides flexibility and conforms to the contours of the body, making it useful for the wounds that are difficult to dress [32].

Nanofiber dressings are made from ultrafine fibers, which often looks like the structure of natural skin. These fibers provide a scaffold, which promotes cell growth and tissue regeneration, making them highly effective for the healing of the wound. It creates a breathable, lightweight, or flexible layer on the wound, which not only allows the air to pass or provides the moisture exchange mechanism but also protects it from the outer bacteria that may cause infection. This kind of breathability, combined with the ability to provide comfort to the wound bed, is good for wounds that require careful and full coverage, such as a deep or irregular shape wound [33].

When we combine the alginate with the nanofibers, it increases or enhances the absorbency and moisture-retention properties of the dressing. Alginate nanofibers absorb extra or more fluid while maintaining a moist wound environment, which is difficult for fast wound healing. The structure is fine that ensures the better integration of the wound bed, and it can reduce the chances of the dressing shifting from its place or causing any irritation. So, the nanofiber dressing is lightweight and can be customized for specific wounds, offering a tailored solution for the complex once [34].

Foam dressings are created to absorb a large amount of wound fluids, while it provides a protective cushion-like structure on the wound. These dressings are sometimes used to treat wounds with moderate to heavy exudate, such as pressure ulcers, venous ulcers, and the post-surgery or postoperative wounds. This foam material traps the wound fluid, protects it from drying out, and maintains the moisture environment that is beneficial for healing. Foam dressing provides insulation and protects the wound from the outer trauma and temperature changes. When it is combined with alginate, the foam dressing is more absorbent as alginate dressings trap fluid and can create a gel when the foam provides structural support. This combination reduces the frequency of dressing changes, as the foam-alginate holds more wound fluid than the traditional one. Foam dressings are non-adherent, meaning they do not stick to that wound bed, making it easy to remove the bandage without any damage or pain. The cushioning effect of that foam dressing protects wounds from more injury, which makes them ideal to use in high-pressure areas.

FOAM DRESSINGS IN CHRONIC WOUND MANAGEMENT

Chronic and non-healing wounds are a global problem that affects millions of people and that costs the healthcare systems significantly. Choosing the right type of dressing is one of the most important aspects for treating it. The main purpose of the wound dressing is maintaining the moist environment, which helps in fast healing. A moist wound allows growth factors to interact, which boost up the new tissue's growth, promotes the formation of new blood vessels, and helps the body to naturally remove dead tissues. Chronic wounds are either highly wet (fluid) or dry [35]. Figure 9.6 shows how foam dressings work in healing the wound by preventing the bacteria and water from entering the wound, which may affect the process of healing.

Wet wounds need absorbent dressings that prevent the surrounding skin from maceration (breaking down). And the dry ones need that type of dressing that keeps the moisture in the wound. Foam dressing is a popular choice because it is very flexible and can be produced with many different levels of stickiness, absorption, and flexibility. These qualities can make the foam dressings suitable for many different

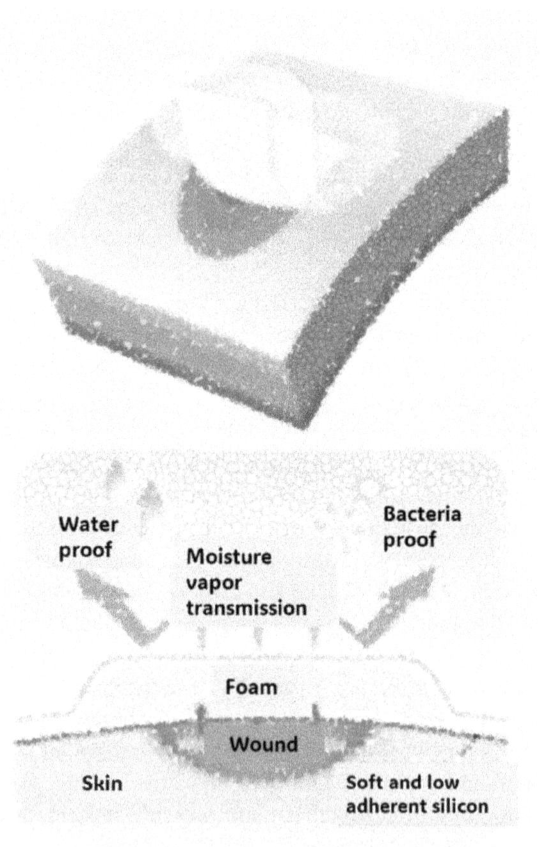

FIGURE 9.6 Foam dressing and working.

types of the wounds, including pressure ulcers, DFUs, and venous ulcers [36]. If the patient is immobile for a long period, then foam dressings help in redistributing the pressure and decreasing the friction. It decreases the pressure mostly at the foot heel area where the majority of wounds develop. It improves health and healing process by decreasing the bacterial infection, bad odor, and the leakage from the wound [23].

History and Innovation in Foam Dressings

The use of dressings was to cover wounds in ancient times. But after that, modern sterile wound dressings become more used commonly in the late 1800s when microorganisms were discovered. Early dressings are like gauze and cotton, and they were designed to absorb wound fluid and prevent infection. However, those materials were stuck to the wound mostly; when the dressing is being changed, it becomes painful and could damage the healing tissues. This then encourages the development of the new materials like polyurethane foam in the mid-20th century. Foam dressings made the revolution in the wound care by absorbing fluids while keeping the wound moist. These foam dressings are not only flexible but also provide cushioning and insulation to the wound. After more innovation and advancements, foam dressings evolved into multilayer dressings that make them easier to remove and decrease the risk of adhesion. Some of the foam dressings also include medications and antimicrobial substances such as silver, which help prevent infections and promote healing [37].

Types of Foam Dressings and Their Uses

Foam dressings should be a popular option in wound care because of their best properties like flexibility, absorbency, and the ability to maintain a moist environment. They are primarily made of polyurethane, a material known for its open-cell shape structure, which allows for both breathability and absorption of wound fluids. There are various types [36] of foam dressings, and their common applications are explained further.

Standard foam dressings are created from a single layer of foam and are primarily used for wounds with the output of moderate to high fluid. These dressings must absorb wound fluid, maintain moisture, and protect the wound from external contaminants. They are commonly used for chronic wounds such as pressure ulcers, DFUs, and venous leg ulcers. Due to the ability to adhere to the wound bed and absorb excess fluid, they must prevent the surrounding skin from getting too wet. It is used for moderate to high fluid wound [36]

These foam dressings have a soft silicone adhesive, which is around the edges to hold them in place without sticking to the wound bed. This decreases the trauma during dressing changes and protects the skin surrounding the wound from damage. That silicone-bordered design helped to secure the dressing while avoiding pain or any disruption to heal the tissue during removal. They are mostly used in pressure ulcers and fragile skin [38].

Silver-impregnated foam dressings are created for wounds that are at risk of infection and are already infected. Mostly, silver has antimicrobial properties, which are then integrated into the foam dressing to help in controlling bacterial growth within the wound bed. These are the dressings used for venous leg ulcers, DFUs, and the other wounds where the infection is concerned. They help prevent wounds from infection and aid in healing by reducing the number of bacteria. It helps in preventing the high-risk wounds that cause any serious kind of infection [39].

Multilayer foam dressings contain several layers, each serving as an absorb fluid, while others act as the moisture barrier, and the next layers add cushioning for protection. These dressings are mostly used for complex wounds that need to enhance protection, moisture management, and cushioning, such as pressure ulcers and surgical wounds. The multiple layers help improve the durability of that dressing and increase the wearing time [40].

Some foam dressings are created to deliver medications directly to the wound site. Foam dressings infused with ibuprofen can help in the management of wound pain; in other cases, dressings may deliver growth factors that stimulate the wound healing. That kind of dressing is especially significant in chronic wounds, where the prolonged healing time and pain are significant concerns. These are used for wounds that need additional medications such as anti-inflammatories and growth factors [35].

Foam dressings are available in both adhesive and non-adhesive types. Adhesive foam dressings have a sticky backing that not only holds the dressing in place but also makes them ideal for the wounds in those areas with a lot of movement. Non-adhesive foam dressing on the other side is considered for wounds that have minimal skin contact or for patients who have sensitive skin types. The adhesive ones are mostly used for those areas like joints, while the non-adhesive ones are used for very sensitive and delicate skin parts [41].

Special foam dressings are produced for use in conjunction with Negative Pressure Wound Therapy (NPWT). These types of dressings help in creating a seal around the wound, while the NPWT device applies suction to remove the fluid, reduce the swelling, and then promote the new tissue growth. They are commonly used for big and deep wounds or for those that have high fluid outcomes. It is mostly beneficial for complex and surgical wounds [42].

ANTIMICROBIAL DRESSING

Antimicrobial dressing is a specialized product that is designed for wound care and protects wounds from infection, which actively manages bacterial growth. Unlike traditional dressings, which serve only to cover and absorb fluid from wounds, antimicrobial dressings combine with agents that not only kill the bacteria but also control the growth of microorganisms like viruses, fungi, and bacteria. This dressing plays an important role in preventing infections in acute wounds, managing chronic wounds that have already been infected, and supporting the healing process by reducing the number of microorganisms in the wound environment. Sometimes, antimicrobial agents are integrated into the dressing material itself, which allows for the sustained release of the agents directly on the wound.

The main function of the antimicrobial dressing is to protect and provide the barrier from harmful pathogens that may enter the wound site and cause serious infections. This is important for those wounds that are at high risk of infection like surgical wounds, burns, and diabetic ulcers. By protecting from microbial contact, it

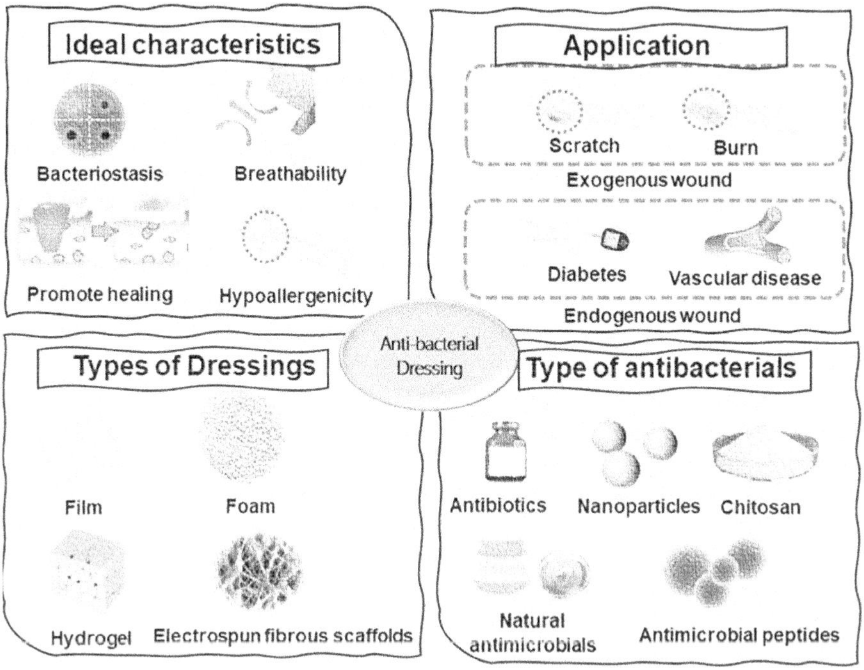

FIGURE 9.7 Antibacterial dressing characteristics, application, and types.

may avoid complications that cause prolonged healing and also increase healthcare costs, mostly in life-threatening cases such as sepsis. Antimicrobial dressing also supports the natural body healing mechanisms by maintaining the moist wound environment, which is important for collagen formation and cell and tissue regeneration [43].

Antimicrobial dressing was created to be versatile and available in different foams like films, foams, hydrogels, and alginates, and each foam suits different types of wounds and different levels of fluids. The selection of each dressing relies on the wound's presence, size, depth, and fluid level. These types of dressings are used in both acute and chronic cases. This is important for patients who have low immune systems or conditions like diabetes, as wound recovery or healing is slow or more prone to infection. Overall, antimicrobial dressings are an important advancement in wound care. Antimicrobial dressing also helps to reduce the need for systemic antibiotics [44]. Figure 9.7 shows the ideal characteristics of an antibacterial dressing like breathability and bacteriostasis, as well as how they benefit in promoting healing, their application for various wounds, and their types and antibiotic agents.

Application of Antimicrobial Dressings

Antimicrobial dressings are widely used in both acute and chronic wound management. Because it performs dual functions: protecting the wound and actively preventing and controlling infections. The primary uses of those dressings are to prevent infections of high-risk wounds, which may be the results of surgery, burns, and trauma. These types of wounds would get contaminated with bacteria due to the open nature of the wound and exposure to external environments, and sometimes, the body compromised barrier function. Using antimicrobial dressings would speed up the healing process while minimizing complications like the delay in the wound closure or reopening of the wound [45].

It is used for DFUs, pressure sores, and venous leg ulcers that are complicated and should be treated properly. It reduces the bacterial load in the wound bed and prevents colonies of bacteria from adhering to the wound surface and breaking down existing biofilms, which are resistant to standard antibiotic treatment. Biofilm breakage is important for effective wound healing, as it reduces inflammation and promotes a healthier wound environment conducive to tissue regeneration. The most sufficient use of antimicrobial dressings is to manage exudative wounds, which create an important amount of fluid. The increased fluid can lead to maceration, which further delays the healing process and increases the risk of infection.

Antimicrobial dressings are very useful for immunocompromised patients, such as those who are undergoing chemotherapy, the transplant recipients for organs, or the person's conditions like HIV/ AIDS. These kinds of patients are at high risk of infection because of their weakened immune systems. Antimicrobial dressings used in those kinds of cases provide an added layer of protection by continuously releasing antimicrobial agents at the wound area. This helps in the prevention of infection, reducing the need for systemic antibiotics and the chances of developing the antibiotic-resistant infections, which is a growing concern in medical care [46].

Antimicrobial Agents in Dressing

The antimicrobial agents are the major active ingredients in antimicrobial dressings, and they work in either killing microorganisms or stopping their growth. These are the agents that are incorporated in the material of dressing and are released over time, which provide continuous infection protection. The most common antimicrobial agents that are used in dressings are antibiotics, iodine, silver, honey, and many other compounds that come from natural and synthetic sources. Every agent has key properties and mechanism of action, making it useful for various types of wounds and microbial threats [47]. Figure 9.8 represents the graphical flow of the antimicrobial agents.

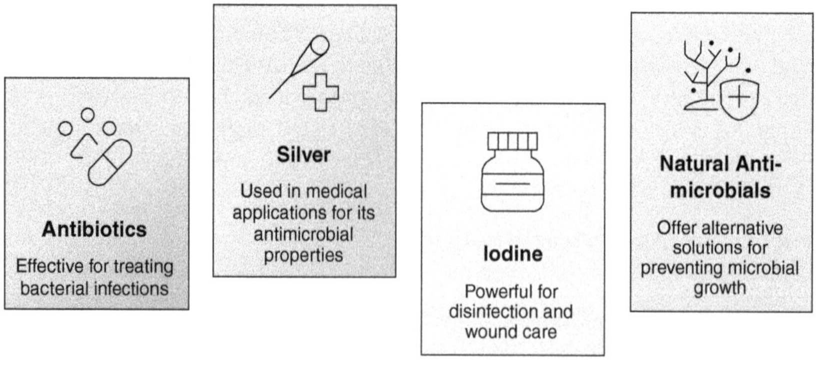

FIGURE 9.8 Antimicrobial agents.

Antibiotics are the most widely recognized antimicrobial agents used in dressings. Pertinent antibiotics, such as gentamicin, bacitracin, and mupirocin, are embedded in dressings to provide the localized antimicrobial activity directly at the wound site. This local treatment decreases the risk of systemic side effects that occur only with oral and intravenous antibiotics or also helps in limiting the development of antibiotic resistance. But the overuse of antibiotic-consisting dressings is very carefully monitored due to the global matter of the antibiotic-resistant bacterial strains. As a result, antibiotics in the wound dressings are generally reserved for wounds that are already infected or at high risk of infection [48].

Silver is the one of most used antimicrobial agents in wound care. Silver ions (Ag^+) are highly effective against a broad spectrum of microorganisms, including both Gram-positive and Gram-negative bacteria, fungi, and viruses. Silver mostly works by disrupting bacterial cell membranes, interfering with microbial respiration, and binding to bacterial DNA, which prevents replication. Silver-based dressing is available in various forms, including foams, hydrogels, and alginates, which provide sustained antimicrobial activity for many days. These are the dressings that are particularly effective in managing chronic wounds and preventing biofilm production, which is a major key challenge in the treatment of non-healing wounds [49].

Iodine is the other important antimicrobial agent that is commonly used in wound dressings, such as those that contain the povidone-iodine and cadexomer iodine, which moves slowly into the wound bed area, killing bacteria, fungi, and viruses. Iodine is effective against a wide range of pathogens and is particularly beneficial in heavy fluid wounds, where it can absorb the properties in helping to manage excessive fluid while delivering the antimicrobial action. So, iodine must be used carefully managed, and the excessive iodine may lead to local irritation or systemic absorption, particularly in patients with thyroid problems [47,50].

Natural antimicrobials such as honey and essential oils are gaining popularity in wound care. Honey, distinctively medical grade Manuka honey, contains natural antimicrobial properties because of the high sugar content, low pH, and production of hydrogen peroxide. The honey-based dressing promotes wound healing by maintaining the moist environment, decreasing inflammation, and providing a broad-spectrum activity of antimicrobials. The essential oils, such as the tea tree or the eucalyptus oil, have antimicrobial properties, and sometimes, they are incorporated with modern wound dressings that enhance efficacy in fighting the infection [51].

BIODEGRADABLE DRESSINGS FOR SUSTAINABLE CARE

Sustainable wound dressings represent a significant advancement in healthcare, aiming to balance clinical efficacy with environmental responsibility. Traditional wound care materials often contribute to environmental degradation due to their non-biodegradable nature and the volume of medical waste generated. In response, the enhancement of sustainable wound dressings focuses on utilizing biomaterials that are both efficient in promoting wound healing and environmentally friendly. Research highlights the incorporation of biodegradable polymers and eco-friendly nanoparticles in the development of these advanced biomaterials. By utilizing these sustainable materials, wound dressings can break down naturally after their intended use, reducing the accumulation of medical waste.

This method not only supports green recovery procedures but also aligns with global sustainability goals, reducing the overall environmental footprint of healthcare practices. Furthermore, sustainable wound dressings incorporate renewable resources and biocompatible substances, ensuring that they are safe for human use while being gentle on the environment. This dual focus on human health and ecological well-being is crucial, especially as the prevalence of chronic wounds, such as diabetic ulcers and pressure sores, continues to rise globally. The convergence of biomedical innovation and sustainable practices marks a pivotal shift in wound care management [52].

Types of Sustainable Wound Dressings

Hydrogel dressings are among the most promising sustainable wound care solutions due to their high biocompatibility, permeability, and three-dimensional structure. These dressings maintain a moist environment conducive to wound healing, which accelerates tissue regeneration and reduces healing time. Hydrogels are typically composed of natural or synthetic polymers that can absorb significant amounts of exudate while maintaining hydration at the wound site. The environmental sustainability of hydrogel dressings is enhanced by their biodegradability. Once their function is fulfilled, these dressings can break down naturally without leaving harmful residues, thereby reducing medical waste [53]

Figure 9.9 shows different considerations of wound dressing designs for different purposes. Additionally, the incorporation of bioactive components such as antimicrobial agents or growth factors can further improve their efficacy, making them suitable for treating a variety of wound types, including burns and diabetic ulcers. However, challenges remain in optimizing the mechanical properties and cost-effectiveness of hydrogel dressings. Ongoing research aims to develop hydrogels with enhanced strength and durability while maintaining their biodegradable nature. Innovations in cross-linking techniques and the use of hybrid polymers are key areas of focus to overcome these limitations and expand the applicability of hydrogel dressings in clinical settings [54].

Electrospun biopolymer nanofibers offer another sustainable option for wound dressings, characterized by their high surface area and porosity. These nanofibers mimic the natural extracellular matrix, providing an optimal scaffold for cell adhesion and tissue regeneration. The electrospinning process allows for the precise control of fiber diameter and morphology, enabling the customization of dressings to meet specific wound healing requirements. Sustainability is achieved through the use of natural biopolymers such as cellulose, chitosan, and alginate, which are renewable and biodegradable. These materials not only support effective wound healing but also minimize environmental impact by reducing the reliance on synthetic, non-degradable polymers [54].

Additionally, the incorporation of nanoparticles like silver or zinc oxide can impart antimicrobial properties, enhancing the clinical efficacy of the dressings without

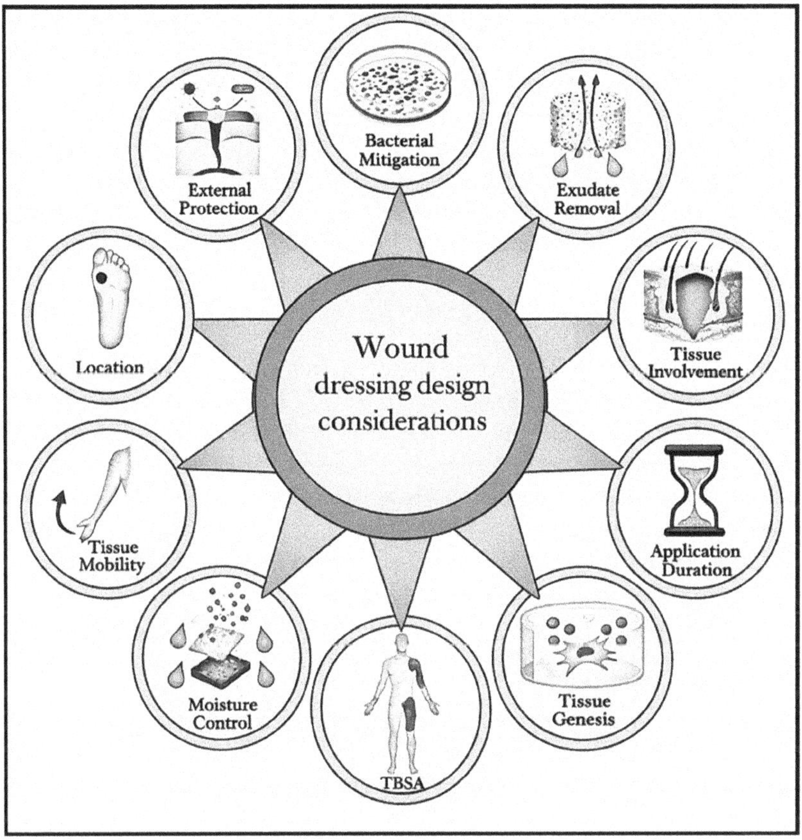

FIGURE 9.9 Some wound dressing design considerations.

compromising their sustainability. Despite their advantages, electrospun nanofibers face challenges related to scalability and mechanical strength. Improving production processes to allow for large-scale manufacturing while maintaining fiber consistency is essential. Moreover, enhancing the mechanical properties of nanofibers without sacrificing their biodegradability remains a critical area for future research, aiming to make electrospun biopolymer nanofibers a mainstream solution in sustainable wound care [55].

Polymeric materials such as foams, hydrocolloids, and alginates are extensively used in sustainable wound dressings due to their versatility and biodegradability. These materials can be tailored to provide specific wound healing environments, such as moisture retention, temperature regulation, and protection from external contaminants. The diversity of polymeric materials allows for the design of dressings that cater to different types of wounds, from minor abrasions to severe ulcers. Sustainable polymeric dressings are often derived from renewable sources, reducing their environmental impact. For example, alginate dressings, sourced from seaweed, offer excellent absorbency and biocompatibility, making them ideal for highly exudative wounds [56].

Similarly, hydrocolloid dressings made from natural polymers provide a gel-like environment that promotes autolytic debridement and minimizes scarring. The main challenges with polymeric materials lie in balancing their mechanical properties with biodegradability. Ensuring that these dressings are strong enough to protect the wound while still being environmentally friendly requires innovative material engineering. Additionally, incorporating bioactive agents into polymeric dressings without compromising their structural integrity is an ongoing area of the research, aiming to enhance both their clinical and environmental effectiveness [57].

Environmental Impact of Sustainable Dressings

Sustainable wound dressing significantly reduces the environmental footprint of wound care by minimizing the generation of non-biodegradable medical waste. Traditional dressings made from synthetic polymers such as polyurethane and polyethylene often persist in the environment, contributing to pollution and waste management challenges. In contrast, sustainable dressings made from biodegradable materials decompose naturally, alleviating the burden on landfills and reducing long-term environmental harm. The use of renewable resources in the production of sustainable dressings further enhances their environmental benefits. Materials like cellulose, chitosan, and alginate are sourced from abundant natural resources, reducing dependency on petrochemicals and promoting the use of sustainable raw materials [58].

By this shift, we do more than just helping the planet. We also start to work by utilizing more resources efficiently and waste to reduce. In addition, the production of sustainable dressings frequently uses less energy and resources than that of their conventional equivalents. Because harmful compounds are not released during the biodegradation process, the materials are returned to the ecosystem in a way that is safe for the environment. Through the implementation of sustainable wound care methods, the healthcare sector may significantly contribute to reducing environmental effects while maintaining high standards of patient care [59].

Clinical Efficacy of Sustainable Dressings

Wound dressings that focus on sustainability aim to do just as well or even better than the usual ones, but they also bring extra perks for the plant. For example, dressings made of hydrogel help wounds heal faster because they keep them moist. They also cut down on how much it hurts and make scars less noticeable. The skill to keep water levels just right plays a big role in making cells grow and moves the way they should. This is important for healing wounds effectively and quickly. Nanofibers made from biopolymers through a process called electrospinning are good for treating wounds. They work well because they act a lot like the natural stuff around our cells. This helps cells to do their job better and makes wounds heal faster. Nanofibers with their tiny spaces and big surface areas make it easier to transport gases and manage fluids from wounds. This lowers the chance of getting an infection and helps wound heal better overall [60].

Furthermore, incorporating antimicrobial nanoparticles into these fibers gives them additional protection against one of the greatest concerns in the treatment of chronic wounds: bacterial cross-contamination. On the other side, polymeric substances like alginates and hydrocolloids also show impressive clinical results. Alginates are quite absorbent and can handle overproduction of exudate, making them suitable for highly exudative ulcers including pressure and DFUs. In contrast, hydrocolloid dressings facilitate autolytic debridement and fend off the penetration of pathogens helping the recovery of wound area [61].

Challenges and Limitations

Although they have considerable advantages, the widespread use and impact of eco-friendly wound dressings have to be enhanced. One of the major barriers is the costs of biobased and green materials being comparatively higher than synthetic polymers. Such cost differences may hamper the harmonious transfer of sustainable dressings, especially in low healthcare resource settings. Another important issue is to adjust the mechanical properties of sustainable dressings. Frequently, biodegradable materials do not have enough toughness and tensile strength for specific wounds, which are prone to motion or pressure [62].

There is an ongoing investigation on how to improve the mechanical strength of these dressings without losing their biodegradable characteristics. Furthermore, more research needs to be done on the incorporation of bioactive substances like antimicrobial agents and growth factors with sustainable wound dressings. The stability of these substances and their controlled and sustained release, with the condition of maintaining the structural integrity of the dressing and its biodegradation, require advanced materials engineering techniques. Furthermore, difficulties in the submission and standardization of new biomaterials can limit the time remaining for sustainable wound dressings to reach the market [63].

Future Directions in Sustainable Wound Care

The advancement of biomaterials and technology is crucial to wound care in the future. Biomaterials technology enables the interdisciplinary development of hybrid materials with various uses. Grafting biodegradable synthetic polymers on natural polymers like chitosan creates effective dressings. However, the progress of materials science as well as nanotechnology enables smarter sustainable dressings into the future. Also important are smart polymers, nanofibers or nanoparticles, and other materials that can respond to the wound environment [64].

It is expected that these advancements will produce dressings that allow for effective doses of drugs to be delivered right to the area of the wound without the need for additional medications and promote wound healing instead. Customized wound dressings are also a focus of further research. By leveraging technologies such as 3D bioprinting, researchers are exploring the creation of custom-fit dressings tailored to the specific needs of individual patients and wound types. This personalized approach can enhance the effectiveness of wound care while minimizing waste, as dressings are produced on demand based on precise specifications. Sustainability will continue to be a guiding principle in the evolution of wound care materials. Future initiatives will prioritize the use of renewable resources, reduction of carbon footprints in manufacturing processes, and the development of fully biodegradable dressings that integrate seamlessly into natural ecosystems. Collaborative efforts among biomedical engineers, environmental scientists, and healthcare professionals will be essential to drive the innovation and implementation of sustainable wound care solutions on a global scale [63].

SMART WOUND DRESSINGS FOR DIABETIC FOOT ULCERS (DFUs)

DFUs are one of the most severe and common complications faced by patients with diabetes. As the global diabetic population grows, so does concern about the rising number of DFUs, which affect around 6.3% of people with diabetes worldwide. DFUs are characterized by ulcerations of the foot, primarily associated with neuropathy or peripheral arterial disease, and they represent a major healthcare burden. The significance of DFUs lies in their potential to lead to lower-extremity amputations if not managed properly, which can drastically impact a patient's quality of life [65].

The economic burden of treating DFUs is substantial due to the long-term nature of the wounds, the need for specialized care, and the high risk of complications. Conventional approaches to DFUs involve educating the patient, ensuring blood glucose levels within control, addressing ischemia by revascularization, offloading/relieving the mechanical pressure, and basic wound care including debridement and infection treatment. Nonetheless, DFUs are still not easy to manage despite improvements in technology and approaches, and their management is complex requiring several avenues. Newer materials and drug forms that act on lesions have some good potential to encourage and speed up the repair of the issue particularly in chronic ulcers or non-healing ulcers [66].

Recent advances in smart wound dressings have focused on the use of new technologies to be able to control wounds more actively. New generation dressings, in addition to covering the defect, are expected to restore the biological deficit of diabetes such as deficiency in angiogenesis and high levels of ROS. Advanced materials like hydrogels are found in some smart wound dressings because they change the humidity of the wound site, accelerate cellular activity, and offer medicines. The significance of creating composite dressings for DFUs cannot be emphasized. Smart dressings, which combine therapeutic delivery with the ability to monitor the wound, may enhance clinical management of DFUs and lead to quicker healing and lower risk of complications. In this regard, it can be said that this is progress in technologies for the management of diabetes-related wounds [67].

Advanced Biomaterials for DFU Treatment

Placenta-derived tissue engineering products were found to be the most advantageous biomaterials in the treatment of DFUs. These products, preserving the native structure of the extracellular matrix, possess important growth factors, chemokines, and cytokines that assist in regulating inflammation and enhancing the healing process. PBTPs enhance tissue repair by facilitating cell migration, reducing angiogenesis, immune rejection, and increasing neovascularization. An important advantage of PBTPs is their potential to be inflammatory nonresponsive, which means they do not cause inflammation, which may slow down the healing process. Amniotic membrane-derived products have been used for over a century in reconstructive surgery with great efficacy in managing chronic ulcers. These products were the most effective of all types in terms of healing the wound with a p-score of 0.90 in comparison to other biological materials [68].

SSLCs made a second ranking, with keratinocytes and fibroblasts included in the DFU healing process. These substitutes reproduce the natural skin structure and provide a scaffold for cells to grow and differentiate. In diabetic wound healing, the skin substitute containing living cells goes to great lengths to enhance dermal tissue repair and cellular repair processes. Nevertheless, their complexity is their weakness as these same products are difficult to make and hard to store. Cells in these grafts, Apligraf and Dermagraft, should continue to survive at given temperatures, which makes it expensive as well as less desirable than other biomaterials. In addition, non-autologous substitutes have a higher chance of having host rejection. With a p-score of 0.70, the SSLCs despite the limitations are a good choice for DFU patients [68].

The third position in the hierarchy of cell sustaining implants is acellular skin substitutes (ASSs), which are simply cut into pieces of tissue devoid of any active living cells but still possess important functional proteins. Nice skin grafts can also be dried or freeze-dried, and they don't need special conditions for their storage, making them cheaper and easier to store and use as compared to SSLCs. Acellular substitutes assist the tissues of the patient in growth during the healing of the parts and in turn decrease infection risk. Graftjacket and fish skin grafts are ASS products that are quite useful and effective in the treatment of DFUs especially in patients who cannot use cellular therapies. The reason why most DFUs were at grade three in healing compared to SSLCs and PBTP was because of a p-score of 0.56 toward SSLC and PBTP healing success, as shown in the meta-analysis. Nevertheless, considering the low cost and ease of usage plus the fact that it has proven to be quite effective ASSs can be used in instance when there are no possible cellular substitutes [69].

Topical Dressings for DFU Treatment

Due to the ease of application and lower costs, advanced topical dressings (ATDs) are widely used for treating DFUs. These dressings include several products including platelet-rich plasma (PRP) gels, honey-infused dressings like Medihoney, and silver nanoparticle gels. ATDs are designed in such a way that they are used to manage the wound environment, promoting moisture balance and protecting against infection. Marked as a valuable option for patients who require non-invasive treatments, still ATDs ranked lower in the meta-analysis with a p-score of 0.34. ATDs are particularly useful for maintaining a healthy wound environment, and they can be incorporated with other therapies to enhance healing properties. Products like PRP gel and ON101 cream have shown positive outcomes, especially when used alongside other biomaterials like skin substitutes [70].

Standard care (SOC) for DFUs typically involves the use of basic wound dressings including paraffin gauze, foam dressings, alginate dressings, and hydrogels.

To protect the wound and manage exudate, these dressings are used in daily or weekly wound care. As SOC is widely accessible and cost-effective, as indicated by the low healing rates in the meta-analysis, it also often falls short in healing chronic or complex DFUs. SOC remains the baseline against which new biomaterials and dressings are compared. More advanced and targeted treatments are required, particularly for patients at risk of amputation or non-healing ulcers [71].

The study intensely emphasizes to search more on head-to-head comparisons of different biomaterials and topical dressings. As the global diabetic population increases rapidly, the demand for effective and accessible DFU treatments will increase. Future studies should focus on cost-effectiveness, patient compliance, and the integration of multiple treatments to enhance healing outcomes. Innovations in biomaterial technology, such as the development of combination therapies that incorporate both cellular and acellular components, may lead to even better healing outcomes for patients with DFUs. Additionally, advancements in personalized medicine, such as tailoring treatment plans based on patient-specific factors, will further improve the management of these challenging wounds [72,73].

MANAGING PRESSURE ULCERS WITH ADVANCED DRESSINGS

Pressure ulcers, commonly known as bedsores, are localized injuries to the skin and underlying tissue resulting from prolonged pressure, typically occurring over bony prominences. They can affect anyone with limited mobility, including elderly individuals, patients recovering from surgery, and those with chronic illnesses. The most common risk factors for developing pressure ulcers include immobility, incontinence, poor nutrition, and certain medical conditions including diabetes and vascular disease. Figure 9.10 shows different stages of pressure ulcers for the management of these wounds with or without cellulitis.

The administration of pressure ulcers is complex and multifaceted, which involves various strategies to relieve pressure, maintain a clean wound environment, and promote healing. Due to their inability to adapt to the dynamic needs of the wound environment, traditional wound care practices often fall short, especially for chronic or deep wounds. Recent advancements in wound care have transformed the approach to managing pressure ulcers, particularly with the introduction of advanced dressings. These dressings not only protect the wound but also actively contribute to the healing process by creating ideal conditions. There are further techniques and methods for managing pressure ulcers, which are explained further below [74].

Moisture-Balancing Dressings: Hydrocolloids and Hydrogels

Moisture is essential in the healing process because a balanced, moist wound environment can accelerate healing, reduce pain, and lower scarring. However, managing moisture in pressure ulcers requires selecting the correct dressing type based on the ulcer's moisture level and exudate production [75]. Hydrogel dressings are primarily composed of water and provide hydration to the wound, making them particularly useful for dry or minimally exuding ulcers. Hydrogel dressings serve several functions, such as maintaining moisture by creating a moist environment that promotes

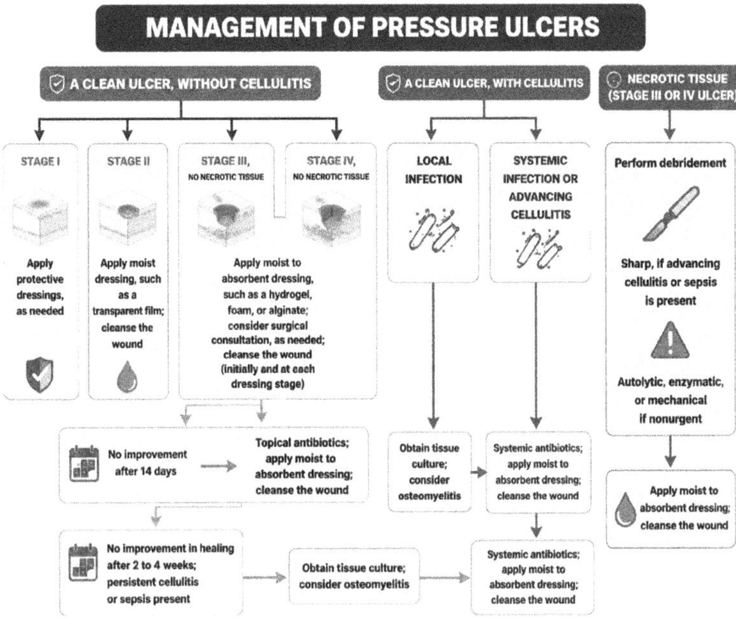

FIGURE 9.10 Management of pressure ulcers.

cell migration and facilitates autolytic debridement, a process by which the dead tissue is naturally removed by the body's enzymes; providing pain relief, as the cooling effect of hydrogel dressings can alleviate pain during dressing changes, making them suitable for sensitive wounds; and being gentle on skin, as they are non-adhesive and do not stick to the wound bed, minimizing trauma during dressing changes [76].

Hydrocolloid dressings are adhesive and composed of materials like gelatin, pectin, or carboxymethylcellulose. They are effective for various wound types due to their unique properties such as moisture management, as hydrocolloids maintain a moist wound environment while absorbing some exudate, which helps prevent maceration of the surrounding tissue; protection against external contaminants, as they provide a barrier to bacteria and other contaminants, thereby reducing the risk of infection; and self-adhesive nature, as these dressings adhere well to the skin without the need for tape or additional adhesives, making them easy to apply and change [77].

Foam dressings are designed to absorb moderate to high levels of exudate. They are composed of a soft, flexible foam material that provides cushioning and protection. Foam dressings have several benefits, such as the ability to absorb a significant amount of fluid, preventing it from pooling in the wound area and reducing the risk of infection; their cushioning nature provides a protective layer that cushions the wound from pressure and friction, which are essential for ulcers located on high-pressure areas; and their moisture-retention property absorbed exudate, which helps to maintain a moist environment necessary for healing [78].

Alginate dressings are derived from seaweed, which are highly absorbent. They are particularly beneficial for wounds with heavy exudate. Key features include high absorbency, which allows alginates to absorb large volumes of fluid and transform into a gel-like consistency that keeps the wound moist while managing exudate levels, and biocompatibility, which is due to the fact that alginates are derived from natural sources and do not cause irritation or adverse reactions. It facilitates healing by the formation of gel during exudate absorption, promotes granulation tissue formation, and supports the healing process [28]. Managing infection is critical in pressure ulcer care, as infection can cause severe complications. Several advanced dressings are designed specifically to address this risk, including materials and technologies that control bacterial growth directly at the wound site [79].

Antimicrobial dressings include those with silver, iodine, or honey, which offer broad-spectrum antibacterial activity. Silver ions, for example, disrupt bacterial cell walls and inhibit microbial growth. Honey-based dressings are also effective as they have natural antibacterial and anti-inflammatory properties and provide a moist environment, aiding in quicker healing. Antimicrobial dressings are recommended for infected wounds or those at high risk of infection, as they create an environment hostile to pathogens while supporting the body's natural defenses [43].

pH levels in a wound are indicators of infection and healing progress. Healthy wounds generally maintain an acidic pH, whereas an alkaline environment may signal bacterial colonization or infection. pH-responsive dressings change color based on the wound's pH level, providing visual feedback on the wound's condition and alerting caregivers to potential complications without requiring dressing removal. These dressings are helpful in both infection prevention and early detection [80].

Necrotic tissue can hinder wound healing, and its removal is often necessary for ulcers. Enzyme-activated dressings facilitate debridement by releasing collagenase or other enzymes that break down dead tissue without affecting healthy cells. For instance, dressings containing proteolytic enzymes target necrotic tissue while sparing viable cells, thus promoting a cleaner wound bed and reducing the need for painful mechanical debridement. These infection-control dressings play a vital role in pressure ulcer management, especially in cases where the ulcer is at high risk of infection or already showing signs of bacterial colonization [81]. Smart dressings integrate sensors that continuously monitor essential biomarkers such as temperature, moisture, pH, and oxygen levels. These metrics are crucial indicators of the wound's healing status, and monitoring them in real time allows for faster interventions and more personalized care [82].

Temperature is a key marker of inflammation or infection. Dressings equipped with temperature sensors can detect subtle increases in wound temperature, which is a common early sign of infection. Some temperature-sensitive dressings also feature color-changing indicators, offering visual feedback without requiring dressing removal. By identifying temperature changes, caregivers can intervene earlier, reducing the risk of complications [83,84]. Oxygen is essential for cellular repair and wound healing because it supports collagen synthesis and new blood vessel formation. Low oxygen levels in a wound can delay healing and increase infection risk. Oxygen-monitoring dressings measure oxygen saturation levels and alert caregivers if levels are too low, enabling targeted oxygen therapy. Some advanced oxygen-monitoring dressings are even capable of releasing oxygen to the wound, supporting tissue repair and cell growth [85].

pH-responsive dressings provide data on the wound's pH level and can release medications when an imbalance is detected. For example, if an ulcer becomes too alkaline (indicating infection), the dressing might release antibiotics to counteract bacterial growth, maintaining a favorable environment and promoting faster healing. By offering real-time data, smart dressing minimizes the need for frequent dressing changes and allows caregivers to monitor wounds remotely. This reduces intervention frequency, cuts healthcare costs, and improves patient comfort [85].

Controlled-Release Drug Dressings

These are the dressings that provide a steady, localized release of medication directly to the wound site, addressing concerns such as pain, infection, or inflammation while minimizing systemic effects. They offer a highly effective solution for managing difficult-to-heal wounds, particularly in patients with chronic ulcers [86]. Antibiotic-infused dressings gradually release antibiotics in controlled amounts, minimizing the need for frequent dressing changes and reducing systemic side effects associated with oral or injectable antibiotics. By ensuring a localized antibiotic presence, these dressings effectively prevent and manage infections [87].

Some dressings contain growth factors such as EGF or PDGF, which help cells grow and repair tissues. These are the special molecules that support the production of collagen, the formation of new blood vessels, and the overall cell repair, helping wounds heal faster [88].

Dressings with pain relievers or anti-inflammatory medicine can help with painful or swollen ulcers. They provide pain relief right at the wound, making dressing changes more comfortable and helping patients rest better, which is important for the healing. These dressings release medicine slowly, targeting the wound directly and improving recovery while reducing side effects and discomfort [89].

Negative Pressure Wound Therapy (NPWT) for Pressure Ulcers

NPWT is an effective and modern way to help wounds heal, especially tough ones such as pressure ulcers. It uses a vacuum system to create the perfect environment for healing. A special foam dressing is placed on the wound and sealed, then connected to a vacuum device that gently removes extra fluids and supports tissue repair. This makes the NPWT an important method in today's wound care [90]. The benefits are explained below.

NPWT is highly effective in managing wound fluids, which, if allowed for accumulation, can slow healing and create an environment for bacterial growth and infection. The therapy gently removes excess fluid, maintaining the right level of moisture to keep the wound clean and promote faster healing. The foam dressing fits snugly into the wound, creating a seal that blocks out the dirt and germs while preventing the wound from becoming too wet. By ensuring a balanced environment, NPWT helps to reduce the healing times and is especially useful for complex or chronic conditions [91].

Another big benefit of NPWT is that it improves blood flow to the wound. The gentle suction from the therapy stimulates blood vessels, bringing more oxygen and nutrients to the area, which are essential for healing. Oxygen helps cells to work properly and grow new tissue, while better blood flow also removes waste and toxins from the wound. This is a process that speeds up tissue repair and helps new blood vessels to form. For people with pressure ulcers, where blood flow is often poor, NPWT can make a big difference by boosting circulation and helping the wound heal faster [92].

Infections are a big concern when treating pressure ulcers and other wounds, but NPWT helps to lower this risk in several ways. The sealed foam dressing keeps the bacteria out of the wound, and the therapy removes extra fluid that bacteria need to grow. By managing moisture, NMPT reduces the chances of infection. It can also help clean the wound by removing bacteria and germs, keeping the area safer for healing. This is especially helpful for wounds that are already infected or at high risk. By maintaining a clean and protected wound site, NPWT supports safer healing with fewer complications [93].

Many studies have shown the NPWT can speed up healing, especially for deep or complicated wounds. Traditional wound care might not be enough for these types of wounds, but NPWT offers a better solution. It is particularly helpful for patients with pressure ulcers, surgical wounds, or injuries that have not healed with the other treatments. NPWT can lead to shorter hospital stays and lower healthcare costs, and patients often feel better as their wounds heal faster. This treatment is especially important in hospitals, where quick and effective wound care is needed to avoid more complications [94].

REVOLUTIONIZING HEALING: HOW SMART DRESSINGS ARE TRANSFORMING WOUND CARE?

Polymer-based materials have changed the way we care for wounds, making dressing stronger, more flexible, and better for the body. Materials like hydrogels, hydrocolloids, and polyurethane foams act like skin and help keep wound moist, which is important for preventing infection and helping tissue heal. For example, hydrogels can absorb extra moisture and keep the right balance around the wound. These materials are safe for the body and don't stick to the skin, making them more comfortable and less painful during dressing changes. New biopolymers like alginates and chitosan have added extra benefits, including fighting infection and helping stop bleeding. Alginate, made from seaweed, forms a gel when it touches the wound, keeping it moist and helping cells grow and heal [63].

Chitosan, made from shells of crustaceans, is biodegradable and helps wounds heal by encouraging collagen production. Scientists are also working on synthetic materials like polyvinyl alcohol and polyurethanes, which can be designed to have specific strength and control how fast they break down. Nanocomposite polymers, which combine tiny nanoparticles with polymers, are becoming a promising option for wound care. These materials offer stronger support, are safe for the body, and can deliver medicines in a controlled way. For example, silver nanoparticles in these materials help fight infection, reducing the risk in long-term wounds. Thanks to the advances in polymers chemistry, these materials can now be customized to control how they break down and release healing agents, which is especially useful for treating complex wounds [95].

Nanotechnology is improving wound care by working at the molecular level to speed up healing. Nanofibers created through electrospinning help cells grow and can be loaded with medicine like antibiotics and growth factors to promote faster healing and reduce infection risks. These fibers release medicine slowly, making them great for chronic wounds. Silver and gold nanoparticles are also used for their strong ability to fight infections [96].

Figure 9.11 shows graphically the different applications of the nanomaterials, which help in wound healing and provide benefits. Silver nanoparticles help prevent infections by disrupting bacteria and promoting healing in infected wounds. Gold nanoparticles can be designed to target specific cells or tissues, offering treatments with fewer side effects. These nanoparticles are used in dressings for continuous antimicrobial protection, especially in tough wounds like DFUs. Nanocarriers, such as liposomes and dendrimers, can carry drugs and release them when triggered by changes in temperature or pH. This helps to treat wounds with high inflammation or infection by delivering medicine directly to the site. These smart nanoparticles make wound care more personalized and effective. [97].

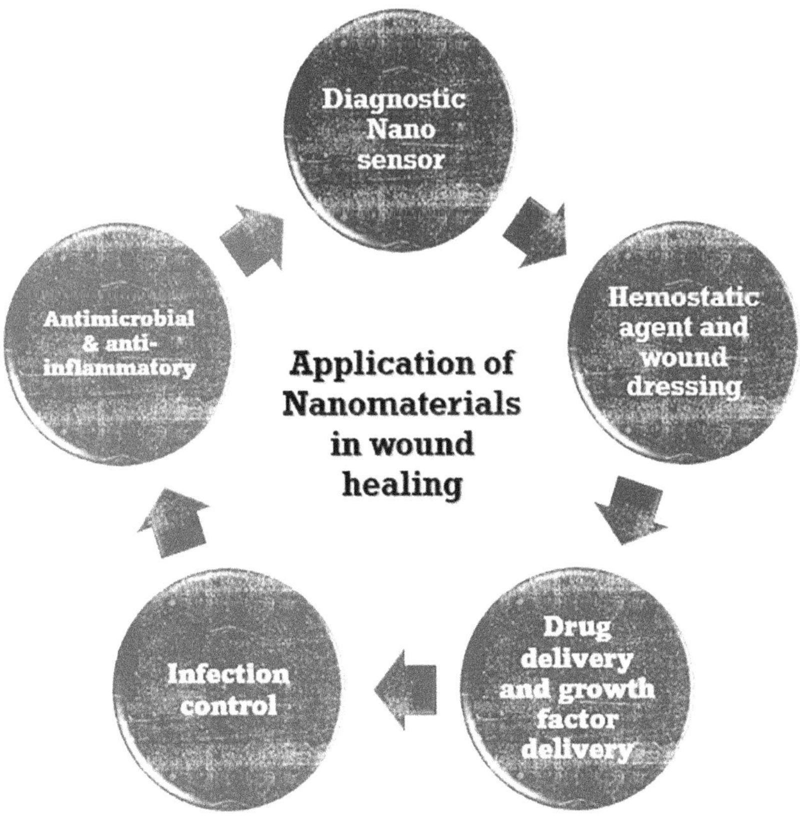

FIGURE 9.11 Applications of nanomaterials in wound healing.

Smart dressings represent a significant leap forward, as they can actively respond to changes in the wound environment. These dressings are designed with sensors or polymers that respond to specific stimuli, such as pH, temperature, or moisture levels. For instance, wounds often become more acidic during infection, and a pH-responsive dressing can release antimicrobial agents only when the pH exceeds a certain threshold, reducing the risk of infection while minimizing unnecessary drug use. Such targeted responses can prevent antibiotic resistance and optimize the healing process. Thermo-responsive dressings are another type of smart dressing, releasing therapeutic agents when the temperature around the wound rises, indicating inflammation or infection [98–100]. Figure 9.12 shows the new emerging trends in wound management, including how intelligent wearable sensors help in the process of healing and real-time monitoring in the management of wound.

These materials often incorporate polymers that undergo a phase change in response to temperature, enabling the controlled release of anti-inflammatory or antimicrobial compounds. Some smart dressings even integrate temperature sensors, providing real-time feedback to healthcare providers about the wound's condition and allowing for timely interventions. Hydrogel-based smart dressings can absorb a lot of fluid while keeping the wound moist, which helps it heal. These dressings can also be enhanced with nanoparticles or healing agents that release medicine over time or in response to changes in the wound. For example, drug-loaded hydrogels can slowly release antibiotics or growth factors, helping chronic wounds heal faster [99].

Bioactive wound dressings are designed to work with the body's natural healing process. They are often infused with compounds like growth factors or peptides that help cells repair and regenerate tissue. For example, epidermal growth factor helps cells to move and grow, which is important for closing the wound. These dressings also promote the growth of new blood vessels to supply oxygen and nutrients. Collagen-based dressings are especially useful since collagen is a key part of tissue repair and helps wounds heal [100].

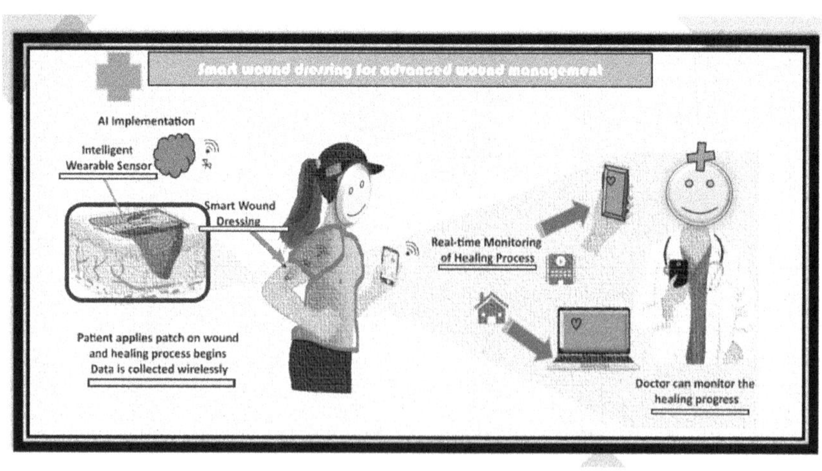

FIGURE 9.12 Emerging trends and future directions of engineering smart dressings for wearable health monitoring.

Collagen-based dressings help cells to attach and grow, supporting the formation of new tissue. They also absorb excess fluid and encourage the growth of new collagen, which reduces scarring and strengthens the wound. Chitosan is another promising material with antimicrobial and clotting properties. Chitosan dressing creates a safe environment for cells to repair the wound, helps retain moisture, and prevents bacteria from growing, lowering the risk of infection [101].

3D printing technology allows for the creation of custom wound dressings designed for each patient's needs. Researchers can use 3D bioprinting to make structures that mimic human skin, helping cells grow and tissues heal. These dressings can be shaped to fit irregular wounds, providing better coverage and reducing discomfort. This is especially useful for burn patients or those with large, unusual, shaped wounds [102].

3D printing also allows for adding different healing agents into the dressing, making them multifunctional. For example, a 3D-printed hydrogel dressing can have both antibacterial agents and growth factors, which help prevent infection and speed up healing. This method allows precise control over how much of each agent is used, making the dressing more effective. It also helps to reduce waste and costs by creating dressings as needed, making it a more sustainable option for personalized care [103].

Combination therapies use multiple treatments to speed up wound healing. For example, dressings with antimicrobial agents, anti-inflammatory compounds, and growth factors can fight infection, reduce swelling, and promote tissue growth. Some dressings also combine physical therapies like NPWT to improve blood flow, reduce swelling, and promote tissue growth. These therapies are especially helpful for tough wounds, such as diabetic ulcers and pressure sores, by addressing the causes of slow healing [104,105].

BREAKING BARRIERS: CHALLENGES IN BRINGING INNOVATIVE WOUND CARE PRODUCTS TO MARKET

The rules for wound care products are complex and differ by region, making things tricky for developers. In the United States, the FDA requires thorough testing and approvals, often treating these products as medium- or high-risk devices. Europe has similar strict rules under the Medical Device Regulation, including detailed safety and clinical tests. While these regulations aim to keep patients safe, they can slow down getting new products to market. Companies must spend time and resources to prove their products are safe, effective, and stable, especially when using new materials like the smart or bioactive dressings [106].

For small companies and startups, dealing with these regulations can be costly and make it harder to launch new products. Working with regulatory experts or contacting authorities early can help but adds extra costs. Innovative products like drug releasing dressings or nanocomposites face stricter checks because they mix drug and device features, requiring them to meet two sets of rules. This makes approvals even harder. Companies need to follow these rules while trying to stay creative, which often slows down progress in wound care innovation [107].

Scaling up the production of advanced wound care materials from laboratory settings to mass production presents numerous challenges. Complex formulations, such as those in bioactive and smart dressings, often involve delicate processes that require precise control over temperature, pressure, and sterility. Scaling these processes while maintaining the quality and consistency of each batch is a technical hurdle, particularly for nanocomposite or 3D-printed materials, which require specialized equipment. Manufacturing bioactive dressings that incorporate growth factors, cytokines, or stem cells is particularly challenging, as these biological agents are sensitive to environmental conditions. Ensuring stability and functionality at a large scale requires sophisticated storage and handling processes, which can increase costs [108].

The risk of contamination is also higher in bioactive and polymer-based dressings, necessitating strict sterile manufacturing conditions to prevent infection risks. Companies face additional logistical challenges when producing combination products that integrate multiple materials, such as hydrogels embedded with nanoparticles or nanofiber scaffolds. These products require multi-step manufacturing processes that can be time-consuming and costly, making it difficult to maintain profitability while scaling production. As a result, many companies partner with established manufacturers with technical expertise to streamline production and reduce costs [109].

Ensuring the biocompatibility of new wound care materials is critical, as materials that provoke immune reactions can delay healing and cause adverse effects. Bioactive materials, especially those derived from animal sources, carry a risk of immune rejection or allergic reactions. For instance, collagen from animal sources may cause allergies in certain patients, while silver nanoparticles, although effective as antimicrobials, can potentially induce cytotoxicity at high concentrations. Balancing efficacy with safety is essential but challenging, particularly for multifunctional wound care products. The safety of nanomaterials, such as nanoparticles and nanofibers, is a subject of ongoing research. While these materials offer significant benefits, including antimicrobial and enhanced wound healing properties, they can also penetrate cellular membranes and potentially lead to cytotoxic effects [110,111].

Using nanomaterials for a long time could affect patient health, thus careful testing is needed to make sure they are safe. Developers must study how toxic these materials might be and figure out safe limits, which takes a lot of time and money. Products like drug releasing dressings also need to ensure that they release medicine at the right pace; too much and too fast can cause side effects, and too little might not work. This is a big challenge, requiring extra safety studies to ensure that the materials are both safe and effective, which adds to the cost and development [111].

Developers must balance innovation with cost-efficiency to make advanced wound care products accessible. Simplifying production and using affordable materials can help but may affect quality. High costs also limit adoption in low- and middle-income countries with tight healthcare budgets. To address these, developers can explore cost-effective materials and methods or partner with NGOs and public health organizations to improve access in resource-limited areas [112].

Consistent quality is crucial for wound care materials, as variability can affect patient outcomes. Ensuring uniformity is challenging especially for bioactive and smart dressings, where small changes can impact performance. Rigorous testing of properties like biocompatibility and drug release rates is essential but adds complexity. Nanocomposites require careful monitoring to prevent nanoparticle clumping, which can reduce effectiveness. The absence of standardized testing protocols further complicates quality control [62].

Traditional dressings are tested for basic properties like absorbency and strength, while smart and bioactive dressings need advanced testing for responsiveness, biocompatibility, and controlled release. Developing these tests is costly and requires specialized tools and expertise. Evolving regulatory standards add to the challenge, requiring companies to adapt processes to stay compliant. This increases costs, slows production, and limits the scalability of advanced wound care materials [113].

Despite advancements in wound care, adopting innovative products in clinical practice is slow. Healthcare providers may hesitate to use unfamiliar materials without strong evidence of their effectiveness. Educating clinicians and patients about the benefits of bioactive and smart dressings is vital but requires investment in training, especially in rural or resource-limited areas. Adoption is further slowed down by the lack of standardized usage protocols for advanced wound care products [114].

Clinicians may struggle with the correct use or frequency of changes for the new dressings, reducing their effectiveness. Clear, user-friendly guidelines and training materials, developed with healthcare experts, can address this. Patient education is also crucial, as adherence impacts wound healing. Advanced dressings, such as drug-eluting or smart types, often require specific instructions. Teaching patients to follow treatment plans, recognize infection signs, and understand how these dressings work can improve outcomes [115]. Figure 9.13 shows different challenges that the market faces in the innovation of the wound care products.

FUTURE TRENDS IN WOUND CARE AND POLYMER MATERIAL DEVELOPMENT

Personalized medicine is reshaping wound care by tailoring treatment plans to the unique needs of individual patients. Wound healing is affected by factors like genetics, age, and conditions like diabetes. Researchers are using biomarkers to identify patients at risk of slow healing and tailor treatments. For example, diabetic patients with poor blood flow might need growth factor-enriched dressings, while those prone to infections may require antimicrobial dressings [116].

Genomic and proteomic profiling helps to identify the molecular pathway involved in a patient's wound healing process [117]. This knowledge enables targeted therapies to address the biological causes of slow healing. Personalized dressings with specific growth factors or anti-inflammatory agents can speed up wound closure and reduce complications, marking a major step forward in patient-centered care. It also opens doors for precision drug delivery in wound care [118].

Smart dressings can release drugs based on wound conditions such as moisture or pH. For example, a pH-sensitive dressing releases antimicrobial agents only when an infection is present, optimizing treatment and reducing drug resistance. This ensures effective treatment while minimizing side effects [119].

AI and machine learning are being used more in wound care to improve diagnosis, monitoring, and treatment. AI can analyze large data to identify patterns and predict

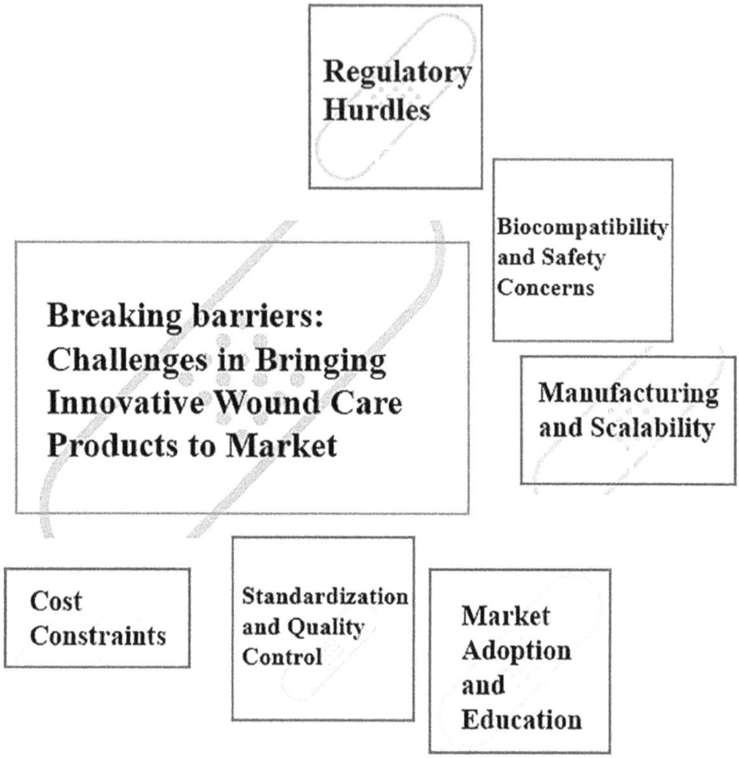

FIGURE 9.13 Breaking barriers in bringing innovative wound care products to market.

healing, helping doctors make better decisions. AI imaging tools can measure wound size, depth, and tissue types, offering accurate data for tracking progress, especially for chronic wounds. Machine learning can also predict risks like infection or slow healing, allowing doctors to personalize treatment and adjust care early [120].

If AI models show a high infection risk, clinicians can use antimicrobial dressings or increase monitoring to reduce the risk. AI decision support systems help improve patient outcomes by guiding targeted treatment. AI can also optimize wound care logistics, analyzing demand patterns to allocate resources and prioritize care, which is especially useful in resource-limited areas. By streamlining workflows, AI can lower healthcare costs and improve access to advanced wound care [121].

Sustainability is becoming more important in healthcare, including wound care. Traditional dressings often create a lot of waste due to frequent changes, especially for high-exudate wounds. Eco-friendly, biodegradable materials like plant-based biopolymers, alginate, cellulose, and chitosan are being developed to reduce environmental impact. These materials decompose naturally, reducing landfill waste. Some biodegradable dressings can even release nutrients as they break down, potentially aiding healing. This is especially important in healthcare facilities that produce large amounts of medical waste [122].

This approach follows eco-design principles, making wound care products environmentally responsible. Research is exploring sustainable sources like agricultural byproducts to create biopolymers for wound care. Cellulose from agricultural waste offers an eco-friendly material for dressings. Using renewable sources reduces environmental impact and can lower production costs, making eco-friendly dressings more affordable. As healthcare focuses on sustainability, the demand for biodegradable wound care products is expected to increase [123].

Advancements in digital health are leading to smart wound dressings with sensors that monitor wound conditions in real time. These dressings track factors like moisture, temperature, and pH, providing important data. Temperature change can indicate infection, allowing for early treatment. The data can be sent to healthcare providers through mobile apps or digital platforms, enabling remote wound care management [124].

Patients can get real-time feedback on their wound's condition without frequent hospital visits, improving convenience and access, especially for those in remote areas or with limited mobility. Integrating AI with monitoring systems can further enhance care by analyzing sensor data to track healing and suggest treatments. This approach supports personalized care tailored to each patient's wound. As digital health technologies advance, smart wound dressings with monitoring features are expected to become standard in chronic wound care [125,126].

Telemedicine has become a valuable tool for remote wound care, especially during the COVID-19 pandemic. It allows patients to consult with specialists via video calls, providing ongoing care without in-person visits. For chronic wounds, telemedicine is a convenient and cost-effective solution, offering guidance on care practices, dressing changes, and infection signs. Digital tools can also help clinicians assess wounds based on photos or data uploaded by patients, enabling accurate monitoring and timely interventions. Telemedicine enhances access to care, especially in rural areas. In the future, AI-driven tools may help automate wound assessments, give care reminders, and alert patients to potential complications, improving outcomes and reducing strain on healthcare facilities [127,128].

Regenerative medicine is becoming more important in wound care, aiming to restore the skin's structure and function. Stem cell therapy, particularly using mesenchymal stem cells (MSCs), shows great promise. MSCs can turn into different cell types, including skin cells, and help promote healing while reducing inflammation, making them ideal for treating chronic wounds [129]. Stem cells can be applied to wounds or added to dressings, where they release growth factors to boost cell growth and tissue repair. Gene therapy, which involves introducing specific genes into wound cells, can help with collagen production and blood vessel growth, aiding healing. Researchers are also working on tissue engineered skin grafts that combine cells and scaffolds to mimic natural skin, making them ideal for large or complex wounds. Advances in biomaterials are improving scaffolds to support cell growth and tissue regeneration. These scaffolds can be engineered to release bioactive molecules that enhance the healing process, creating an environment conducive to cell migration and proliferation. As regenerative medicine technologies advance, they are expected to provide new solutions for chronic and complex wounds that are resistant to conventional treatments [130].

CONCLUSION

The skin, as the body's primary defense, undergoes a complex healing process involving hemostasis, inflammation, proliferation, and remodeling, which advanced wound dressings effectively support. Hydrocolloid dressings maintain a moist healing environment, while alginate dressings are particularly effective for managing high-exudate wounds. Foam dressings provide cushioning, and antimicrobial dressings prevent infections using agents such as silver, iodine, and honey. Biodegradable and natural polymer-based dressings offer sustainable solutions, combining clinical efficacy with environmental benefits, although challenges such as cost and regulatory barriers persist. Smart dressings, equipped with biosensors and controlled drug-release mechanisms, are transforming care for chronic wounds, including DFUs and pressure ulcers, by enabling real-time monitoring and precise treatment. Innovations in biomaterials, nanotechnology, and polymers are enhancing infection control and sustainability, paving the way for multifunctional dressings that address both clinical and environmental needs. Despite existing market challenges, these advancements are reshaping wound care, promising improved outcomes and a more sustainable future for healthcare.

REFERENCES

1. T. Lagoa, M. C. Queiroga, and L. Martins, "An overview of wound dressing materials," *Pharmaceuticals*, vol. 17, no. 9, p. 1110, 2024, doi:10.3390/ph17091110.
2. A. Abtin et al., "Perivascular macrophages mediate neutrophil recruitment during bacterial skin infection," *Nat Immunol*, vol. 15, no. 1, pp. 45–53, 2014, doi:10.1038/ni.2769.
3. E. A. Lenselink, "Role of fibronectin in normal wound healing," *Int Wound J*, vol. 12, no. 3, pp. 313–316, 2015, doi:10.1111/iwj.12109.
4. W. Alam, J. Hasson, and M. Reed, "Clinical approach to chronic wound management in older adults," *J Am Geriatr Soc*, 2021, doi:10.1111/jgs.17177.
5. T. Serena, R. Yaakov, S. Aslam, and R. Aslam, "Preventing, minimizing, and managing pain in patients with chronic wounds: challenges and solutions," *Chronic Wound Care Management Res*, vol. 3, pp. 85–90, 2016, doi:10.2147/cwcmr.s85463.
6. "Pressure sores and pressure-decreasing," 1994.
7. N. Cullum et al., "Preventing and treating pressure sores," *Qual Health Care*, vol. 4, pp. 289–297, 1995.
8. S. Lee et al., "A fabric-based wearable sensor for continuous monitoring of decubitus ulcer of subjects lying on a bed," *Sci Rep*, vol. 13, no. 1, 2023, doi:10.1038/s41598-023-33081-7.
9. R. A. Angelova and D. Sofronova, "E-textile for non-invasive control of the body movement of bedridden patients," *IOP Conf Ser Mater Sci Eng*, vol. 1031, pp. 01209, 2021, doi:10.1088/1757-899X/1031/1/012029.
10. D. Sofronova, R. A. Angelova, and Y. Sofronov, "Design and development of an e-textile mat for assuring the comfort of bedridden persons," *Materials*, vol. 14, no. 18, 2021, doi:10.3390/ma14185437.
11. R. Kumar et al., "Burn injury management, pathophysiology and its future prospectives," *J Res Appl Sci Biotechnol*, vol. 1, no. 4, pp. 78–89, 2022, doi:10.55544/jrasb.1.4.10.
12. Z. Wang et al., "Metabolic reprogramming in skin wound healing," *Burns Trauma*, 2024, doi:10.1093/burnst/tkad047.
13. "Wound Healing and Repair," 2024.

14. D. M. Monroe and M. Hoffman, "What does it take to make the perfect clot?" *Arterioscl Thromb Vasc Biol,* 2006. doi:10.1161/01.ATV.0000193624.28251.83.
15. J. M. Reinke and H. Sorg, "Wound repair and regeneration," 2012. doi:10.1159/000339613.
16. A. Cioce, A. Cavani, C. Cattani, and F. Scopelliti, "Role of the skin immune system in wound healing," 2024, doi:10.3390/cells13070624.
17. M. Wei, X. He, N. Liu, and H. Deng, "Role of reactive oxygen species in ultraviolet-induced photodamage of the skin," 2024, doi:10.1186/s13008-024-00107-z.
18. Y. Firmansyah, V. M. Sidharta, L. Wijaya, and S. T. Tan, "Unraveling the significance of growth factors (TGF-β, PDGF, KGF, FGF, pro collagen, VEGF) in the dynamic of wound healing," *Asian J Med Health*, vol. 22, no. 3, pp. 49–61, 2024, doi:10.9734/ajmah/2024/v22i3992.
19. The Skin, 2024. www.wiley.com/go/buote/wounds.
20. C. J. Zhou and Y. Guo, "Mini review on collagens in normal skin and pathological scars: current understanding and future perspective," 2024, doi:10.3389/fmed.2024.1449597.
21. P. Chudaman Bhamare et al., "Potential role of collagen and its supplements in treatment of skin ageing", 2024.
22. Y. L. Luo, S. F. Luo, L. Luo, M. Ou, and M. L. Tang, "Effect of hydrocolloid dressing on pressure ulcer in patients with non-invasive positive pressure ventilation: a meta-analysis," *Int Wound J*, vol. 21, no. 2, 2024, doi:10.1111/iwj.14442.
23. M. Saco, N. Howe, R. Nathoo, and B. Cherpelis, "Comparing the efficacies of alginate, foam, hydrocolloid, hydrofiber, and hydrogel dressings in the management of diabetic foot ulcers and venous leg ulcers: a systematic review and meta-analysis examining how to dress for success," *Dermatology*, 2016, https://doi.org/10.5070/D3228032089.
24. O. L. Cortés et al., "Impact of hydrocolloid dressings in the prevention of pressure ulcers in high-risk patients: a randomized controlled trial (PENFUP)," *Sci Rep*, vol. 13, no. 1, 2023, doi:10.1038/s41598-023-47483-0.
25. J. C. Dumville, S. Deshpande, S. O'Meara, and K. Speak, "Hydrocolloid dressings for healing diabetic foot ulcers," 2013, doi:10.1002/14651858.CD009099.pub3.
26. J. Wang, Q. Gao, X. Feng, and Y. Chen, "Role of hydrocolloid dressing in preventing face pressure ulcers from non-invasive ventilation and facilitating postoperative wound healing in maxillofacial surgery: a meta-analysis," *Int Wound J*, vol. 21, no. 3, 2024, doi:10.1111/iwj.14780.
27. C. Wang, R. Li, X. Su, J. Zhang, and Z. Liu, "Effect of hydrocolloid dressings on preventing air leakage when applying negative pressure wound therapy to the perineum, buttocks, and sacrococcygeal region," *Wound Repair Regen*, vol. 32, no. 1, pp. 74–79, 2024, doi:10.1111/wrr.13136.
28. N. Qosim, Y. Dai, G. R. Williams, and M. Edirisinghe, "Structure, properties, forming, and applications of alginate fibers: a review," *Int Mater Rev*, vol. 69, no. 5–6, pp. 309–333, 2024, doi:10.1177/09506608241280419.
29. B. A. Aderibigbe and B. Buyana, "Alginate in wound dressings," 2018, doi:10.3390/pharmaceutics10020042.
30. P. Nezhad-Mokhtari, M. Hasany, M. Kohestanian, A. Dolatshahi-Pirouz, M. Milani, and M. Mehrali, "Recent advancements in bioadhesive self-healing hydrogels for effective chronic wound care," 2024, doi:10.1016/j.cis.2024.103306.
31. K. Yasuda, M. Ogushi, A. Nakashima, Y. Nakano, and K. Suzuki, "Accelerated wound healing on the skin using a film dressing with β-glucan paramylon," *In Vivo (Brooklyn)*, vol. 32, no. 4, pp. 799–805, 2018, doi:10.21873/invivo.11310.
32. A. Tanaka, T. Nagate, and H. Matsuda, "Acceleration of wound healing by gelatin film dressings with epidermal growth factor," *J Vet Med Sci*, vol. 67, pp. 909–913, 2005.
33. T. Li, M. Sun, and S. Wu, "State-of-the-art review of electrospun gelatin-based nanofiber dressings for wound healing applications," *Nanomaterials*, vol. 12, no. 5, p. 784, 2022, doi:10.3390/nano12050784.

34. L. Cremar et al., "Development of antimicrobial chitosan based nanofiber dressings for wound healing applications," *Nanomed J*, vol. 5, no. 1, 2018, doi:10.22038/nmj.2018.05.002.
35. A. Hargis, M. Yaghi, N. M. Bermudez, and A. Gefen, "Foam dressings for wound healing," 2024, doi:10.1007/s13671-024-00422-2.
36. K. Fogh and J. Nielsen, "Clinical utility of foam dressings in wound management: a review," *Chronic Wound Care Manag Res*, p. 31, 2015, doi:10.2147/cwcmr.s50832.
37. D. Queen, H. Orsted, H. Sanada, and G. Sussman, "A dressing history," *Int Wound J*, vol. 1, no. 1, pp. 59–77, 2004, doi:10.1111/j.1742-4801.2004.0009.x.
38. N. Chaiken, "Reduction of sacral pressure ulcers in the intensive care unit using a silicone border foam dressing," *J Wound Ostomy Contin Nurs*, vol. 39, no. 2, pp. 143–145, 2012, doi:10.1097/WON.0b013e318246400c.
39. P. M. Kharkar, S. N. Osborne, S. L. Stern, A. Pleitner, K. M. Wiencek, and K. M. Kieswetter, "Assessment of silver levels in a closed-incision negative pressure therapy dressing: in vitro and in vivo study," *Adv Wound Care (New Rochelle)*, vol. 9, no. 8, pp. 462–471, 2020, doi:10.1089/wound.2019.0997.
40. M. Yoshimura et al., "The incidence of intraoperatively acquired pressure injuries in the park-bench position was reduced by applying soft silicone multilayer foam dressings," *Int Wound J*, vol. 21, no. 2, 2024, doi:10.1111/iwj.14407.
41. S. Leonard, P. McCluskey, S. Long, V. Butters, R. Winter, and G. Smith, "An evaluation of Allevyn™ adhesive and non-adhesive foam dressings," *Wounds UK*, vol. 5, pp. 17–28, 2009.
42. L. Téot, F. Boissiere, and S. Fluieraru, "Novel foam dressing using negative pressure wound therapy with instillation to remove thick exudate," *Int Wound J*, vol. 14, no. 5, pp. 842–848, 2017, doi:10.1111/iwj.12719.
43. Y. Gou, L. Hu, X. Liao, J. He, and F. Liu, "Advances of antimicrobial dressings loaded with antimicrobial agents in infected wounds," 2024, doi:10.3389/fbioe.2024.1431949.
44. B. Boonkaew et al., "Development and characterization of a novel, antimicrobial, sterile hydrogel dressing for burn wounds: single-step production with gamma irradiation creates silver nanoparticles and radical polymerization," *J Pharm Sci*, vol. 103, no. 10, pp. 3244–3253, 2014, doi:10.1002/jps.24095.
45. F. Yousefian et al., "Antimicrobial wound dressings: a concise review for clinicians," 2023, doi:10.3390/antibiotics12091434.
46. S. Parham et al., "Antimicrobial synthetic and natural polymeric nanofibers as wound dressing: a review," 2022, doi:10.1002/adem.202101460.
47. Y. Gou, L. Hu, X. Liao, J. He, and F. Liu, "Advances of antimicrobial dressings loaded with antimicrobial agents in infected wounds," 2024, doi:10.3389/fbioe.2024.1431949.
48. L. Miranda-Calderon et al., "Combinatorial wound dressings loaded with synergistic antibiotics in the treatment of chronic infected wounds," *Chem Eng J*, vol. 476, 2023, doi:10.1016/j.cej.2023.146679.
49. A. May, Z. Kopecki, B. Carney, and A. Cowin, "Antimicrobial silver dressings: a review of emerging issues for modern wound care," 2022, doi:10.1111/ans.17382.
50. Y. Jiang et al., "Effectiveness of silver and iodine dressings on wound healing: a systematic review and meta-analysis," *BMJ Open*, vol. 14, no. 8, p. e077902, 2024, doi:10.1136/bmjopen-2023-077902.
51. J. Yupanqui Mieles, C. Vyas, E. Aslan, G. Humphreys, C. Diver, and P. Bartolo, "Honey: an advanced antimicrobial and wound healing biomaterial for tissue engineering applications," 2022, doi:10.3390/pharmaceutics14081663.
52. A. Saxena, R. J. Anandhi, K. Rashmi, N. Singh, D. Kumar Yadav, and R. S. Zabibah, "Biomedical materials for sustainable wound care: a review of environmental impact and clinical efficacy," *E3S Web Conf*, 2024, doi:10.1051/e3sconf/202455201060.

53. X. Liang et al., "Natural hydrogel dressings in wound care: design, advances, and perspectives," 2024, doi:10.1016/j.cclet.2023.109442.
54. Y. Yang, P. Wang, G. Zhang, S. He, and B. Xu, "Inorganic-nanomaterial-composited hydrogel dressings for wound healing," 2024, doi:10.3390/jcs8020046.
55. Y. El-Ghoul, A. S. Altuwayjiri, and G. A. Alharbi, "Synthesis and characterization of new electrospun medical scaffold-based modified cellulose nanofiber and bioactive natural propolis for potential wound dressing applications," *RSC Adv*, vol. 14, no. 36, pp. 26183–26197, 2024, doi:10.1039/d4ra04231j.
56. H. Zhang, X. Lin, X. Cao, Y. Wang, J. Wang, and Y. Zhao, "Developing natural polymers for skin wound healing," *Bioact Mater,* 2024, doi:10.1016/j.bioactmat.2023.11.012.
57. M. Kuddushi, A. A. Shah, C. Ayranci, and X. Zhang, "Recent advances in novel materials and techniques for developing transparent wound dressings."
58. S. O. Oselusi, N. R. S. Sibuyi, M. Meyer, and A. M. Madiehe, "Phytonanotherapeutic applications of plant extract-synthesized silver nanoparticles in wound healing—a prospective overview," 2024, doi:10.1007/s12668-024-01535-5.
59. Y. Lv et al., "PLLA-gelatin composite fiber membranes incorporated with functionalized CeNPs as a sustainable wound dressing substitute promoting skin regeneration and scar remodeling," *J Mater Chem B*, vol. 10, no. 7, pp. 1116–1127, 2022, doi:10.1039/d1tb02677a.
60. M. Somogyi Škoc, N. Stevelić, and I. Rezić, "Development and characterization of sustainable coatings on cellulose fabric and nonwoven for medical applications," *Sustainability (Switzerland)*, vol. 16, no. 2, 2024, doi:10.3390/su16020857.
61. S. Alven and B. A. Aderibigbe, "Chitosan-based scaffolds incorporated with silver nanoparticles for the treatment of infected wounds," 2024, doi:10.3390/pharmaceutics16030327.
62. L. Teot and N. Ohura, "Challenges and management in wound care," *Plast Reconstr Surg*, vol. 147, no. 1 S-1, pp. 9S–15S, 2021, doi:10.1097/PRS.0000000000007628.
63. P. Sanjarnia et al., "Bringing innovative wound care polymer materials to the market: challenges, developments, and new trends," 2024, doi:10.1016/j.addr.2024.115217.
64. R. Kumar et al., "Burn injury management, pathophysiology and its future prospectives," *J Res Appl Sci Biotechnol*, vol. 1, no. 4, pp. 78–89, 2022, doi:10.55544/jrasb.1.4.10.
65. J. R. Hilton, D. T. Williams, B. Beuker, D. R. Miller, and K. G. Harding, "Wound dressings in diabetic foot disease." https://academic.oup.com/cid/article/39/Supplement_2/S100/327419
66. L. Yazdanpanah, "Literature review on the management of diabetic foot ulcer," *World J Diabetes*, vol. 6, no. 1, p. 37, 2015, doi:10.4239/wjd.v6.i1.37.
67. J. C. Dumville, M. O. Soares, S. O'Meara, and N. Cullum, "Systematic review and mixed treatment comparison: dressings to heal diabetic Foot ulcers," 2012, doi:10.1007/s00125-012-2558-5.
68. A. C. Y. Chen, Y. Lu, C. Y. Hsieh, Y. S. Chen, K. C. Chang, and D. H. Chang, "Advanced biomaterials and topical medications for treating diabetic foot ulcers: a systematic review and network meta-analysis," *Adv Wound Care (New Rochelle)*, vol. 13, no. 2, pp. 97–113, 2024, doi:10.1089/wound.2023.0024.
69. M. Ríos-Galacho, D. Martínez-Moreno, E. López-Ruiz, P. Gálvez-Martín, and J. A. Marchal, "An overview on the manufacturing of functional and mature cellular skin substitutes," 2022, doi:10.1089/ten.teb.2021.0131.
70. A. C. Y. Chen, Y. Lu, C. Y. Hsieh, Y. S. Chen, K. C. Chang, and D. H. Chang, "Advanced biomaterials and topical medications for treating diabetic foot ulcers: a systematic review and network meta-analysis," *Adv Wound Care (New Rochelle)*, vol. 13, no. 2, pp. 97–113, 2024, doi:10.1089/wound.2023.0024.

71. L. Gerdesmeyer et al., "Topical treatment is effective and safe for acute ankle sprains: the multi-center double-blind randomized placebo-controlled TRAUMED Trial," *J Clin Med*, vol. 13, no. 3, 2024, doi:10.3390/jcm13030841.
72. R. K. Chan et al., "A prospective, randomized, controlled study to evaluate the effectiveness of a fabric-based wireless electroceutical dressing compared to standard-of-care treatment against acute trauma and burn wound biofilm infection," *Adv Wound Care (New Rochelle)*, vol. 13, no. 1, pp. 1–13, 2024, doi:10.1089/wound.2023.0007.
73. M. Saco, N. Howe, R. Nathoo, and B. Cherpelis, "Comparing the efficacies of alginate, foam, hydrocolloid, hydrofiber, and hydrogel dressings in the management of diabetic foot ulcers and venous leg ulcers: a systematic review and meta-analysis examining how to dress for success," *Dermatology*, 2016, doi:10.5070/d3228032089.
74. D. Bluestein, "Pressure ulcers: prevention, evaluation, and management," 2008, www.aafp.org/afp.
75. C. Wiegand, U. Wesenberg, and J. Heggemann, "A moisture-balancing hydropolymer gel dressing with a tissue boost effect—experimental and clinical evidence," *Chronic Wound Care Manag Res*, vol. 10, pp. 11–21, 2023, doi:10.2147/cwcmr.s422493.
76. P. Nezhad-Mokhtari, M. Hasany, M. Kohestanian, A. Dolatshahi-Pirouz, M. Milani, and M. Mehrali, "Recent advancements in bioadhesive self-healing hydrogels for effective chronic wound care," 2024, doi:10.1016/j.cis.2024.103306.
77. O. L. Cortés et al., "Impact of hydrocolloid dressings in the prevention of pressure ulcers in high-risk patients: a randomized controlled trial (PENFUP)," *Sci Rep*, vol. 13, no. 1, 2023, doi:10.1038/s41598-023-47483-0.
78. A. Hargis, M. Yaghi, N. M. Bermudez, and A. Gefen, "Foam dressings for wound healing," 2024, doi:10.1007/s13671-024-00422-2.
79. X. Yang, "Research on strategies for wound healing and infection control in skin disease nursing," *SHS Web Conf*, vol. 200, p. 02011, 2024, doi:10.1051/shsconf/202420002011.
80. Z. Xu et al., "Cellulose-based pH-responsive janus dressing with unidirectional moisture drainage for exudate management and diabetic wounds healing," *Adv Funct Mater*, vol. 34, no. 3, 2024, doi:10.1002/adfm.202307449.
81. G. Kakar, S. Pathak, and H. Krishnani, "Therapeutic advances in wound healing."
82. B. Gupta, R. Agarwal, and M. S. Alam, "Textile-based smart wound dressings," 2010.
83. X. Li, X. Xue, and P. Xie, "Smart dressings and their applications in chronic wound management," 2024, doi:10.1007/s12013-024-01402-w.
84. Y. Wang, H. Li, L. Xu, J. Yan, and X. Y. Wang, "Preparation and properties of temperature-sensitive silver-loaded antibacterial sericin/poly (N-isopropylacrylamide) hydrogel," *J Macromol Sci B* Phys, vol. 63, no. 10, pp. 889–908, 2024, doi:10.1080/00222348.2023.2290803.
85. K. Youssef, A. Ullah, P. Rezai, A. Hasan, and A. Amirfazli, "Recent advances in biosensors for real time monitoring of pH, temperature, and oxygen in chronic wounds," 2023, doi:10.1016/j.mtbio.2023.100764.
86. Z. Zhang, H. Liu, D. G. Yu, and S. W. A. Bligh, "Alginate-based electrospun nanofibers and the enabled drug controlled release profiles: a review," 2024, doi:10.3390/biom14070789.
87. C. Wu, H. Ren, Y. Zhang, D. Jian, Y. Gao, and J. Wu, "pH-responsive nanofiber membranes for superior controlled release of poorly water-soluble drug and its release mechanism study," *Colloids Interface Science Commun*, vol. 57, 2023, doi:10.1016/j.colcom.2023.100750.
88. J. A. Mullin, E. Rahmani, K. L. Kiick, and M. O. Sullivan, "Growth factors and growth factor gene therapies for treating chronic wounds," 2024, doi:10.1002/btm2.10642.
89. Z. Yuan et al., "Multi-functional fibrous dressings for burn injury treatment with pain and swelling relief and scarless wound healing," *Adv Fiber Mater*, vol. 5, no. 6, pp. 1963–1985, 2023, doi:10.1007/s42765-023-00320-5.

90. A. Orlov and A. Gefen, "Effective negative pressure wound therapy for open wounds: the importance of consistent pressure delivery," *Int Wound J*, vol. 20, no. 2, pp. 328–344, 2023, doi:10.1111/iwj.13879.
91. A. Gefen et al., "Fluid handling by foam wound dressings: from engineering theory to advanced laboratory performance evaluations," *Int Wound J*, vol. 21, no. 2, 2024, doi:10.1111/iwj.14674.
92. Y. Tang et al., "Negative pressure wound therapy promotes wound healing of diabetic foot ulcers by up-regulating PRDX2 in wound margin tissue," *Sci Rep*, vol. 13, no. 1, 2023, doi:10.1038/s41598-023-42634-9.
93. V. Jones, J. E. Grey, and K. G. Harding, "ABC of wound healing wound dressings."
94. S. Baek and J. H. Park, "Negative pressure wound therapy (NPWT) after hybrid reconstruction of occipital pressure sore using local flap and skin graft," *Medicina (Lithuania)*, vol. 59, no. 7, 2023, doi:10.3390/medicina59071342.
95. T. Sharma, R. Mittal, and P. Kaushik, "Advances in polymer-based scaffolding for enhanced wound healing: a comprehensive review," 2024, doi:10.1080/00914037.2024.2367208.
96. A. Ullah, M. Ullah, G. J. Lee, and S. I. Lim, "A review of recent advances in nanotechnology for the delivery of therapeutics in wound healing," 2024, doi:10.1007/s40005-024-00692-9.
97. S. Nasra, S. Pramanik, V. Oza, K. Kansara, and A. Kumar, "Advancements in wound management: integrating nanotechnology and smart materials for enhanced therapeutic interventions," 2024, doi:10.1186/s11671-024-04116-3.
98. X. Li, X. Xue, and P. Xie, "Smart dressings and their applications in chronic wound management," 2024, doi:10.1007/s12013-024-01402-w.
99. Y. Dong, S. Fu, J. Yu, X. Li, and B. Ding, "Emerging smart micro/nanofiber-based materials for next-generation wound dressings," 2024, doi:10.1002/adfm.202311199.
100. Z. Yuan et al., "Anti-inflammatory, antibacterial, and antioxidative bioactive glass-based nanofibrous dressing enables scarless wound healing," *Smart Mater Med*, vol. 4, pp. 407–426, 2023, doi:10.1016/j.smaim.2023.01.001.
101. S. M. Tatarusanu et al., "New smart bioactive and biomimetic chitosan-based hydrogels for wounds care management," *Pharmaceutics*, vol. 15, no. 3, 2023, doi:10.3390/pharmaceutics15030975.
102. S. Li et al., "High self-supporting chitosan-based hydrogel ink for in situ 3D printed diabetic wound dressing," *Adv Funct Mater*, 2024, doi:10.1002/adfm.202414625.
103. O. Kammona, E. Tsanaktsidou, and C. Kiparissides, "Recent developments in 3D-(bio) printed hydrogels as wound dressings," 2024, doi:10.3390/gels10020147.
104. R. P. Rathna and M. Kulandhaivel, "Advancements in wound healing: integrating biomolecules, drug delivery carriers, and targeted therapeutics for enhanced tissue repair," 2024. doi:10.1007/s00203-024-03910-y.
105. H. Jangid, S. Singh, P. Kashyap, A. Singh, and G. Kumar, "Advancing biomedical applications: an in-depth analysis of silver nanoparticles in antimicrobial, anticancer, and wound healing roles," 2024, doi:10.3389/fphar.2024.1438227.
106. R. Laurano, M. Boffito, G. Ciardelli, and V. Chiono, "Wound dressing products: a translational investigation from the bench to the market," 2022, doi:10.1016/j.engreg.2022.04.002.
107. X. Tang et al., "Wound healing driver gene and therapeutic development: political and scientific hurdles," 2021, doi:10.1089/wound.2019.1143.
108. C. Wang et al., "Wound management materials and technologies from bench to bedside and beyond," *Nat Res*, 2024, doi:10.1038/s41578-024-00693-y.
109. J. Nandhini, E. Karthikeyan, and S. Rajeshkumar, "Nanomaterials for wound healing: current status and futuristic frontier," *Biomater Trans*, 2024, doi:10.1016/j.bmt.2023.10.001.

110. J. Butler, R. D. Handy, M. Upton, and A. Besinis, "Review of antimicrobial nanocoatings in medicine and dentistry: mechanisms of action, biocompatibility performance, safety, and benefits compared to antibiotics," *ACS Nano*, vol. 17, no. 8, pp. 7064–7092, 2023, doi:10.1021/acsnano.2c12488.
111. D. C. Aduba and H. Yang, "Polysaccharide fabrication platforms and biocompatibility assessment as candidate wound dressing materials," 2017, doi:10.3390/bioengineering4010001.
112. V. Gounden and M. Singh, "Hydrogels and wound healing: current and future prospects," 2024, doi:10.3390/gels10010043.
113. A. Gefen et al., "How should clinical wound care and management translate to effective engineering standard testing requirements from foam dressings? mapping the existing gaps and needs," 2024, doi:10.1089/wound.2021.0173.
114. L. Van Rijswijk, "Back to the future in wound care: a view from here," *J Wound Ostomy Contin Nurs*, vol. 51, no. 1, pp. 17–18, 2024, doi:10.1097/WON.0000000000001050.
115. G. K. Srivastava et al., "Progress in wound-healing products based on natural compounds, stem cells, and MicroRNA-based biopolymers in the European, USA, and Asian markets: opportunities, barriers, and regulatory issues," 2024, doi:10.3390/polym16091280.
116. S. Khan, V. Rai, S. Srivastava, S. Agarwal, N. Bano, and Y. Gupta, "Nano medicine in healing chronic wounds: opportunities and challenges," *J Res Appl Sci Biotechnol*, vol. 3, no. 1, pp. 12–16, 2024, doi:10.55544/jrasb.3.1.3.
117. L. E. Lindley, O. Stojadinovic, I. Pastar, and M. Tomic-Canic, "Biology and biomarkers for wound healing," *Plast Reconstr Surg*, vol. 138, no. 3, pp. 18S–28S, 2016, doi:10.1097/PRS.0000000000002682.
118. L. A. Damiati, D. Durand-Herrera, and M. El Soury, "Editorial: the future of modern medicine: cells, scaffolds, and biofactors," 2024, doi:10.3389/fmed.2024.1434760.
119. X. Li, X. Xue, and P. Xie, "Smart dressings and their applications in chronic wound management," 2024, doi:10.1007/s12013-024-01402-w.
120. R. Encarnação, T. Manuel, H. Palheira, J. Neves-Amado, and P. Alves, "Artificial intelligence in wound care education: protocol for a scoping review," *Nurs Rep*, vol. 14, no. 1, pp. 627–640, 2024, doi:10.3390/nursrep14010048.
121. "WINT-14-2_12–15_Heerschap".
122. E. Moshkbid, D. E. Cree, L. Bradford, and W. Zhang, "Biodegradable alternatives to plastic in medical equipment: current state, challenges, and the future," *J Compos Sci*, vol. 8, no. 9, p. 342, 2024, doi:10.3390/jcs8090342.
123. J. Nandhini, E. Karthikeyan, and S. Rajeshkumar, "Eco-friendly bio-nanocomposites: pioneering sustainable biomedical advancements in engineering," 2024, doi:10.1186/s11671-024-04007-7.
124. N. Kasoju et al., "Digital health: trends, opportunities and challenges in medical devices, pharma and bio-technology," *CSI Trans ICT*, vol. 11, no. 1, pp. 11–30, 2023, doi:10.1007/s40012-023-00380-3.
125. M. Dabas, D. Schwartz, D. Beeckman, and A. Gefen, "Application of artificial intelligence methodologies to chronic wound care and management: a scoping review," 2023, doi:10.1089/wound.2021.0144.
126. M. U. Tariq, "Advanced wearable medical devices and their role in transformative remote health monitoring," In: M.B. Garcia, R.P.P. de Almeida, editors, *Transformative Approaches to Patient Literacy and Healthcare Innovation*, IGI Global, 2024, pp. 308–326. https://doi.org/10.4018/979-8-3693-3661-8.ch015.
127. K. A. McLean et al., "Evaluation of remote digital postoperative wound monitoring in routine surgical practice," *NPJ Digit Med*, vol. 6, no. 1, 2023, doi:10.1038/s41746-023-00824-9.

128. N. Babaei et al., "Barriers to the implementation of virtual care programmes for patients with chronic wounds: qualitative empirical research," *Nurs Open*, vol. 10, no. 11, pp. 7301–7313, 2023, doi:10.1002/nop2.1983.
129. D. Huang et al., "Role of mesenchymal stem cell-derived exosomes in the regeneration of different tissues," 2024, doi:10.1186/s13036-024-00431-6.
130. A. M. Jorgensen, N. Mahajan, A. Atala, and S. V. Murphy, "Advances in skin tissue engineering and regenerative medicine," *J Burn Care Res*, vol. 44, no. 1, pp. S33–S41, 2023, doi:10.1093/jbcr/irac126.

10 AI-Based Advancement in Wound Care

Muhammad Abbas Haider Alvi,
Muhammad Qamar Khan, and Ick Soo Kim

INTRODUCTION

The management of wounds is a cornerstone of medical practice, but the problems associated with wound management are greatly influenced by one distinction that can be critical: the distinction between acute and chronic wounds. The textbook definition of how the body can take care of itself is through an acute wound [1]. Consider a small cut or a surgical incision, or a clean cut. There is a rational, orderly progression of healing of these wounds that occurs in a timely and efficient manner in four specific stages, including hemostasis, inflammation, proliferation, and remodeling. The process is a rather viscerally designed biological ordeal that will normally occur within four weeks with few complications. But there is an utterly different and much more disturbing terrain when it comes to chronic wounds. These are the wounds that do not follow the usual course of healing, and they take a long time to heal, usually over four to six weeks. The most typical ones, such as diabetic foot ulcers (DFUs), pressure sores (bedsores), and venous leg ulcers, appear to be not just surface-level damage. Rather, they are deep signs of a health problem with the system. As an example, a diabetic ulcer most likely occurs due to the lack of proper circulation and neuropathy [2], which causes a diabetic ulcer because it does not permit the required nerve signals and blood flow to reach the location of the wound. On the same note, a pressure sore implies prolonged pressure that has led to local death of the tissue. These injuries get stalled at the inflammatory stage, where they do not transition to the proliferative stage, and new tissues do not grow. The biological stagnation causes a vicious loop of tissue injury and failure to heal, transforming a manageable injury to become a chronic, debilitating condition. The number of patients affected by chronic wounds all over the world is a big challenge, and it is also increasing on the healthcare system. Not only are they painful for the patient, but they also result in a massive surge in the cost of management of the patients, a prolonged stay in hospitals, as well as an enhanced occurrence of severe and dire complications such as severe infections, gangrene, and, in the worst-case scenario, amputation. It is dismal to note that this crisis spells a stark necessity of providing superior and smarter wound care technologies. The management of all forms of wounds, whether new or old wounds, has in the past decades been based on passive dressings to the extent that their level of care is used. Products such as gauze, hydrogels, foams, and alginates have been the labor of wound care, and they have served well. They are useful in

DOI: 10.1201/9781003616726-12

offering a shield, soaking up extra fluid, and keeping an open wound wet, which is essential for healing.

Nevertheless, these conventional dressings come with one basic drawback [3], i.e., passivity. They are a universal remedy to a situation that is far more complex. A foam dressing, when applied once, cannot dissipate in this close environment, as a chronic wound is very dynamic and constantly changing. It is not capable of real-time response to critical healing parameters, including the pH levels, temperature, signs of infection, or oxygenation. Clinicians are left to depend on visual inspections, which are generally uncommon and subjective, and wait until they notice signs of the problem before taking measures. This responsive treatment causes a wound-affected condition to become worse without the observer knowing what goes on under the dressing, followed by delayed interventions, poor patient outcomes, and repetitive dressing and visits to the clinic for patients. The reason that many people today view chronic wound management as a long, arduous, and often unsuccessful process boils down to the lack of intelligence in these materials. The stark contrast between the level of complexity that is central in chronic wounds and the level of simplicity that defines traditional care has necessitated the need to change the care paradigm. The future of wound management is in proactive, personalized, and adaptive management. These two disciplines are advanced biomaterials and artificial intelligence (AI), which are driving the current transformation [4]. The current age of smart wound management is now about getting away from the basic wound cover to a smart, interactive system. Biomaterials are being developed such that they have inbuilt biosensors that can capture the most important physiological indicators in real time. These smart bandages can monitor things such as temperature, pH (which can indicate whether they have an infection), or the presence of certain biomarkers. However, the real jump can be achieved thanks to the incorporation of AI. The smart dressings are run by AI, which is the brain behind them.

It will be able to draw conclusions about the large amount of information gathered by the sensors, detect minute patterns that cannot be seen by the human eye, and offer meaningful suggestions to its clinicians. This synergy is possible to revolutionize care: from early diagnostics, in which AI algorithms are capable of analyzing the images of wounds and correctly diagnose the wound, the wound type, and forecasting the healing trends, to personalized treatment schemes, in which AI can suggest the most effective treatment based on the real-time data of the wound. In the end, such incorporation will result in the shift of the wound care paradigm, shifting it to a highly predictive and individualized approach, making it possible to heal wounds faster, with lower costs, and improve the quality of life of millions of patients around the world with chronic wounds.

The Fundamentals of Wound Healing and Its Interruption

In order to truly appreciate the possibilities of intelligent wound care, it is necessary to first get to know the fine art of the events that make up normal healing. The process itself is not an instance but a cascade of four successive overlapping and highly controlled phases, which have a definite purpose.

This stage is the initial defense in the body, and it is known as hemostasis. Damaged blood vessels constrict in times of injury to reduce blood loss [5]. At this point, platelets are then brought to the area, creating a clumpy plug. The stability of this blood clot is due to the platelet plug and the action of clotting factors. This has two crucial roles: it stops bleeding and becomes a temporary matrix, or scaffold, on which the next protagonists of the game can develop. After that, the inflammatory phase is initiated after the bleeding has been under control. The blood vessels surrounding the wound open up to raise the blood flow that can reach the injury and grant access to immune cells. The main actors here include neutrophils and macrophages, which are the cleaning crew of the body. They consume and kill bacteria, remove corpses of dead cells, and secrete a plethora of signaling molecules that sterilize the wound bed to accomplish rebuilding. This develops clinically in the form of the classic signs of inflammation, redness, heat, swelling, and pain. Although inflammatory response is necessary to heal, it occurs in optimal conditions and is the most frequent spot of failure in chronic wounds. The wound gets trapped in a degenerative cycle, thus failing to move to the next stage in case this phase is sustained longer by an ongoing infection or other causes. This is the wound healing stage, also known as proliferation, in which the wound is rebuilt. Fibroblasts start moving into the wound to form a new structure of collagen, a form of extracellular matrix (ECM) that is the main protein constituting the structure of the skin. This newly formed robust red tissue, which is known as the granulation tissue, is a clear indication of healing. At the same time, the growing tissue requires oxygen and nutrients, so it is connected to new blood vessels by the formation of blood vessels through a process known as angiogenesis. Lastly, wound edge epithelial cells start moving toward the center, hence forming a new layer that covers the wound. The last and longest phase is Remodeling, which may last months or even years. New tissue is to be built upon and hardened here. The collagen fibers are initially organized randomly, then reorganized and linked together in crosses, rendering the new tissue tensile stronger. Cellular action is reduced, and the wound site is reduced and hardened to a scar with less vasculature. It will take time for this new tissue to be as strong as the actual skin, but this stage makes the wound as strong and usable as possible.

The Barriers to Healing: When the Process Fails

Once this well-orchestrated process is disrupted, a wound may enter into a pathogenic status. This non-healing condition is a multifactorial concern that is caused by a mixture of local and systemic factors. DFU [2] is one of the most successful examples of numerous impediments in action. Neuropathy means that the patient cannot have the primary injury, and poor circulation as a result of atherosclerosis reduces the availability of oxygen and nutrients, which the injury requires to heal. The most frequent obstacles on the pathway to healing can be classified, as presented in Table 10.1.

TABLE 10.1
The Most Common Impediments to Healing

Impediment	Description	Clinical Example	Impact on Wound
Infection	A high load of the pathogenic bacteria overpowers the immune system and extends the inflammatory period	A pus-filled, filthy stench surgical cut	Causes chronic inflammation, tissue destruction, and delayed healing
Poor perfusion	Poor blood supply to the wound, which is usually caused by the underlying conditions	Venous leg ulceration in a patient with peripheral artery disease	Denies oxygen and nutrients to the wound, which deprives it of being rebuilt at the cellular level
Biofilms	An intricate, viscous collection of exceedingly antibiotic-resistant bacteria	A pressure sore that is chronic, with a yellowish, slimy coating that is difficult to debride	Protect bacteria against immune system and antibiotics, leading to long-term inflammation
Moisture imbalance	An overdried or a moist wound	A scabby, hard, dry (desiccation) or red, softened (maceration) edged wound	A dry wound cannot facilitate cell migration, whereas a wet wound will lead to a breakdown of the early skin, enlarging the wound
Underlying diseases	There are systemic conditions that interfere with the healing capacity of the body	An unhealing wound of a patient who has unregulated diabetes or a weak immunity	It interferes with the way the cell functions, blood circulation, and the immune response to develop effective healing

The Power of Real-Time Monitoring: A Paradigm Shift

These impediments used to be identified reactively in the past, whereby a nurse would observe the change in temperature or exudate color during the scheduled dressing change, which might be days away. It might be the case that the complication would have already progressed by the time they diagnose it. That is where the AI and biosensors are establishing a mega talent shift in paradigm. The affinity to permanently incorporate more advanced and sensitive biosensors into the dressings of the wounds enables real-time monitoring of the wound space [6].

How It Works in Practice

Temperature Sensors

The presence of a temperature elevation in a specific location is one of the cardinal signs of inflammatory and infectious processes. A smart bandage will be able to monitor the temperature of the wound 24 hours a day, and once there is a drastic increase in temperature, it can alert the smartphone or iPad of the clinician. This enables us to be able to act directly and with pinpoint accuracy, such as a change of antibiotic therapy far in advance of the infection, conferring its cytotoxic effects in a clinical situation.

pH Sensors

A normal, healing wound is slightly acidic (usually pH 5.5–6.5). Nevertheless, as an inflammatory process occurs, the organism increases the pH to a more alkaline level (pH > 7.5). This change can be sensed by a colorimetric or an electrochemical sensor in the dressing. An example of this would be the transformation of a color-changing hydrogel, which could change color from blue to red, thus giving a clear visual indication to the patient or care receiver of the need to seek a consultation.

Exudate Composition Sensors

The draining fluid in a wound (exudate) is rich in information. Certain enzymes, such as matrix metalloproteinases (MMPs) that break down tissue, are at high levels in chronic wounds. Smart dressings may be fitted with sensors that sense these particular biomarkers, which can give a detailed biochemical picture of the healing state of the wound. Such information can help the clinician determine whether the wound is indeed taking the right direction or needs to be planned otherwise. The transition to continuous assessment and real-time monitoring enables to identify the complications early enough, makes individual adjustments to care, and, as a result, considerably decreases the amount of time needed to cure a chronic wound.

Overview of Artificial Intelligence in Healthcare

The healthcare community is embracing the use of AI with much enthusiasm, with early systems that are both experimental and theoretical, giving way to more achievable clinical applications. AI, in its basic form, is a wide collection of algorithmic techniques intended to imitate the behavior of human intelligence. Among the larger area, Machine Learning (ML) and Deep Learning (DL) have emerged as especially effective and useful, especially when it comes to processing large and complex datasets, such as medical images and real-time sensor data, as well as huge amounts of clinical data. Choosing the particular parameters to follow is done automatically by the ML algorithms without being programmed. They find trends, make forecasts, and adjust their performance according to what they read in greater measure. DL is a specific form of ML that resorts to the multilayered artificial neural networks designed after the human brain. These networks are exceptionally good at identifying complex patterns in unstructured data, such as images and raw sensor signals, and are thus perfect to use on complex diagnostic tasks. When merged, these technologies enable AIs to process piles of information and find insights that can transform care provision to patients much faster and more effectively than what human brains on their own can achieve [7]. The potential in the use of AI in wound care holds a lot of potential in terms of resolving most of the issues that have plagued the field of wound care historically. The use of AI is being developed in several major areas (Figure 10.1).

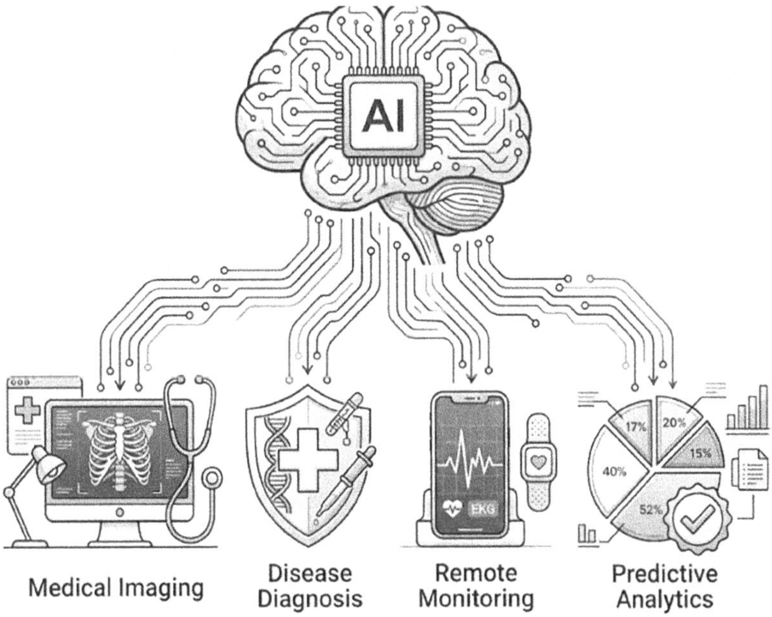

FIGURE 10.1 The rule of AI in healthcare.

Automated Diagnosis and Image-Based Classification

AI in wound care is one of the most direct and immediate applications of AI in wound image-based diagnosis and classification. The conventional process of wound assessment may be based on subjective visual examination by the caregivers, which has the same issue of imprecision and delay in the determination of the key aspects of the wound. AI, with its powerful computer vision (CV) algorithms, creates the possibility of a more objective and accurate alternative [8].

Ultra-Accurate Measurement and Characterization

AI software can process high-resolution pictures of wounds to precisely measure their length, width, depth, and modifications in surface area over time, as well as build a 3D topology of wounds. This numerical information is vital so that it can be used to track the healing process as well as measure treatment efficacy. As an example, an AI system can exactly determine the percentage amount of various tissue types within a wound bed—healthy granulation tissue, necrotic tissue (dead tissue) or slough—and then give a detailed picture of how healthy the wound is [9].

Automated Classification

DL models have the potential to become a powerful tool that can be used to classify the types of wounds (e.g., diabetic ulcer, pressure injury, and surgical wound) and even identify early signs of wound complications owing to a large dataset of wound images that can be used to train the ML/DL models. The possibilities are endless with a smartphone application that a patient or caregiver may take a picture of a wound, and AI automatically recognizes potential warning signs of an infection or imperative wound healing based on minute visual stimuli such as a change in color, exudate characteristics, or periwound skin changes. This will help intervene early, therefore, minimizing the chances of contracting severe complications and better patient outcomes.

Prognostic Modeling and Personalized Treatment

In addition to diagnosis, AI is already a lifesaver in terms of predicting wound healing patterns and being able to provide patients with personalized treatment options.

Achieving Good Results at Healing

Combining image data and the rest of clinical records (patient demographics, medical history, and comorbidities such as diabetes and prior responses to treatment), a comprehensive prognostic model can be developed by AI algorithms. These models have the capability of predicting the outcome of a particular wound (will it be healed within a given time or not?) or a risk that a patient may develop a non-healing wound. As an example, AI would evaluate the blood glucose levels, wound size development, and the existence of particular biomarkers to predict the likelihood that a DFU will heal in less than 12 weeks. This predictability can enable the clinicians to be pre-emptive in arousing change in treatment approach and make better use of resources as well as need-based patient expectations (Figure 10.2).

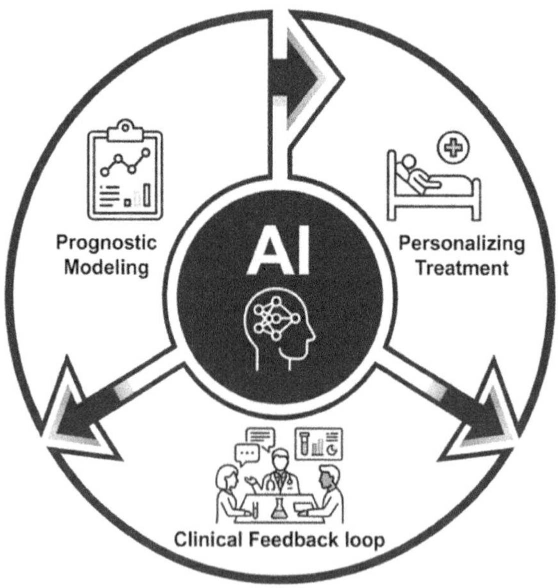

FIGURE 10.2 Prognostic modeling and personalized treatment.

TABLE 10.2
AI's Applications in Wound Care

AI Application Area	Description	Impact on Wound Care
Automated diagnosis	AI enables the measurement (size, depth, and tissue type) of the wound and determination of its main features	Objective reproducible wound measurement; minimizes human error; provides remote monitoring
Image-based classification	The AI models identify the types of wounds (e.g., acute, chronic, diabetic ulcer, and pressure sore) and show the early signs of complications	Accelerates early triage; alerts high-risk wounds; allows preventive action in time
Prognostic modeling	AI estimates the paths to healing and forecasts which patients are at danger of not healing using multi-modal information	Allows effective planning of care; the best use of resources; establishes realistic expectations with patients
Personalized treatment	AI suggests individualized interventions (type of dressing, medication, and debridement) depending on wound data in real time and the profile of a patient	Makes treatment as effective as possible; minimizes trial and error; increases the speed of the healing process

Personalized Interventions

The final objective, then, is to go beyond broad-based protocols to highly personalized treatments that AI can achieve. Depending on the real-time sensor data of smart bandages and prognostic models, one can suggest the best type of dressing, propose a certain debridement method, or just recommend the best dressing frequency. In another scenario, when smart bandage identifies that there is a rise in wound pH and temperature, which are indicative of early infection, the AI system may suggest a certain antimicrobial dressing, or a shift in antibiotic regimen to stretch machine specific to the particular patient and depending on the current condition of the wound. Such a dynamic course of action means that a patient is always treated in the best interests, and this once again increases the likelihood of healing success. Table 10.2 illustrates a summary of the uses of AI in wound care.

Medical AI is an enormous promise, but it also presents formidable ethical and regulatory obstacles on the way to deployment. It is all the more so to guarantee a safe, fair, and responsible usage of these exceptionally potent technologies.

Data Security and Privacy

AI works best when its many data inputs are diverse, and there is a need to secure various datasets that patients can provide, such as medical records, photos, and genetic data. How to secure this information against theft and abuse is a very important issue. Data protection regulations such as Health Insurance Portability and Accountability Act (HIPAA) in the United States and General Data Protection Regulation (GDPR) in Europe afford a basis upon which data protection can be derived, yet the vastness of data and the intricacy of it being processed by AI require an attentive eye and an effective form of cybersecurity. The correct patient consent regarding data collection and data usage is also a very important, and, at the same time, complex issue.

Transparency and Explainability ("The Black Box Problem")

Most ML models are transparent and explainable, especially DL networks, which can be described as a black box because it is hard to understand the inner workings of such AI systems. Such a lack of transparency in healthcare, where minor misjudgments of medical decisions can turn out to be life or death, can damage the trust on both sides, the clinicians and the patient. Healthcare professionals are required to know the reasons why an AI system came up with a specific recommendation to confirm that the AI system is correct and will not jeopardize patient safety. The solution to this is the development of Explainable AI (XAI) to make AI decisions more interpretable.

Fairness and Algorithmic Biases

An AI model is trained using data; whatever is in the training data will end up in the model. If it mirrors historic inequalities or under-represents certain groups of the population (e.g., particular ethnic groups, gender, and socioeconomic background), AI can reproduce or even increase the inequalities that existed before, leading to unfair healthcare outcomes. A hypothetical example would be to train an AI precision medical device on image data biased to be lighter-skinned and find that the AI precision medical device would work less accurately on darker skin tones, misdiagnosing some groups of people or delaying care. Strict bias detection and a variety of datasets, as well as continuous auditing, are the necessary components to achieve fairness.

Clinical Validation and Regulatory Approval

AI-powered medical devices will not be used widely unless they can pass through rigorous clinical validation to demonstrate how good, safe, and generalizable they have become in the actual world. This usually entails large-scale clinical trials, which show the capability of AI over a large and heterogeneous patient set and multiple clinical conditions. Regulatory agencies, including the Food and Drug Administration (FDA) in the United States and the EMA in Europe, are currently working on regulations regarding the validation of AI-based medical devices with the emphasis on proper testing, post-market surveillance, and clear documentation of the AI application's potential and limitations. It is crucial to address these ethical and regulatory aspects not as just a compliance effort; it is central to the realization of trust, alignment with equitable care, and the complete potential of AI in transforming wound care to become more universal and widely accepted. All the critical considerations are shown in Table 10.3.

Smart Wound Dressings: Evolution and Components

The drawbacks of the conventional ways of wound dressing have led to a paradigm change to smart dressing of wounds. Not just passive coverings but multifunctional biomedical machines are designed to monitor responsively and even aid in the

TABLE 10.3
Ethical/Regulatory Considerations of AI in Wound Care

Ethical/Regulatory Considerations	Description	Impact on AI in Wound Care
Data privacy & security	Preventing unauthorized persons from accessing sensitive patient information (medical records, images)	Proper patient trust and legal adherence (HIPAA, GDPR) require comprehensive cybersecurity
Transparency & explainability	Knowing more about the origins of the decisions made by AI algorithms ("black box" problem)	Vital to acceptance and responsibility of clinicians; permits the destiny of AI suggestions
Fairness & algorithmic bias	Preventing the introduction or even increasing known biases of the training datasets into AI models	Does not allow biased results of the treatment; needs numerous diverse datasets and constant audits
Clinical validation & approval	Strict testing of AI, which proves its safety, efficacy, and generalizations in real-life clinical conditions	Makes sure AI is trustworthy and efficient; this is a requirement to be accepted by the regulations and to become widely used

healing process on a real-time basis. Its development is supported by the combination of the most innovative materials science, enhanced sensing, and microfluidic technology. The essence of smart wound dressings is that they replicate or supersede the natural healing environment and, in that regard, present a sub-optimal microclimate to tissue regeneration, as well as unprecedented visibility into the physiologic condition of a wound. The smartness of these new dressings is due to the creativity of the material used, which is no longer the plain gauze but rather an adhesive layer [10] (Figure 10.3).

Hydrogels

These could be the most noticeable advanced materials in smart dressing. Hydrogels are three-dimensional polymer networks with the ability to absorb and retain large quantities of water, to provide a moist environment that is essential for cell migration and repair of the tissue. They are biocompatible and made of soft, flexible materials, making them suitable for direct touch with fragile wound beds. They are stimuli-responsive, which makes them smart. This is in the sense that they will be able to alter their properties (e.g., swelling, permeability, and drug release) in the presence of particular stimuli of the wound environment.

pH-Responsive Hydrogels

A key factor in determining the state of a wound and possible infection is pH. Healthy skin has a slightly acidic pH between 4.0 and 6.0, whereas chronic and infected wounds themselves are often more alkaline (>7.0) pH. When the pH becomes shifted

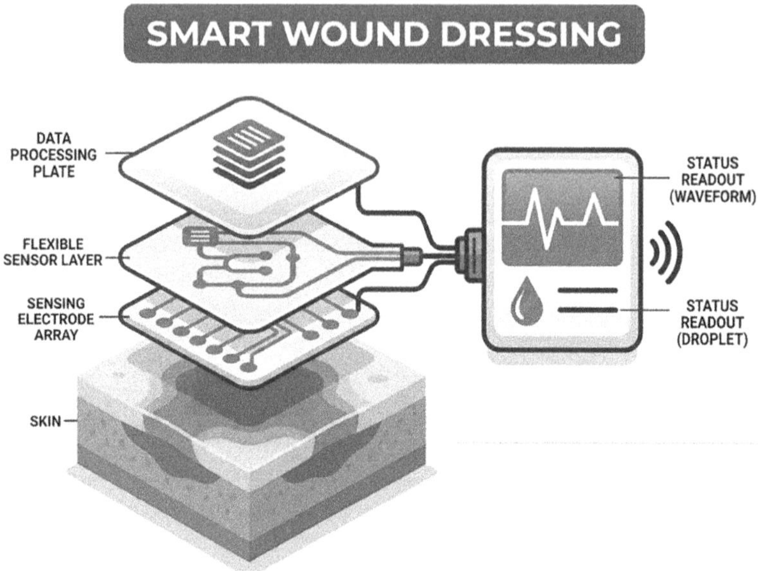

FIGURE 10.3 Smart wound dressing.

to an alkaline range, hydrogels can be designed to swell or release encapsulated therapeutics (such as antimicrobials), actively seeking out an infection. As an example, the drug can be incorporated within a hydrogel and be released only at wounds with an increased pH, which means bacteria interact in the wound.

Temperature-Influenced Hydrogels

A rise in temperature of wounds could indicate the incidence of inflammation or infection. In some hydrogels, there is a special design so that the temperature changes cause changes in structure, which is a mechanism for delivering the medication or other healing processes. This makes it possible to treat them on a localized and on-demand basis using the thermal signature of the wound.

Redox-Responsive Hydrogels

Oxidative stress in a wound leads to an increase in the redox (reduction-oxidation) state, which is high in chronic wounds. Hydrogels may also be developed to respond to these changes and release antioxidants or other factors to re-establish balance in the wound and favor healing [11].

Nanofibers

These are very fine fibers usually made using methods such as electrospinning, and they resemble the natural ECM of the skin. Their low surface-area-to-volume ratio, interconnected porous design, and their mechanical properties make them ideal for the applications mentioned.

Mimicking ECM

Giving them a scaffold that helps the cells adhere, proliferate, and migrate so as to speed the regrowth of tissues.

Controlled Drug Delivery

Nanofibers can be loaded with a variety of therapeutic agents (e.g., antibiotics, growth factors, and anti-inflammatory drugs) and optimized to release them over a certain period or under specific conditions and ensure that there is always a constant presence of a therapeutic agent at the wound site. This is a selective delivery that reduces the systemic side effects and maximizes the efficacy of the location.

Exudate Management

They have good porosity, which helps in the absorption of exudate, yet provide a breathable environment to the wound without causing maceration and giving optimum moisture content.

Microfluidics

Microfluidics is the field of microscale fluid processing within a dressing or on the order of the channels within the dressing. Microfluidic features in smart dressing can play a significant role:

Exudate Management and Sampling

The smart dressing can include a microchannel network that efficiently wicks hyper-exudate off the wound face, thus preventing fluid accumulation, and this can also have a sample function. More importantly, they can constantly exchange the wound fluid with new ones on the biosensors to ensure the data that is obtained is reflective of the current condition of the wound and not the stagnant liquid.

Localized Drug Delivery

It can be adapted to deliver small, controlled amounts of therapeutics locally to particular regions of wounds; this would grant specificity and eliminate waste.

Lab-on-Skin Capability

Smart dressings with embedded microfluidic channels coupled with biosensors can become tiny diagnostic laboratories in the form of a dressing on skin, where complex assays of wound biomarkers can be performed, removing the need to resort to conventional laboratory instrumentation.

The sophisticated biosensors, which are the key elements that turn a passive dressing into an intelligent monitoring system, are embedded in the advanced material platforms. These sensors are made to sense and measure certain amounts of biological or chemical identifications (biomarkers) in wound exudate that can give real-time objective information on the health of the wound. Table 10.4 presents a detailed description of the markers that are critically monitored and their corresponding method of detection by the biosensors [10,12].

TABLE 10.4
Key Markers Monitored and How Biosensors Detect Them

Biomarker	Clinical Significance	Sensor Type and Detection Mechanism
pH	Inflammation/Infection Indication: Healthy healing lesions are acidic (5.5–6.5 pH range). A rise of pH to an alkaline condition (pH value greater than 7.5) is a good indication of bacterial infection, as many bacteria form alkaline end products	Colorimetric Sensors: The dressing contains dyes that alter in color to indicate when there is a change in pH. Electrochemical Sensors: Detect the variation of electrical potential or flow because of the concentration of ions, which corresponds to pH
Moisture/exudate levels	Optimal Healing Environment: Dryness discourages cell migration; a wet environment has maceration issues and results in difficulty with infection	Conductivity/Impedance Sensors: Detect the levels of electrical conductivity or impedance of the dressing, which varies with the moisture level. Gravimetric Sensors: They measure weight changes associated with fluid absorption
Oxygen (O_2)	Tissue Viability and Healing Potential: Oxygen plays a vital role in cell metabolism, the formation of collagen, and combating infection. Poor perfusion and healing arrest are observed when low oxygen (hypoxia) occurs	Optical Sensors (e.g., Phosphorescent): Sensory materials have light to be quenched by oxygen; the rate of phosphorescent decay varies with the level of O_2. Electrochemical Sensors: Measure the Reduction current of oxygen
Nitric oxide (NO)	Inflammation and Infection Response: NO has both low-level and high-level meaning—low levels can mean impaired healing, and high sustained levels can point to chronic inflammation or infection. It also plays a part in vasodilation and antimicrobial protection	Electrochemical Sensors: These make use of electrodes that react with NO to give an electrical response that can be measured Optical Sensors: Probes that are fluorescent and are intensity-sensitive to NO
Hydrogen peroxide (H_2O_2)	Oxidative Stress and Infection: Oxidative stress is an increased state of oxidation in the body that occurs as a consequence of immune system action. H_2O_2 is a reactive oxygen species (ROS) generated by immune cells to combat pathogens. An increase in concentration may signal high oxidative stress and chronic infection, especially open wounds	Enzymatic Electrochemical Sensors: Apply enzymes (e.g., horseradish peroxidase) to catalyze the reaction between H_2O_2 to create a current that is detectable. Colorimetric Sensors: Reagents use a color change with H_2O_2
Temperature	Inflammation and Infection: Early diagnosis and evidence of inflammation or infection, a local increase in temperature is a dependable sign	Thermistor/Thermocouple Sensors: Electronic components that change resistance or generate voltage with temperature, providing precise readings. Nanodiamonds: They can be embedded in fibers to provide highly precise, contactless temperature sensing

The supreme strength of smart wound dressings is manifested in the complete interaction of these more advanced materials and biosensors. Using the previous example, a hydrogel-based dressing could incorporate pH sensors so that the antimicrobial agent is released when they detect an alkaline shift. At the same time, integrated microfluidic channels sample new exudate constantly and ensure that the pH values are reliable and, in turn, transport any current fluid to other sensors that measure oxygen levels or particular protease activity. This data could then be wirelessly sent to a smartphone or a cloud-based system, where AI algorithms run against the data and track trends, warning clinicians about any possible complications. Such a holistic manner changes wound management to a data-based, proactive, and tremendously personalized intervention, which is no longer guesswork-driven. Smart dressings allow the clinician to make informed decisions earlier according to objective information provided continuously into the microenvironment of a wound, and thus, they result in a much faster healing process, elimination of any complications, and a dramatic reduction in patient morbidity.

AI Integration in Wound Dressing: The Intelligent Frontier

The actual revolution in modern wound care is the smooth connectivity between high-tech smart wound covering with AI. In a way, AI is not an auxiliary tool but rather an advanced analytical machine that will turn raw and continuous data provided by biosensors and visual inputs into clinical intelligence that can guide action. Such deep integration makes it possible to achieve a new degree of accuracy, customization, and intervention outside the realm of feasibility in the historical, frequently subjective approaches to managing wounds. With the support of unending wound monitoring, interpretation, and prediction, AI allows healthcare workers to stay informed and make informed decisions that help a wound heal much faster and reduce complications. CV is one of the most visually transformative fields of AI that has been applied to wound care: with CV, the computer can see and interpret the images. This ability lies at the center of the Convolutional Neural Networks (CNNs), a type of DL algorithm. Such networks excel in visual information processing and learning about hierarchical features directly in terms of raw pixels, as well as finding complex patterns that the human eye may not behold.

Automatic Wound Segmentation and Area Measurement: It's More Than Just a Ruler

Measurement of the size of a wound has been determined manually for decades and sometimes inconsistently through the use of rulers, transparent grids, or even by digital planimetry. The methods had high inter-observer reliability and measurement errors, particularly in imperfectly round wounds or wounds that are on body locations that are not quite round. CNNs, however, have provided a breakthrough to this. This type of network, when trained on large datasets of manually annotated wound images, can be employed to automatically outline the confines of a wound. This comes in the form of separating the affected wound part from the healthy skin and background surroundings with high precision. The result is a map of the wound at a pixel level, and based on this information, length, width, and area can be determined with great repeatability and accuracy [13].

Take the situation into account of a home healthcare nurse or even patient (with instructions) who takes a smartphone photo of a pressure ulcer. This image immediately undergoes analysis with AI, which gives objective values of dimensions and monitors the tiniest alterations in size in several days or weeks. This ability is not only able to normalize reporting but can be used to supply reliable, quantitative measures that are key to determining the status of healing over time.

Classification and Quantification of Tissue Type of Granular Type: Under a Microscope

In addition to size, wound bed composition should be considered as a priority in wound treatment. Most healthy healing wounds have a vibrant red granulation tissue, which is an indication of new blood vessel formation and tissue growth. By contrast, the non-healing wounds frequently appear with different percentages of one of the following: slough—a yellowish, soft, fibrinous tissue; necrosis—black, devitalized tissue. Indicatively and precisely estimating such tissue types is crucial in advancing debridement plans and assessing therapy efficiency. CNNs are taught to do this complicated task. Through the examination of colors, textures, and color and structure patterns within segmented wound area, they can classify and quantify to the percentage of each tissue type. As an example of the report presented by an AI, it may include the following items: The wound bed contains 75% healthy granulation tissue, 15% non-viable slough, and 10% necrotic tissue. The goal of consistent evaluation enables clinicians to make informed judgments, including whether debridement is needed or not, or whether the present dressing is active to encourage healthy tissue formation [14].

Early Detection of Minute Changes: The Unseen Being Seen

The sensitivity of some visual cues is probably one of the most important benefits of AI, its ability to analyze the image. The early manifestation of complications may also be overlooked due to human observation, especially when they are seen at an uncommon clinic visit. By continually analyzing large amounts of data on the images taken over time, AI has the potential to identify even very small changes in the color of the wound, even small changes in the composition of exudate, or minor changes in the condition of the skin around the wound (the so-called periwound skin). Another instance is that an extremely small amount of redness change or shift in the hue of the wound bed can be a signal of impending infection or halting the inflammatory stage. These initial indications, which are not noticeable to the naked eye, are the ones that help to change the situation before a small problem becomes a big problem that may take weeks or even months to heal.

Predictive Modeling: Forecasting Healing Trajectories and Infection Risk

The real vision that AI has in wound care is its ability to do predictive analytics. The combination of multiple data sources, such as the objective data provided by the image analysis, with the continuous monitoring of the patient by the biosensors in the smart dressing, and an extensive clinical history, helps AI models to create very powerful predictions on the future of a wound.

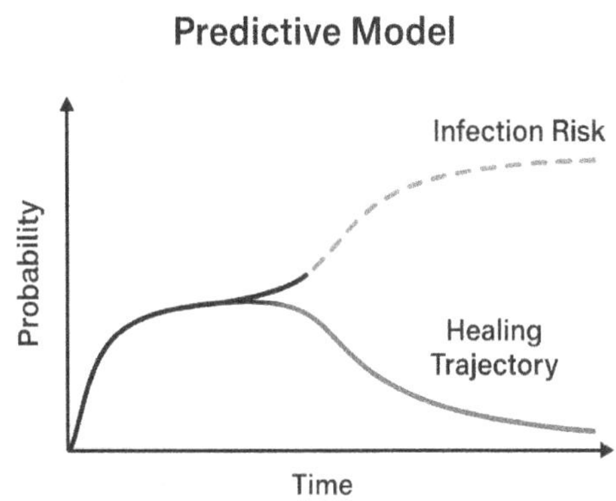

FIGURE 10.4 Predictive modeling.

The Future Prognosis of Healing Diagnosis: Not Following the Linear Trend

Chronic wound healing is never linear. The AI algorithms are trained on large amounts of historical data of wound progression to predict the wound healing rates of a particular wound. Such models take into account a wide variety of influential aspects: the size, depth, and nature of the wound, the age and pre-wounding health condition of the patient, whether they have other ailments (diabetes, peripheral vascular disease, autoimmune diseases), nutritional levels, their medical treatment plan, and most importantly, the live biometric data (e.g., pH, temperature, oxygenation, and specific biomarkers levels) that is gathered with the use of smart dressings. If the actual progression of a wound go down a far different path than the expected course, the AI can alert the doctor to a stalled wound, such as when a DFU is displaying less than 20% reduction in size after two weeks, which is a common indicator of non-healing. The useful feature of the proactive alert system is that it requires a clinician to reconsider the current treatment plan and make timely changes. This functionality is especially important in chronic wounds that regularly fail to progress over time and have no evident clinical manifestations, threatening to cause extended pain and hyper-spending of economic resources [13,15] (Figure 10.4).

Detecting Risk of Infection: Active Protector

Although biosensors can be used to determine whether an infection occurs, AI does an even greater task of analyzing the chances of infection in the future. An example would be when there is a history of consistently high blood glucose levels, and there are the slightest changes in temperature in the wound that are noticed in the smart dressing, where the AI would notice an increased risk of bacteria multiplication even before any visible signs of infection (like pus or unpleasant smell) appear. This forecasting ability can be used to take prophylactic action, to apply an antimicrobial dressing, or even sooner, topical antimicrobial intervention before the full-blown manifestation of an infection that may go so far as to hamper wound healing greatly, admit the patient to hospital, or result in an amputation.

Early Intervention Planning: Reactive to Proactive

The deep understanding created with the help of AI gives clinicians the possibility to change the direction of their focus toward proactive intervention rather than reactive problem-solving. The ability to predict the future is invaluable because, instead of waiting to observe a wound to worsen or to rely on a laboratory test to determine that something is wrong, healthcare providers will be able to intervene early and change the treatment plan based on predictions of the future. This is not only an effective solution to the problem of complications resulting in an adequate improvement of patient outcomes but also has the positive effect of decreasing the cost and burden of care since extended treatments, hospitalization, and surgical interventions, which may be prescribed otherwise by the physician, would have been avoided as well. The end game of the potential of AI wound care is the capacity to use it to develop fully personalized methods of treatment. In the realization that not all wounds and all patients are treated in identical ways or represent an identical biological and clinical refinement, AI algorithms are able to interpolate and assimilate all quantifiable input to provide highly specific and optimized interventions. This goes further than overgeneralized protocols.

Best Dressing Type Selection

The dressing type of wound is of utmost importance. Depending on the current level of exudate of the wound, the type of specific tissues that occur in it (e.g., the large percentage level of slough/healthy granulation), and the risk it poses to become infected, the AI can advise the most suitable covering of a potentially infinite number of dressing types. As an example, a wound with substantial exudate and elevated risk of infection may bring about the suggestion of an antimicrobial alginate dressing, which is also especially bioabsorbent and delivers localized antimicrobial activity. On the contrary, a dry wound in the case of healthy granulation tissue could indicate the use of a moisture-donating hydrogel to achieve the best epithelialization.

The dressing choice is dynamic and evidence-based, which keeps trial and error to a minimum while also avoiding the need to compromise the wound environment.

Optimization of Doses and Frequency of Therapy

In the case of active interventions, AI may optimize the doses and the frequency of therapy. This may entail advising on the exact dosage of a topical antimicrobial, the most suitable negative pressure drainage of wound vacuum-assisted closure or the most suitable dressing change frequency. These suggestions are calculated by AI and are continuously revised with the real-time reaction of the wound, through the sensors of the smart dressing, and are therefore as effective as possible, with limited wastage or discomfort to the patient.

Steering Higher-Order Management (Electrical/Antimicrobial)

In case AI identifies ongoing inflammation, the development of antibiotic-resistant biofilm, or early resistance indicators of bacteria by analyzing the biomarker, then this may pre-emptively recommend the implementation of further intercessionary measures. This may involve the suggestion of adjunctive treatments such as electrical stimulation (which has demonstrated its ability to induce tissue growth, improve blood perfusion, and lower the bacterial burden) or a certain systemic antibiotic, depending on the likely pathogen susceptibility. This will make sure that treatment plans are appropriately tailored to the dynamically changing requirements of the wound, which guides effective therapies at crucial time points during wound healing. It is a level of individualization that is incomparable to any other; it is the AI-powered personalization that enables every patient to have the most effective and efficient treatment, with the least that could be done on unnecessary procedures, waste, and healthcare costs; and, most importantly, it allows them to complete the journey of wound healing much faster than before. Table 10.5 depicts the big picture of the transformative adaptation of AI into wound dressing.

TABLE 10.5
Transformative Adaptation of AI Into Wound Dressing

AI Capability	How AI Works (Mechanisms and Technologies)	Key Data Inputs	Impact on Wound Dressing and Treatment (Benefits)
Objective image analysis	Utilizes **Computer Vision** and **Convolutional Neural Networks (CNNs)** for: **Semantic Segmentation**: Pixel-level identification of wound boundaries and tissue types (granulation, slough, necrosis, and epithelialization). **Quantitative Measurement**: Precise calculation of wound length, width, area, and volume; percentage of different tissue types	High-resolution digital images (e.g., smartphone cameras and specialized wound imaging devices)	Replaces subjective visual assessment with highly precise, consistent, and quantitative data. Enables standardized documentation, remote monitoring, and objective tracking of healing progression or regression. Reduces inter-observer variability
Predictive analytics	Employs **Machine Learning (ML)** algorithms (e.g., Random Forests, Gradient Boosting, Recurrent Neural Networks). **Pattern Recognition**: Identifies complex correlations between diverse data points. **Risk Stratification**: Calculates the probability of non-healing or complications. **Trajectory Forecasting**: Predicts future wound status based on current and historical data	Real-time sensor data (pH, temperature, oxygen, specific biomarkers), patient demographics, medical history (diabetes, vascular disease), medication lists, previous treatment responses, and wound history	Allows for proactive intervention, identifying stalled wounds or potential infections *before* they become critical. Optimizes resource allocation by prioritizing high-risk cases. Enables clinicians to set more realistic expectations for patients

(*Continued*)

TABLE 10.5 (*Continued*)
Transformative Adaptation of AI Into Wound Dressing

AI Capability	How AI Works (Mechanisms and Technologies)	Key Data Inputs	Impact on Wound Dressing and Treatment (Benefits)
Personalized treatment recommendations	Leverages **AI algorithms** (e.g., Reinforcement Learning, Expert Systems, Collaborative Filtering) to: **Contextual Decision-Making**: Synthesizes all available data to understand the unique wound-patient context. **Optimal Selection**: Recommends the most suitable dressing type, debridement method, or adjunctive therapy. **Parameter Optimization**: Suggests precise dosing for topical agents or optimal settings for devices (e.g., negative pressure, electrical stimulation)	Output from Objective Image Analysis and Predictive Analytics; patient-specific needs; available treatment options; cost-effectiveness data	Moves from "one-size-fits-all" to highly individualized care, maximizing treatment efficacy and accelerating healing. Reduces trial and error, minimizes unnecessary interventions, and improves patient comfort
Continuous monitoring and alerts	AI systems constantly process incoming real-time data from smart dressings and integrated platforms. **Anomaly Detection**: Identifies deviations from expected healing patterns or normal biomarker ranges. **Automated Notifications**: Triggers immediate alerts to clinicians (e.g., via mobile app, EHR integration) when critical changes or risks are detected	Real-time streams of pH, temperature, moisture, oxygen, and specific biomarker data from embedded biosensors	Ensures timely intervention, even between scheduled visits, by providing continuous oversight. Reduces the need for frequent manual dressing changes, minimizing patient discomfort and infection risk Prevents complications from escalating

The Internet of Things (IoT) and Remote Monitoring

Severely disrupting the wound care industry is the concept of Internet of Things (IoT) that is revolutionizing the closed-loop ecosystem between devices, data, and clinicians. The paradigm shift transfers wound management out of the clinic and into the home of the patient, allowing the provision of a continuous feedback loop, which is very individual and proactive. The fundamentals of the IoT system in wound care are a set of three significant elements: a smart bandage as a data-capturing device, a communication protocol including wireless transfer of data, and a telehealth system that plays the role of the intelligent interface in relation to its analysis and clinical monitoring [16].

Wireless Smart Bandages

The smart bandages are the building block of IoT in wound care. They are not like the conventional, passive dressings, but highly complex bioelectronic devices where a set of flexible sensors is embedded in the dressing itself. The sensors are intended to continuously supply real-time data on the wound measurements at a specific part of the body where the naked eye cannot see. The information that they gather is a holistic computer encryption of the microenvironment of the wound [17] (Figure 10.5).

Physiological and Biochemical Biomarkers

A normal healing wound has a particular physiological balance. On smart bandages, sensors measure the levels of specific biomarkers or indicators, and they give special attention to the following factors:

pH

Healthy skin maintains an acidic level (pH 4–6), which prevents the growth of bacteria.

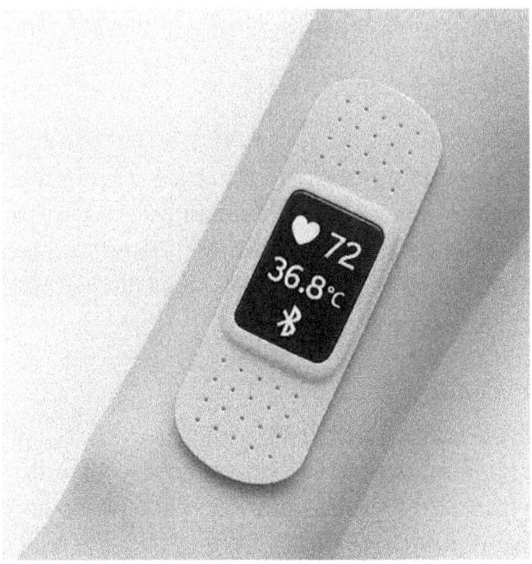

FIGURE 10.5 Wireless smart bandages.

Rise of Alkalinity

Rise of alkalinity (e.g., to a pH of 7.4 or above) indicates a strong presence of inflammation or a forming bacterial infection.

Temperature

Regions of temperature changes can indicate inflammation or infection. One of the trademarks of physiological reaction to pathogens is the elevation of the wound bed temperature that continues over time.

Moisture and Oxygenation

The cell movement and tissue development require the maintenance of the ideal moisture. The measurement of exudate level is possible with sensors, thus avoiding excessive drying of the wound (hindrance in the healing process) or excessive moistening (enhancement of maceration and infection). On the same note, it is important to monitor the oxygen tension because a hypoxic state (low oxygen) may be a severe factor in the healing process.

Biochemical Markers

Current smart bandages can go beyond the traditional parameters to track very specific biochemical markers. Researchers have started to include the measurement of uric acid (UA), which is a metabolite whose high level may indicate the occurrence of inflammation and tissue destruction. The rest of the prototypes monitor the presence of inflammatory cytokines like Interleukin-6 (IL-6) and Interleukin-10 (IL-10) to determine the inflammatory status of the wound directly and in real time [18].

Wireless Communication Protocols

The data gathered by these sensors in real time should be forwarded to a central processing unit via wireless communication, which in most cases is a smartphone or dedicated gateway. There are two main protocols of communication employed such as:

Bluetooth Low Energy (BLE)

BLE has become the overwhelming solution to these requirements because its power usage and mode of operation is so low, and it can be used in spaces where long-term continuous monitoring can be done with minimal battery replacement. It can enable smart bandages to stream data to the smartphone of the patient, which in turn transfers the data to a secure cloud solution.

Near-Field Communication (NFC)

In smaller designs that do not require battery power, NFC is a promising technology. A patient or a clinician can just tap his smartphone on the dressing to turn on the sensor and prompt a transfer of stored data. The data available on demand is ideal to cut on the power consumption and a low-cost and user-friendly option to BLE when constant streaming is unnecessary.

Telehealth Platforms and On-Device AI: The Command Center

The information obtained by the smart bandage is only a beginning. Its actual worth will be achieved when it is analyzed and consolidated into one full functional telehealth platform. These platforms function as the intelligence nerve center, combining the information provided by the sensors, the information that is visualized by the camera found on the device, and the information that is reported by the patient to create a complete picture of the wound.

On-device AI is used in many current products, including the conceptual product of Wound AI Assist and the commercial product Swift Medical. This implies that a shallow model in the DL system has been embedded directly into a cell phone app. This enables instant client processing of images, which are taken using smartphone camera. Using the example of wound, a patient can use his phone to capture an image of his wound, and the on-device AI can immediately perform a segmentation, dropping the borderlines of the wound and determining the area of the wound. It gives a quick and objective measurement without being required to be networked. The process of uploading the data is followed by the cloud-based telehealth platform. An advanced AI engine processes all of the information, real-time changing trends in the biomarkers captured by the smart bandage, objective measures provided by the on-device AI, and self-reported symptoms (e.g., pain, discomfort). This AI will produce a full report to the clinician, which is easy to read. The platform gives physicians a safe dashboard where they can:

- Store their information.
- Remotely track the changes of the wound over the period.
- Install automated fire alarms on high-risk indicators (e.g., an instant sudden change in temperature or pH).
- Make virtual consultations and exchange images safely.
- Fine-tune treatment plans, using detailed, data-driven knowledge of the behavior of the wound.

These platforms allow patients or carers to record and observe wounds in the comfort of their homes, therefore taking up a proactive role in their care. This not only increases the continuity of care but also decreases both the logistic and financial cost burden through reduced need to continuously visit the clinic in person.

Advanced Sensor Technology

Skin trauma and consequent skin trauma and frequent, even painful, sensor retrieval have been a critical issue to smart bandage design. New solutions to this are emerging lately with breakthroughs in material science and engineering.

The second line of smart bandages is achieved by the creation of biodegradable elements of sensors. Such sensors, which may be produced out of material that can be broken down by the body or absorbed into the vital systems without any side effects, are not to be removed. It would especially be beneficial in cases of delicate wounds and patients with sensitive skin because the probability of mechanical trauma will also be reduced during dressing changes. The other major development occurs in the growth of non-invasive and contactless forms of sensing technologies. This technique sets the sensing mechanism aside without actual contact with the wound bed. An excellent example is the utilization of the contactless gas sensing systems that are capable of tracking volatile organic compounds (VOCs) being evaporated by the skin, including the wound bed. Variations in the profile of the VOC indicate good evidence of growth and infection by bacteria.

Alternatively, as in the high-tech iCares device designed by Caltech and USC researchers, it can take the form of a microfluidic design. This system may be used to extract fluid using wound fluid through a channel that has sensors so that the sensor will not come in contact with the healing tissue and thus biomarkers may be analyzed in real time. This is not only likely to reduce trauma but also enhance biocompatibility and long-term stability of the device. A combination of sensor technology (such as these), the capability of IoT, and AI are ushering in a new age of proactive and personalized wound care. This leads to an uninterrupted feedback loop that provides the most efficient treatment at each therapy phase in the healing process and results in drastic patient improvement and greater life quality [16,18] (Table 10.6).

TABLE 10.6
Summary of Key IoT and Remote Monitoring Capabilities

Component	How it Works (Mechanisms and Technologies)	Key Data Inputs	Impact on Wound Care (Benefits)
Wireless smart bandages	Integrates flexible bioelectronic sensors directly into the dressing. Utilizes ultra-low-power electronics to measure and store data	Real-time pH, temperature, moisture, oxygenation, and specific biomarkers (e.g., uric acid, IL-6/10) from the wound bed	Provides continuous, objective data on the wound's microenvironment. Enables the early detection of inflammation and infection. Reduces the need for frequent, manual inspections
Communication protocols	**BLE**: Streams data continuously to a mobile device **NFC**: Enables on-demand, battery-free data transfer when a smartphone is tapped near the bandage	Sensor data (pre-processed or raw) from the smart bandage	Facilitates remote data collection and monitoring. BLE is ideal for long-term, continuous tracking; NFC is efficient for quick, on-demand checks, reducing power consumption

(*Continued*)

TABLE 10.6 (*Continued*)
Summary of Key IoT and Remote Monitoring Capabilities

Component	How it Works (Mechanisms and Technologies)	Key Data Inputs	Impact on Wound Care (Benefits)
Telehealth platforms	Cloud-based or mobile-first platforms (e.g., Wound AI Assist, Swift Medical) that provide a dashboard for clinicians and a user interface for patients	Smart bandage sensor data, patient-captured images, on-device AI analysis, and patient-reported symptoms	Centralizes all wound-related data for a holistic view. Enables remote physician oversight and virtual consultations. Streamlines documentation and communication between care teams
On-device AI	Lightweight deep learning models integrated into a mobile app. Performs immediate analysis of patient-captured photos	High-resolution images of the wound from a smartphone camera	Provides instant, objective wound assessment (e.g., automated segmentation and area measurement). Enables reliable tracking of wound size without network dependency. Empowers patients with real-time feedback
Advanced sensor tech	**Biodegradable**: Sensors made of materials that dissolve or are absorbed by the body **Contactless**: Non-invasive methods like gas sensing or microfluidic designs that prevent direct sensor-wound contact	Data from sensors that don't require direct physical contact with the wound	Eliminates the risk of skin trauma and pain associated with sensor removal. Improves patient comfort. Reduces the risk of infection from dressing changes. Ensures biocompatibility and device stability

Advanced Wound Care: Case Studies and Recent Innovations

Wound care is the area that is revolutionized by advanced materials, microfluidics, biosensors, and AI. Such inventions are changing the scenario of reactive wound management to proactive treatment options, which allow detecting problems at an early stage and specific therapy plans with an individual approach. There are three high-profile case studies and recent innovations that illustrate this change [19–22]:

iCares Smart Bandage (Caltech)

The iCares smart bandage is a revolutionary lab-on-skin device that enables real-time wound monitoring of chronic wounds to be continuously monitored, a product developed by a team led by Professor Wei Gao at the California Institute of Technology (Caltech).

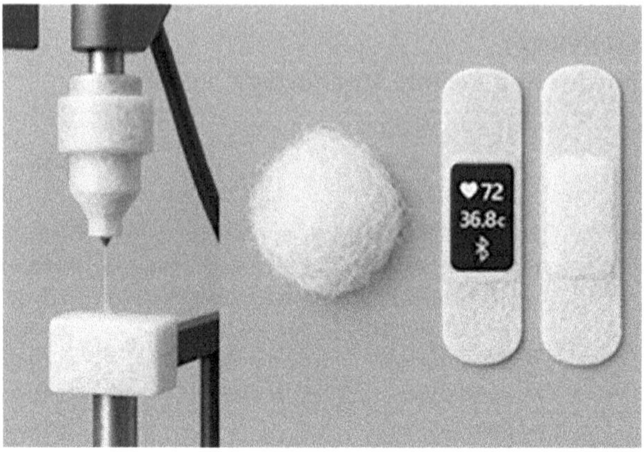

FIGURE 10.6 Smart bandage.

It has crossed the bridge from animal to human clinical trials and proved that it will change wound management (Figure 10.6).

Core Technology and Mechanism

The iCares system is a fusion of three key technologies:

Bio-Inspired Microfluidics The device has a highly advanced microfluidic system based on the microstructures shown in the vascular system of plants. It contains multiple channels and modules to continuously sample new wounds and exudate—the liquid that leaks out of a wound—without getting it mixed with older stagnant fluid. This will make data gathered accurate and representative of the existing wound scenario. In addition, moisture is controlled, with any surplus fluid eliminated to encourage optimal healing conditions.

Nanoengineered Biosensor Array The bandage has a disposable sensor array, which is 3D printed to be the most cost-effective means of manufacture. This slide can sense several biomarkers concurrently, and these are:

- **Nitric oxide (NO)**: A measure of inflammation.
- **Hydrogen peroxide (H_2O_2)**: One of the big indicators of the possibility of infection.
- **pH and temperature**: The wound microenvironment broad classification indicators.
- **Oxygen**: A biomarker indicating the ability to heal. Utilization of electrochemical detection that allows the measurement of small electrical flows reduces the material cost of the device while retaining a thin and flexible form factor.

Artificial Intelligence (AI) and Machine Learning The data obtained with the help of the sensors is transferred to any type of smartphone or any other device wirelessly. This multi-parameter data is then fed through a bundled Machine Learning algorithm to give a personalized representation of the wound. The model is capable of properly categorizing the type of wounds and, most importantly, can predict with great accuracy (as high as 94%), the length of time it takes to heal.

Primary Innovations and Clinical Implications

The major strength of iCares smart bandage lies in the early warning system that it enables. It can detect high levels of inflammatory biomarkers and infectious biomarkers, including nitric oxide and hydrogen peroxide, three days before the onset of symptom visibility. Such early detection is the key in time intervention, which can prevent the development of a minor wound into a grave complication and avoid chances of readmission of patients to the hospital. It is also a data-supported device that provides objective information whose quality could be up to the precision of the expert clinical decision.

BITS Pilani Smart Bandage (Hyderabad)

A team of researchers at BITS Pilani Hyderabad has designed a smart bandage that includes both an active mode of wound care (by eradicating bacterial infection) as well as a passive mode of wound care (a distinct visible distinction to show the presence of a wound). The innovation will be vital, especially in combating antimicrobial resistance (AMR), since no conventional antibiotics will be used.

The Principle and Mechanism

The multilayered smart bandage has been developed to be proactive in terms of treating wound infection:

Antibiotic-Free Bactericidal

The bottom layer of the band layer is made out of special fibers that are coated with silver nanoparticles. One example is silver, which is a renowned antimicrobial agent that effectively kills multiple bacteria and destabilizes their cellular functions. This method is an alternative to the use of traditional antibiotics to respond to the evolving risk of antibacterial resistance.

Visible Colorimetric Detection

A gel layer is set above the antimicrobial layer, which serves as the sensor. In the case of wound infection, when there are bacteria in the organism, they can synthesize particular substances, which spread into the gel. This reaction causes a gel color change and gives an easy, visible detection of infection. The color change is readily identifiable by the clinicians or patients, making it suitable for use at the bedside or at home.

Companion Color Analysis App

A user-friendly mobile application was also developed to make the visual assessment more precise by eliminating subjectivity in its performance. The smartphone dressing can be photographed by the users: the application includes an algorithm to process the color change in the photograph and gives a precise, objective judgment about the presence and severity of infection.

Key Innovations and Clinical Impact

BITS Pilani smart bandage is offering an easy, economical and proficient methodology regarding the point-of-care wound management. It has the advantage of using antibiotic-free bacteria destruction with a colorimetric and visual sensor to provide a strong early intervention and remedy to wound infections. Its ease of use, i.e., enablement using an accompanying app, makes it suitable to use in healthcare-professional circles as well as patient communities, albeit in poor resource conditions. The bandage is at the human trials stage and is set to be availed to address diabetic ulcers, post-surgical infections, and burns.

Multi-Analyte Swab-Based System

This is a merged unit of diagnostics that was aimed to resolve the high stakes of non-healing DFUs by integrating 3D-printed assays, a specific mobile app, and CV. It is an evidence-based quantitative mechanism to evaluate the severity of wounds that is not reliant on visual assessment [23].

Core Technology and Mechanism

The system is a complete system having two major parts:

- **Multi-analyte assays**: An important diagnostic feature is a low-cost, 3D-printed base with multiple swabs in it. The swabs have enzymatic tests impregnated to identify wound exudate particular biomarkers. As a demonstration, lactate-sensing swabs were developed, which are made of lactate oxidase body secretions. Swab pretreatments and drop-coatings also prevent enzyme leaching, allowing more sensitive and stable assays. The assays are designed in such a way that they can be detected through colorimetric methods (i.e., the presence and level of a biomarker trigger a color or density change on the swab).
- **iOS App with computer vision**: An iOS app is an important component of the system called Wound Sensor. It will guarantee controlled image acquisition with the zoom minimized as well as adjusting to different lighting conditions commonly techniques found in a home-based wound photography. The severity of the wound can be automatically and objectively identified by studying the change in density of the swabs, by means of which the app can identify the severity of the wound.

Key Innovations and Clinical Impact

It is an objective and relatively straightforward diagnostic tool presented by this system to a significant clinical challenge. It addresses the non-healing DFUs; therefore, it addresses a condition that may result in high expenses and amputation. The combination of 3D-printed assays and a mobile program has become a point-of-care solution, which could be addressed by both healthcare professionals and patients. Using CV to quantify the colorimetric change gives a repeatable, quantitative measure of wound state, something that is greatly lacking with the current commonly used method of visual assessment of wounds, which is both subjective and highly debatable. It is potentially able to make more specific and immediate changes in treatment since it is essential in real-time tracking of the healing progress and vital

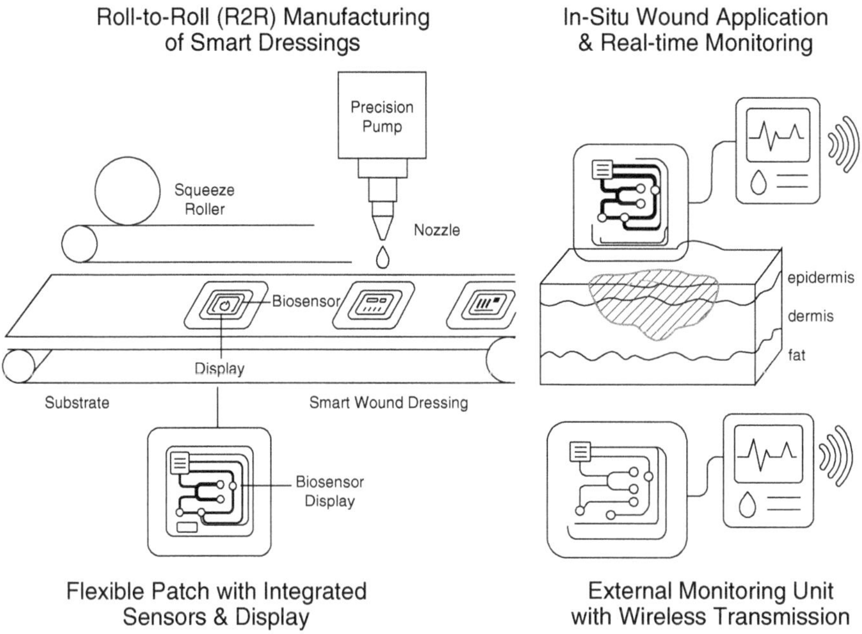

FIGURE 10.7 Schematic diagram of the manufacturing mechanism of the next-generation smart wound dressing in real time.

parameters, and the final goal is ultimately to have higher healing rates and fewer chances of complications occurring (Figure 10.7).

Challenges and Limitations of Smart Bandage Technology

The smart bandage and other more sophisticated forms of wound supervision technologies do promise a lot, but the way they are going to be used effectively in clinics is full of numerous issues in various sectors. The following barriers should be overcome in a way that these devices become not just effective but also safe, accessible, and ethically clean [24].

Data Security and Ethics

The sustained accumulation of patient-sensitive inferences by intelligent bandages brings complicated problems of privacy, safety, and ethical utilization.

Connected medical devices, such as smart bandages, are subject to more stringent laws such as the HIPAA in the United States and the GDPR in Europe. The high-frequency and continuous data (e.g., wound temperature, pH levels, and biofluid composition) should be well encrypted and secured to avoid data breaches and unauthorized access. This data is continuously changing, unlike the medical record, which is mainly static; thus, it forms a bigger attack surface when it comes to cyberthreats. Informed consent under continuous monitoring means that the ethical framework is further complicated. Those concerned ought to be made fully informed about the kind of information being treated, the uses of the information, to whom their information is being shared, and how long it will take. This should be made presentable as understandable, especially to patients whose health literacy levels are low or those who have low cognitive abilities. Smart bandages are characterized by the analysis of wound data and the forecast of healing trajectories using AI and ML. Nevertheless, such algorithms are trained using past data, which is unlikely to reflect the diverse population of patients. In the case of training datasets without enough information within specific racial or socioeconomic, or ethnic groups, the developed algorithms can be less valid about the respective groups. Such minority bias may hurt patients (either directly by misdiagnosis or delayed treatment, or indirectly by the inability to access treatment resources) and thus reinforce healthcare disparities.

Power and Miniaturization

It is an engineering problem because combining power sources and electronic components on a flexible, biocompatible bandage is technically a challenging project.

Often several days or weeks are spent with a bandage on and the power source used must be small, lightweight, and be able to operate the full time; the bandage is in use without the need of using a bulky external battery pack. The conventional batteries that carry heavy metals are mostly non-biocompatible, and leaking batteries or absorbed battery pose a toxic liability. This has seen the other power systems being researched on to include:

- Devices that can extract power sources on the body itself, e.g., some power from the body heat, some from the movement of a patient, and some through the chemical energy of the biofluids of a wound.
- Scientists are working on making the batteries of non-toxic, bioabsorbable materials such as zinc-molybdenum or other polymers to allow safe degradation of body when their functional life ends. Nevertheless, this type of system suffers from a short working life (several days to a few weeks), and the energy content until now is low, which is a significant drawback to supplying more advanced sensors and wireless transceivers.

The whole electronic system, comprising sensors, microprocessors, wireless communications modules (such as Bluetooth), and the energy source, should be downsized and reduced into a thin, flexible, and stretchable substrate. This involves micromanufacturing technologies that are highly advanced, specialized tooling, and managing the material constraints so that the device stays comfortable and functional on an always-moving section of the body.

Clinical Validation and Regulation

The introduction of a new medical device to the market is a process that can be characterized by tough and time-consuming clinical validation and regulatory clearance.

The majority of smart bandage prototypes are under early or preclinical development, with most animal models or lab-based experiments being focused on. A great deal of quality, peer reviewed clinical evidence of human trials is required to demonstrate their harmlessness, effectiveness, and clinical value. Smart bandages are considered either Class III or Class II medical equipment in the United States, depending on the functions achieved. A plain bandage is considered Class I, whereas a bandage that proactively detects and administers therapeutic measures (such as electrical stimulation or drug release) is a more sophisticated device, the clearance of which envisages demanding data to be approved by the U.S. FDA. This may be costly and time-consuming; according to this, a lot of documentation is involved, and quality management systems such as ISO 13485 apply. Also, there is a need to change the traditional practice in wound care when smart bandages are used. Most medical efficiency systems are based on the visualization of wounds and the unevenness of data collection. The implementation of new technology that gives constant, objective information will require the redesigning of current standards, educating healthcare professionals, and formulating new uniform clinical practice.

Cost and Patient Adherence

The practical and economic aspects of smart bandages may pose some inhibitions to the adoption and utilization of the same, especially for patients.

Smart bandages are much more costly to manufacture than conventional bandages because they employ high-tech materials, complex microfabrication processes, and combine several sensors into the product. Such high prices may restrict their application to special clinics or well-to-do patients, further spiraling healthcare disparities. There is also a large question mark as to whether these devices are insurable, and insurance coverage for these gadgets will play a dominant role in having them penetrate the market. Although smart bandages are made to be more convenient, they involve some form of patient engagement. Patients, particularly older patients or those with poor technical literacy, may have difficulty with the related usage instructions, such as connecting the device to a smartphone, diagnosing connectivity problems, or interpreting the data displayed on a companion app. Low usability causes a digital divide whereby the advantages of the technology are not shared equally. There is also the risk of trauma or pain associated with applying or removing the device to/or on the skin, as well as the skin irritation that may be caused by sensors or adhesives [21–25].

Future Perspectives and Opportunities in Smart Wound Care

The wound care sector is taking the next technological leap toward intelligent active healing platforms instead of being passive, reactive dressings. The three areas of AI, advanced materials, and bioelectronics are converging to establish a new paradigm for treating chronic and acute wounds. This report expounds on four important areas that steer this change [25,26].

Predictive Wound Care

The biggest change in the future wound care direction will be the transition to predict and prevent rather than cure. The focus point of this change is AI.

With tremendous amounts of wound images, patient histories, and clinical outcomes being fed into the AI model, it will have the incredible ability to get the wound healing trajectory right in most of the wound cases. They can examine visual data (the size of the wound, its color, and the type of tissue), physiological parameters (temperature, pH, and biomarkers), and patient-specific parameters (age, medical history, and comorbidities such as diabetes) to predict the probability of successful wound healing or the possibility of complications. Instead of waiting until infection is visibly displayed, AI-enabled systems will be able to anticipate something going wrong one to three days before symptoms appear clinically. As an example, a sharp increase in a biomarker of infection, e.g., hydrogen peroxide, or an increase in nitric oxide levels (which indicates inflammation) would awaken the alert. The early warning would enable clinicians to start using antibiotics or any other procedures long before the bacteria would have significant progression, which would greatly improve healing and decrease the risk of amputation among patients with chronic wounds. Using such predictions, AI might propose or even automatically provide custom treatment options. This may involve suggesting a given variant of higher-powered dressing, altering the rate of dressing change schedule, or cueing a bioelectronic element to administer a treatment dosage of medication or electric polarity [27].

Bioelectronic Convergence

Smart bandages of the future will not simply be sensors but will be a self-contained, autonomous system that monitors and treats. This is what, according to this definition, is called the convergence of biology and electronics to be able to facilitate self-adaptive healing.

The integration of smart bandages with soft robotics and even the so-called robot skin will enable gadgets that can sense as well as shape and adapt to the wound location. These systems might squeeze gently to aid control of bleeding, flex to fit swelling, or even do gentle debridement of necrotic tissue. Bio-bandages will have low-level electrical currents switched on and used on the wound area. The procedure referred to as electrotherapy can decrease the duration of tissue healing, enhance blood viscosity, and have antimicrobial properties [10]. This bandage will contain sensors to track the condition of the wound and regulate the scope and intensity of the electrical stimulation according to the best effect. In these platforms, arrays of painless and tiny needles will be added, which are microscopic in size that have the surface to penetrate through the outer skin layer to provide therapeutics to the wound. The built-in sensors and AI will decide when and in what dosage to administer drug delivery to ensure that antibiotics, growth factors, or anti-inflammatory drugs will be used at the right moment in the area where they make the most sense to act. The bandages, in turn, will be composed of so-called smart materials, which are capable of instantaneous transition in their properties, like responsive hydrogels. A hydrogel could expand to sop up excess water (exudate) present and then shrink to administer a drug in, all of which is pH/moisture dependent on the wound.

Multi-Modal Sensing

Future wound assessment will entail a comprehensive, multi-modal paradigm that will provide a comprehensive picture of the microenvironment of the wound. Rather than using one piece of data, such systems will monitor an entire package of parameters. In addition to pH and temperature, next-generation sensors shall be able to detect a broad array of biomarkers at molecular and cellular levels. These involve, among others, measuring the presence of certain proteins that signal inflammation

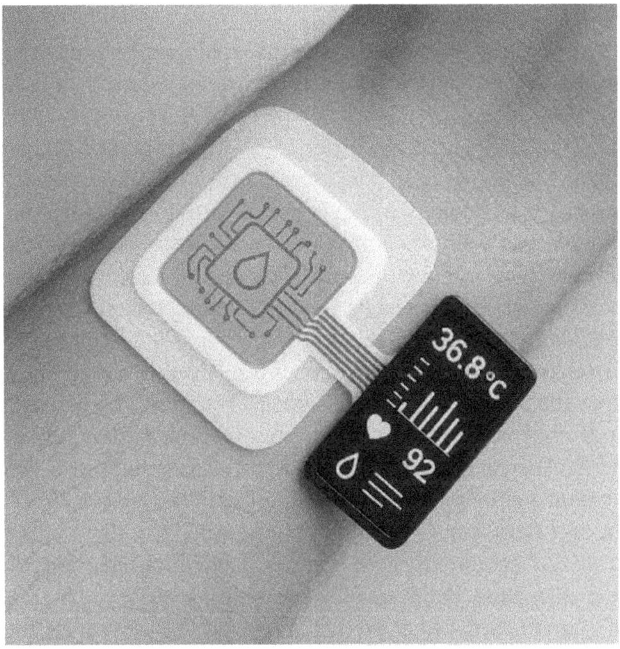

FIGURE 10.8 Multi-modal sensing.

(e.g., cytokines), enzymes contained within the presence of tissue response to damage (e.g., MMPs), and gaseous emissions that indicate the maturation and multiplication of bacteria [28] (Figure 10.8).

Physical and chemical parameters: A single dressing was capable of monitoring:

- **pH**: pH degree, which is either alkaline (infection) or healthy environment (acidic).
- **Moisture**: Keeping the wound hydrated and not too wet.
- **Temperature**: A localized feeling of heat may indicate inflammation or infection.
- **Pressure**: Patients who are at risk of developing pressure sores, their continual pressure monitoring will mean that bedsores will be averted at an early stage because the caregivers will know when to rotate them to a new position.
- **Oxygen and gas emissions**: A key level of determining the wound's health would be the achievement of oxygen saturation in the tissue and gases such as hydrogen sulfide, which is unfortunately formed by a few bacteria.

Combining these disparate data can help to form a wound profile that, through an AI-driven ML algorithm, will provide a significantly greater level of detail and diagnostic capability that is not currently available.

Interdisciplinary Collaboration

The design of such highly developed solutions would not be limited to one area. It needs a teamwork ecosystem in which various disciplines are built in mutually beneficial ways.

Clinicians: They play an essential role in offering profound information on the practical problems in wound care. They specify the clinical requirements, establish the usefulness of the technology in the practical setting, and make the end product secure, easy to use, and that can comfortably fit in current healthcare processes.

AI researchers: They are the ones who will design the complex algorithms that collect, analyze, model, and control data. They furnish clinical interpretations out of the intricate biological data of the sensors.

Materials scientists: The applied sciences involved in designing the high-tech elements within the project, the flexible screens, responsive hydrogels, and biocompatible materials that provide the foundation to the whole system, would come under material experts. They address such obstacles as sensor stability when placed in a damp environment and long-term biocompatibility of the material.

Co-design and iteration: It is rather important to have the co-design, in which these experts will collaborate from the first day. It avoids the emergence of a high-end technologically innovative but practically inapplicable device. This rightest way of collaboration guarantees the final product to be not only advanced but also affordable, scalable, and makes a substantive contribution to the improvement of the treatment of patients [26,27].

CONCLUSION

The transformation of wound care management/care tools from passive dressings to smart, AI-based systems is a paradigm shift that will lead to a paradigm shift from reactive care to proactive, more personalized, and highly effective care. With the advent of highly precise sensing technologies, predictive analytics, and therapy in response, a new age where wound healing is not such an agonizingly slow unknown process and is now an optimizing adaptive journey has dawned. Conventional dressings are meant to accomplish a fixed end: they are meant to cover the wound and to absorb exudate. However, smart dressings are bioelectronic platforms that take part in the healing process through monitoring and controlling. Upgradable biosensors allow continuous measurements of key biomarkers, including pH, temperature, hydration, and important enzymes, to give a real-time, quantitative measurement of the microenvironment of the wound. This constant observation helps to discover such complications as infection or inflammation in their initial stages and immediately provide intervention before the adverse condition gets worse. Seasonal sensing and delivery of responsive therapies is also possible beyond passive sensing in these next-generation dressings. The interpretation of sensor data could activate specific response actions, including the release of antimicrobials locally to counter infection, or the electrical stimulation of tissue to induce cell migration and tissue regeneration. The sensing, analysis, and treatment over and over again is known as the closed-loop system, which has been proven through studies to greatly speed up wound healing, the production of scar tissue, and vascularization. The flexibility to tailor the care applied to fill the wound to the precise condition in terms of its status at any given time is a key principle that cuts healing periods and attendant chances of complications that cause further distress and related expenses.

Wounds, such as DFUs and pressure injuries, present a meteoric, logistical, and financial challenge to healthcare systems around the globe at an annual cost of billions of dollars on treatments, hospitalization, and nursing time. Smart dressings are likely to relieve such burdens significantly since they help to make care more efficient and decrease the number of expensive interventions. Although smart dressing can be economically higher than a conventional one at the beginning of the process, its long-term cost-effectiveness is higher. These technologies involve significant savings since they reduce the time taken for healing, infections, dressing changes, and follow-up expenses. Such digital wound care technologies are already shown to cut average healing rates by more than a third, highlighting how they can reduce patient suffering and lower the overall cost of care. This change in economic modeling, from the value of a single product to the value of the whole process of healing, must occur to prove the worth of these evolutions.

This new paradigm cannot be designed in isolation but is something that has had an intense cross-disciplinary collaboration. This need involves integration of materials science knowledge to develop biocompatible and flexible electronics, AI and data science knowledge of constructing reliable predictive models, and clinical medicine knowledge of establishing the effectiveness and safety of the gadgets. To be transitioned into a standard of care, these innovations will involve in-depth clinical testing and require regulatory permission to get off the laboratory bench and into the clinic. More importantly, the effective implementation of smart dressings should be fair. These technologies should not deprive few of the advantages of these technologies. To make it widely and easily accessible, considerable effort must be put to mitigate the limitations related to its affordability, data transportation infrastructure, and educating medical staff. Engaging different stakeholders, including researchers and clinicians, policymakers, and community health advocates alike, will allow us to design, develop, and implement these life-altering innovations in a way that serves all populations and can, thus, bring about a future of more efficient, personalized, and equitable wound care to everyone.

REFERENCES

1. C. T. Hess, *Clinical Guide to Skin and Wound Care*, 7th ed., Lippincott Williams & Wilkins, 2012. https://books.google.com.pk/books?hl=en&lr=&id=KpmQOfSpSHMC&oi=fnd&pg=PR1&dq=The+textbook+definition+of+how+the+body+can+take+care+of+itself+is+through+an+acute+wound.&ots=dEo6jypmTR&sig=OfjlHPZcRGnHEwxt5I0oqPb5ncs&redir_esc=y#v=onepage&q&f=false (Accessed August 5, 2025).
2. P. Laing, "The development and complications of diabetic foot ulcers," *The American Journal of Surgery*, vol. 176, no. 2, pp. 11S–19S, 1998, doi:10.1016/S0002-9610(98)00182-2.
3. E. Rezvani Ghomi, S. Khalili, S. Nouri Khorasani, R. Esmaeely Neisiany, and S. Ramakrishna, "Wound dressings: Current advances and future directions," *Journal of Applied Polymer Science*, vol. 136, no. 27, p. 47738, 2019, doi:10.1002/APP.47738.

4. M. Mozafari, "How artificial intelligence shapes the future of biomaterials?" *Next Materials*, vol. 7, p. 100381, 2025, doi:10.1016/J.NXMATE.2024.100381.
5. R. N. Mitchell and F. J. Schoen, "Blood vessels," In: V. Kumar, A. K. Abbas, and J. Aster (Eds.), *Robbins & Cotran Pathologic Basis of Disease*, 8th ed., pp. 487–528, Saunders Elsevier, 2010.
6. R. Malviya, S. Sundram, R. Kumar Dhanaraj, and S. Kadry (Eds.), *Digital Transformation in Healthcare 5.0: Volume 1: IoT, AI and Digital Twin*, Walter de Gruyter GmbH & Co. KG, 2024. https://books.google.com.pk/books?hl=en&lr=&id=j2EDEQAAQBAJ&oi=fnd&pg=PA67&dq=The+Power+of+Real-Time+Monitoring:+A+Paradigm+Shift+wound+healing&ots=c8ezAJzHiP&sig=yRKQlUPZTM-bYWK36Zzts2MNUeeM&redir_esc=y#v=onepage&q&f=false (Accessed August 5, 2025).
7. P. Amisha, P. Malik, M. Pathania, and V. Rathaur, "Overview of artificial intelligence in medicine," *Journal of Family Medicine and Primary Care*, vol. 8, no. 7, p. 2328, 2019, doi:10.4103/JFMPC.JFMPC_440_19.
8. F. Li, H. Chen, Z. Liu, X. Zhang, and Z. Wu, "Fully automated detection of retinal disorders by image-based deep learning," *Graefe's Archive for Clinical and Experimental Ophthalmology*, vol. 257, no. 3, pp. 495–505, 2019, doi:10.1007/S00417-018-04224-8.
9. E. U. Haq, J. Huang, L. Kang, H. U. Haq, and T. Zhan, "Image-based state-of-the-art techniques for the identification and classification of brain diseases: a review," *Medical & Biological Engineering & Computing*, vol. 58, no. 11, pp. 2603–2620, 2020, doi:10.1007/S11517-020-02256-Z.
10. S. O'Callaghan, P. Galvin, C. O'Mahony, Z. Moore, and R. Derwin, "'Smart'wound dressings for advanced wound care: a review," *Journal of Wound Care*, vol. 29, no. 7, pp. 394–406, 2020, doi:10.12968/JOWC.2020.29.7.394.
11. M. Farahani and A. Shafiee, "Wound healing: from passive to smart dressings," *Advanced Healthcare Materials*, vol. 10, no. 16, 2021, doi:10.1002/ADHM.202100477.
12. S. Baptista-Silva et al., "A view on polymer-based composite materials for smart wound dressings," In: A. K. Bhowmick, R. K. Gupta, & S. Thomas (Eds.), *Smart Polymeric Materials for Biomedical Applications*, Springer, pp. 425–456, 2022, doi:10.1007/978-3-030-70266-3_14.
13. M. Dabas, D. Schwartz, D. Beeckman, and A. Gefen, "Application of artificial intelligence methodologies to chronic wound care and management: a scoping review," *Advances in Wound Care,* vol. 12, no. 4, pp. 205–240, 2023, doi:10.1089/WOUND.2021.0144.
14. S. Karnehed, I. Larsson, L. Petersson, L. K. Erlandsson, and D. Tyskbo, "Navigating artificial intelligence in home healthcare: challenges and opportunities in nursing wound care," *BMC Nursing*, vol. 24, no. 1, 2025, doi:10.1186/S12912-025-03348-7.
15. E. Rezvani Ghomi, M. Niazi, and S. Ramakrishna, "The evolution of wound dressings: From traditional to smart dressings," *Polymers for Advanced Technologies*, vol. 34, no. 2, pp. 520–530, 2023, doi:10.1002/PAT.5929.
16. H. Sattar et al., "An IoT-based intelligent wound monitoring system," *IEEE Access*, vol. 7, pp. 144500–144515, 2019, doi:10.1109/ACCESS.2019.2940622.
17. P. Mostafalu, W. Lenk, M. R. Dokmeci, B. Ziaie, A. Khademhosseini, and S. R. Sonkusale, "Wireless flexible smart bandage for continuous monitoring of wound oxygenation," *IEEE Transactions on Biomedical Circuits and Systems*, vol. 9, no. 5, pp. 670–677, 2015.
18. H. Derakhshandeh, S. S. Kashaf, F. Aghabaglou, I. O. Ghanavati, and A. Tamayol, "Smart bandages: The future of wound care," *Trends in Biotechnology*, vol. 36, no. 12, pp. 1259–1274, 2018.

19. R. Ghosh, P. Singh, A. H. Pandit, U. Tariq, B. K. Bhunia, and A. Kumar, "Emerging technological advancement for chronic wound treatment and their role in accelerating wound healing," *ACS Applied Bio Materials*, vol. 7, no. 11, pp. 7101–7132, 2024, doi:10.1021/ACSABM.4C01064.
20. G. Garcia, "An expanded focus in advanced wound care for geriatric emergency management nursing: a case study analysis," *British Journal of Nursing*, vol. 33, no. 15, pp. S16–S26, 2024, doi:10.12968/BJON.2023.0232.
21. M. A. Weigelt et al., "Advanced wound diagnostics: toward transforming wound care into precision medicine," *Advances in Wound Care*, vol. 11, no. 6, pp. 330–359, 2022, doi:10.1089/WOUND.2020.1319.
22. Q. Saifullah and A. Sharma, "Current trends on innovative technologies in topical wound care for advanced healing and management," *Current Drug Research Reviews*, vol. 16, no. 3, pp. 319–332, 2023, doi:10.2174/0125899775262048230925054922.
23. U. S. Jayapiriya and S. Goel, "Body-worn enzymatic biofuel cell with automated pencil drawn bioelectrodes for energy harvesting from human sweat," *Journal of Micromechanics and Microengineering*, vol. 32, no. 4, p. 044002, 2022, doi:10.1088/1361-6439/AC5428.
24. P. Mostafalu et al., "Smart bandage for monitoring and treatment of chronic wounds," *Small Methods*, vol. 14, no. 33, 2018, doi:10.1002/SMLL.201703509.
25. A. McLister, J. McHugh, J. Cundell, and J. Davis, "New developments in smart bandage technologies for wound diagnostics," *Advanced Materials*, vol. 28, no. 27, pp. 5732–5737, 2016, doi:10.1002/ADMA.201504829.
26. A. Madh and N. Sing, "Textiles," In: A. K. Bhowmick, R. K. Gupta, and S. Thomas (Eds.), *Smart and Sustainable Approaches for Wound Care*, Taylor & Francis, pp. 395–426, 2025, https://doi.org/10.1201/9781003651697-13.
27. Y. Sharma, S. Ghatak, C. K. Sen, and S. Mohanty, "Emerging technologies in regenerative medicine: The future of wound care and therapy," *Cell and Tissue Research*, vol. 102, no. 12, pp. 1425–1450, Dec. 2024, doi:10.1007/S00109-024-02493-X.
28. S. Probst, G. Gethin, and P. Bobbink, "Practical implications for wound care," In: J. Smith, R. Brown, and L. Johnson (Eds.), *Advanced Wound Management*, pp. 135–143, 2024, doi:10.1007/978-3-031-53230-6_15.

11 Challenges in Advanced Wound Dressing Development

Muhammad Abbas Haider Alvi
and Muhammad Qamar Khan

INTRODUCTION

Wound healing is a highly sophisticated biological process that is highly coordinated, helping to re-establish the structure and function of injured skin and underlying tissue. It involves four overlapping phases: hemostasis, inflammation, proliferation, and remodeling (shown in Figure 11.1) [1]. After the injury, hemostasis causes clot formation to prevent hemorrhage. The Inflammatory Phase follows, where the immune cells, including neutrophils and macrophages, clear pathogens and cellular debris. In the proliferative phase, tissue is regenerated, i.e., re-epithelialization, angiogenesis, and fibroblast activity [2]. Finally, in the remodeling phase, the extracellular matrix (ECM) is remodeled, and tissue is given tensile strength back. Although acute wounds tend to follow the same pattern and heal within a period that is expected, chronic wounds including diabetic foot ulcers, venous leg ulcers, and pressure sores tend to become stuck in one of the early phases due to such factors as infection (for example, as a result of diabetes, poor blood circulation, or other systemic diseases).

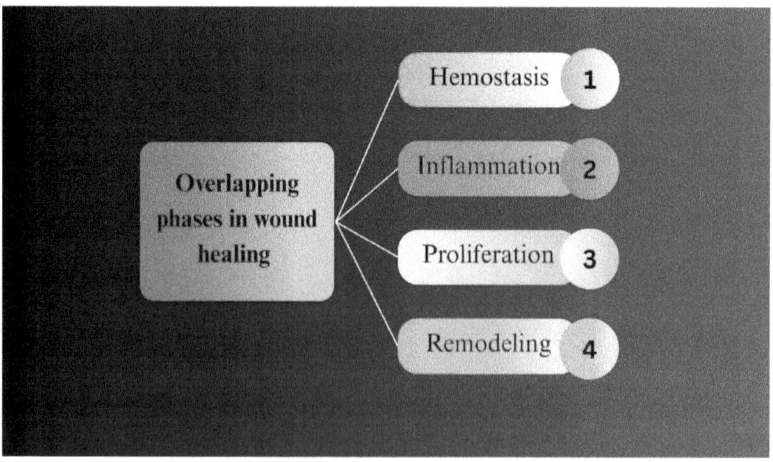

FIGURE 11.1 Overlapping phases in wound healing.

DOI: 10.1201/9781003616726-13

These forms of wounds pose serious clinical challenges and a significant amount of morbidity and healthcare costs to the patients [3].

Traditional wound dressings that comprise gauze, cotton pad, and basic bandage have, for a long time, been used as the norm when it comes to wound care. Such materials mainly provide passive cover and act as physical barriers against environmental pollutants and the exudate of wounds. Nevertheless, they are inadequate in providing for biological requirements of a healing wound. They do not encourage the growth of tissues, cannot hold moisture, and provide no antimicrobial protection. In addition, much of the traditional dressings stay on the wound bed and can potentially cause pain and additional tissue damage once removed. Of the utmost importance is their ineffectiveness in the control of chronic wounds, where infection control, moisture balance, and stimulation of tissue regeneration have gained significance, precluding them from clinical use. The limitations have called for an increased need for improved wound care options [4].

The emergence of nanotechnology has brought in a revolutionary concept of managing wounds. Unguided by their physical chemistry, chemical, or biological characteristics, their reactions with other nanomaterials or their distinct chemical characteristics are determined by the size of 1–100 nm, attributed to the high surface area/volume ratio and quantum effect. In wound care, nanotechnology allows the creation of highly sophisticated dressings, which, in addition to covering and protecting, also interact with the wound microenvironment to promote faster healing. For example, metallic nanoparticles—silver and zinc oxide—offer mighty antimicrobial effects by interfering with the membranes of microbes and creating oxidative stress. Various nanocarriers like liposomes and polymeric nanoparticles can be designed to deliver drugs/growth factors/anti-inflammatory agents specifically to the wound site in a controlled manner. Electrospun nanofibers can copy the architecture of the ECM, thus providing support for cellular migration and regeneration of tissue. Moreover, the combination of nanosensors with wound dressings has allowed the production of "smart" dressings that can monitor the characteristics of wounds (pH, moisture, and bacterial load) in real time. These developments are promising in terms of enhancing the outcomes in wound healing, particularly for chronic and infected wounds. However, the broad clinical embracement of nanotechnology-based wound dressings suffers from a number of setbacks, including safety issues, regulatory issues, the feasibility of their mass production, and affordability. Such developments deserve implementation as their properties are of vital importance in determining the real implications of nanotechnology in contemporary wound care [5].

THE ROLE OF NANOTECHNOLOGY IN WOUND HEALING

Nanotechnology has redefined the prospect in wound management as it has brought about materials that are involved in actively interacting with the wound environment at the cellular and molecular levels. Unlike traditional materials, nanomaterials have some special properties, including increased reactivity, a high surface-area-to-volume ratio, and crossing/breaking biological barriers. Such characteristics render them particularly efficient in solving critical problems associated with wound healing, such as prevention of infection, restoration of tissue, and controlled delivery

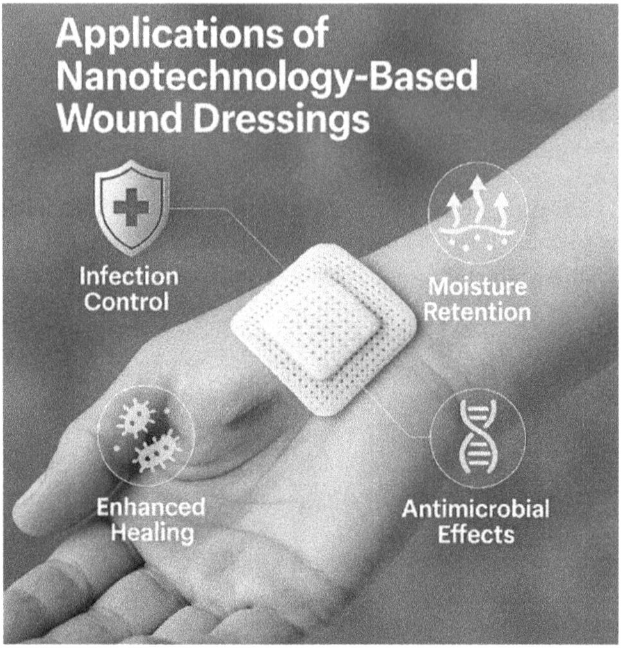

FIGURE 11.2 The role of nanotechnology in wound healing.

of drugs. The incorporation of nanostructures into wound dressings turns them into bioactive systems that can elicit and expedite the process of wound healing [6] (Figure 11.2).

Numerous nanomaterials have been tested for wound care applications, and this category of nanomaterials presents various advantages. Metallic nanoparticles, such as Ag, ZnO, and Au, are among the most intensively studied because of their high and broad-spectrum antimicrobial activity. For example, silver nanoparticles can disrupt bacterial membranes, obstruct metabolic pathways, and produce reactive oxygen species (ROS), so they are very effective against antibiotic-resistant strains. Likewise, ZnO nanoparticles display antimicrobial effects and also support epithelialization and angiogenesis. In addition to metals, polymeric nanoparticles produced from materials, including chitosan, poly(lactic-co-glycolic acid) (PLGA), and polyethylene glycol (PEG), have excellent biocompatibility and biodegradability. These polymeric carriers can encapsulate bioactive molecules and slowly release them over several days/weeks, ensuring therapeutic drug levels at the wound site [7].

The other significant class of nanomaterials applied to wound dressings is nanofibers. Sourced mainly through electrospinning, these ultrafine fibers replicate that of the ECM, allowing for an excellent scaffold for cells to adhere, proliferate, and migrate. Nanofibrous mats can be laced with the antimicrobial agent, anti-inflammatory agents, or growth factors, and the micropore characteristics allow for controlled moisture retention as well as gas diffusion, which is very important for optimal reach of the wound. Besides, more and more uses of lipid-based nanocarriers, including liposomes and solid lipid nanoparticles, in the delivery of hydrophobic drugs and delicate biological agents (peptides and nucleic acids) are found nowadays. These carriers shield the payload from degradation, facilitating penetration into skin layers [8].

The effectiveness of nanotechnology-improved wound dressings goes well beyond just drug delivery. Most of these systems are created to react to alterations in the wound microenvironment. For example, pH-sensitive nanocarriers can unload their therapeutic load upon exposure to an acidic environment that is a characteristic of infected wounds. Similarly, temperature- or enzyme-sensitive systems allow site- and time-specific release. Some sophisticated regimens are being combined with nanosensors to be able to monitor bacterial load, pH changes, or the level of moisture in real time, thus allowing for the early detection of infection and timely therapeutic action.

DESIGN AND FABRICATION STRATEGIES

There is indeed more to the successful development of nanotechnology-based wound dressings than the type of nanomaterial employed, but rather other methods employed to incorporate these nanomaterials into functional, stable, and clinically effective dressings. Different processing techniques have been examined to enhance the therapeutic efficacy of nanomaterials while being biocompatible, mechanically stable, and easy to apply. These modes will help build a single dress care platform that can incorporate various functions like antimicrobial action, drug delivery, and "responsive" behavior into a single dress, for specific wound type, healing phase, etc. [9] (Figure 11.3).

The most common method applied in the production of nanostructured wound dressings is electrospinning. This method generates a nanofiber with diameters of tens to hundreds of nanometers, similar to the native ECM. Electrospun nanofibrous mats provide superb surface area, high porosity, and potential for incorporation of

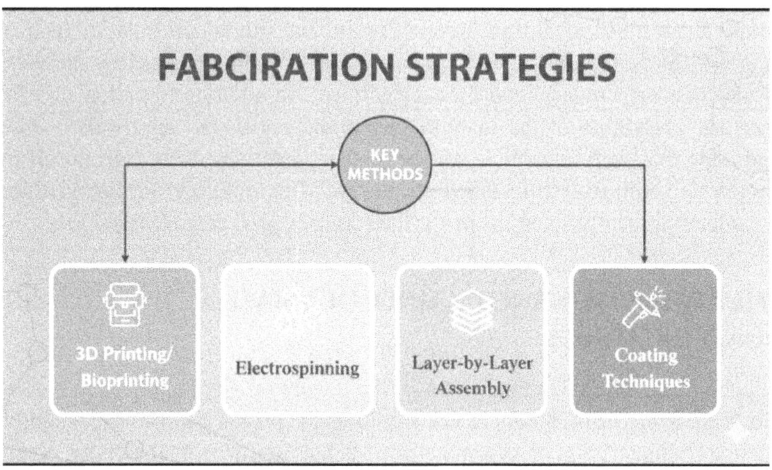

FIGURE 11.3 Technical processes used to create the dressings.

various therapeutic agents during the spinning process. Such properties are important in making electrospun scaffolds perfect in supporting cell attachment, migration, and proliferation, hence delivering antimicrobial agents, growth factors, or anti-inflammatory drugs in a controlled manner. Adjustability in composition, alignment, and mechanical properties of the fibers further increases their appropriateness for wound healing purposes.

Another promising method is layer-by-layer (LbL) assembly; it consists of the deposition of oppositely charged materials in a growing multilayered nanocoating. This approach allows for fine-tuned regulation of the thickness, composition, and kinetics of drug elution of the entrapped agents. LbL-assembled dressings can integrate antimicrobial nanoparticles, cytokines, or enzymes into certain layers that will provide spatial and temporal regulation of therapeutic delivery [10].

Both 3D printing and biofabrication techniques have found increased application in advanced wound dressings as well. Such approaches provide the possibility of developing patient-specific constructs of designed geometries with integrated functionalities. 3D-printed dressings loaded with drugs, cells, or nanofibers in conjunction with nanomaterials are capable of cell regeneration. For example, hydrogels loaded with silver nanoparticles and nanocapsules can be printed in specific wound architectures, which would offer antimicrobial defense and their structural prowess. Such systems can also be designed to deteriorate slowly, eliminating the necessity of dressing changes and reducing discomfort for patients.

The introduction of smart wound dressings is among the most futuristic developments that have been made in the field. These dressings involve the use of nanosensors and stimuli-responsive materials for monitoring in real-time and adaptive therapy. For instance, dressings containing pH-sensitive nanoparticles could detect the bacteria developing an infection and therefore release antibiotics. Others may be colorimetric indicators that change with temperature, moisture level, or presence of bacteria, where, visually, clinicians or patients will get a cue. Such intelligent systems are a major step toward personalized and active wound care. Although great progress has been made with regard to fabrication techniques, optimism is still uncertain about the clinical translation of optimized single-cell isolation techniques. Among various factors that need to be taken into account are sterility, shelf-life stability, mechanical strength, and user-friendliness, in addition to biological efficacy. Further, the scalability of the manufacturing and regulatory approvals is essential to guarantee that such innovative wound dressings are able to be introduced from a laboratory to a clinical setting. However, the growing toolbox of fabrication methods is an epidemiologically sound basis for the future wound care toolbox [11].

APPLICATIONS OF NANOTECHNOLOGY-BASED WOUND DRESSINGS

Nanotechnology-based wound dressings find a wide range of applications (shown in Figure 11.4): from the treatment of acute injuries to chronic non-healing wounds. The distinctive characteristics of nanomaterials, such as antimicrobial activity, controlled drug release, and improved capacity of tissue regeneration, make them ideal for all

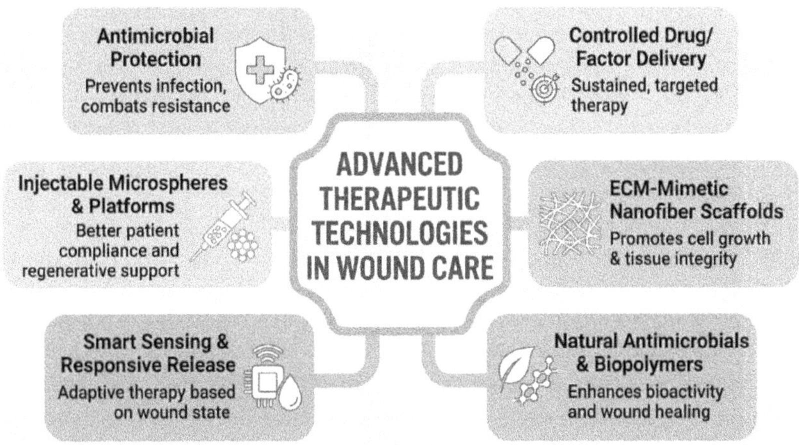

FIGURE 11.4 Applications and their key benefits.

types of wounds. The adaptability of these dressings has generated new opportunities in wound care; more effective, personalized, and efficient treatment is possible, particularly for sickly or chronically affected patients [12]. For acute wounds (such as surgical incisions, cuts, and abrasions), nanotechnology-incorporated dressings serve to facilitate a rapid recovery. For instance, the application of dressings with the incorporation of silver nanoparticles or nanocomposites into them can ensure immediate but non-invasive antimicrobial protection from infection while the wound heals in a moist environment, which is crucial for tissue regeneration. Further, nanofiber mats or hydrogels loaded with growth factors can encourage cellular activity as well as accelerate re-epithelialization, minimizing the chances of scar formation and time taken to recovery. The fact that these dressings are capable of creating an optimal balance between moisture and oxygen levels in the wound furthers the body's natural healing process.

Specifically, the use of nanotechnology-based dressings has proved to be quite promising in the treatment of chronic ulcers, which describes an ulcer that does not progress through the normal healing phases. The common case examples are diabetic foot ulcers, venous leg ulcers, and pressure ulcers, which frequently involve obstacles such as poor circulation, infection, or prolonged inflammation. Chronic wounds have a notorious history of being hard to treat since conventional dressings do not address the problem of infection control, inflammation, and regenerating tissues. However, Nanomaterials could offer answers with continuous antimicrobial action, less inflammation, and also induce angiogenesis, as a result of the delivery of growth factors. For example, it is possible to use silver nanoparticles impregnated into a hydrogel or foam dressing, which will allow for both infection control and a moist environment at the same time, or nanofibrous scaffolds to stimulate the movement of fibroblasts and keratinocytes and repair the dermal layer quickly [13].

Burn wounds associated with tissue damage and high risks of infections also benefit from nanotechnology-based dressings. Commonly, traditional burn treatments work with occlusive dressings that do not provide enough protection from microbial colonization. Some nanoparticles, such as silver, when combined with dressings, play an important role as powerful antimicrobial agents that can prevent common infections that are known to create infections in burn wound regions. Furthermore, this type of dressing is moisture appropriate for faster epithelialization, and the fact that it regulates the microclimate of the wound (e.g., by controlling moisture levels and temperature) makes the overall wound healing process easier. Besides, nanomaterials can help in pain management because of a non-invasive barrier that will reduce pain and discomfort during dressing changes [14].

For an infected wound, the introduction of nanomaterials to wound dressings can be game-changing. The employment of nanoparticles to target and kill bacteria via routes such as membrane disruption, ROS production, and interference with the formation of microbial biofilms offers a potent piece of equipment in the fight against chronic infection. Silver nanoparticles, specifically, have good reports of broad-spectrum antimicrobial activity that includes those such as MRSA (Methicillin-resistant *Staphylococcus aureus*) and VRE (Vancomycin-resistant *Enterococcus*). Moreover, in the development of nanoparticle-based systems, design can be incorporated to allow for the gradual release of antibiotics or antiseptics with a steady therapeutic concentration at the wound site while reducing the chance of rejecting the medicine. This form of controlled release also alleviates concerns about the need to change dressing frequently, providing segregation on the part of the patient in controlling the abdomen more freely [15].

One of the most promising prospects of the use of nanotechnology in the care of wounds is the creation of so-called "smart" wound dressings, under the influence of which the injury will be monitored and will react in real time to changes in the environment of the wound. These dressings use the nanosensors that detect indicators such as pH, temperature, moisture content, and the presence of bacteria. For instance, a dressing loaded with pH-sensitive nanoparticles can sense the acidic pH and accordingly release an antimicrobial. Similarly, dressings with a color change indicate bacterial activity for clinicians or patients to take appropriate action, such as the application of topically prescribed antibiotics or changing the dressing. The true-time loop strategy of smart dressings not only improves the accuracy of wound management practices, but it may also present an opportunity to develop customized and variable care protocols.

CHALLENGES AND LIMITATIONS

Although the prospect of nanotechnology-based wound dressings is promising, developing and applying them in a clinical environment presents many challenges and constraints. These issues apply to a wide variety of fields, from biocompatibility, scalability in production, regulatory challenges, and economic appropriateness. Having overcome these obstacles would significantly contribute to the successful translation of nanotechnology from the laboratory to the clinic and the implementation on a large scale.

Biocompatibility and safety are two of the greatest issues shown in Figure 11.5 related to nanotechnology-based wound dressings [16]. Although various nanomaterials have distinct therapeutic properties, their interaction with human tissues and

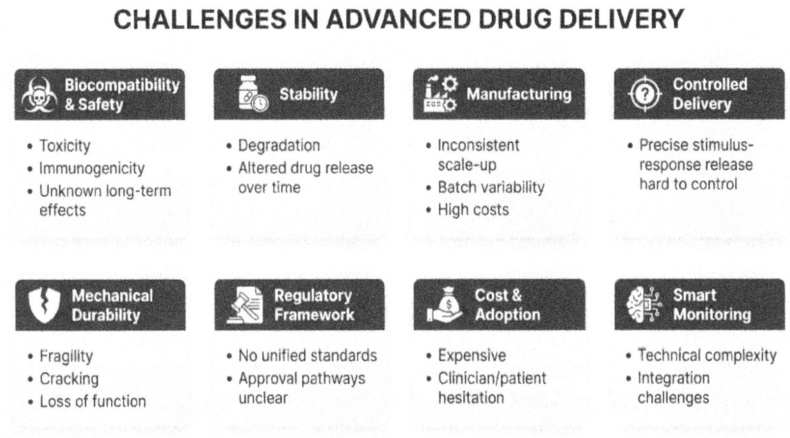

FIGURE 11.5 Challenge areas and their key issues.

biological systems is not clearly defined. The size and surface area of nanoparticles are small and large, respectively, which allows them to infiltrate cells and bodies and trigger odd biological reactions. For instance, particular nanoparticles may be cytotoxic, or induce inflammation, or oxidative stress, which may yield adverse effects in healthy tissue. There is still ongoing research into the long-term implications of human health from the holistic impacts of nanomaterials and their potential to build up in organs. Making sure that nanomaterials are safe for short- and long-term use involves massive in vitro and in vivo testing, determining possible toxicity and negative reactions on humans. In addition, it is important that nanotechnology-based dressings do not cause allergic reactions or hypersensitivity in patients.

Another major challenge would be the stability and degradation of nanoparticles. Most nanomaterials, especially those used for drug delivery, are liable to instability when placed in the biological environment. For instance, the release of drugs or other active agents from nanoparticles can be affected due to factors such as pH, temperature, or ionic strength, thus causing nonuniform or premature drug release. Sometimes, nanomaterials may degrade too fast or not at all, thus impacting their performance. It is vital to balance the stability that nanoparticles have with their regulated degradation over time to optimally set the efficacy in the case of nanotechnology-based dressings. Additionally, the degradation products of nanoparticles need to be biocompatible and non-toxic, not to harm the surrounding tissues [17].

Other barriers to commercialization include manufacturing and scalability. Extrapolation of Laboratory production of nanomaterials, however, to a manufacturing level is both technically and economically challenging. Synthesis of nanomaterials in high quantities should be cost-effective while retaining the quality and homogeneity needed for clinical use. Moreover, existing manufacturing methods may not be ideal for manufacturing complex multifunctional dressings, which combine various nanomaterials, drugs, and sensors. The creation of the standardizable and reproducible processes of producing nanomaterials on an industrial scale is essential to provide uniformity and cut costs. Without the possibility of scalable production, the price of such advanced dressings is cost-prohibitive, thereby limiting access to the product in constrained settings.

Another major barrier to nanotechnology-based wound dressings is regulatory approval. The pathways for clearing medical devices or wound care products are complicated, and this may change from region. Numerous regulatory agencies (e.g., USA Food and Drug Administration, USA FDA, USA FDDA; FDA, US FDA, US FDDA) and the European Medicines Agency, EMA, do not adequately address the evaluation of nanomaterials in medical use (in vivo applications) to the extent they are needed. This lack of regulatory clarity has quite often contributed to delays in the approval process and delayed the timely availability of new ways in which to treat wounds. Furthermore, due to the fact that nanomaterials are often handled differently than traditional materials, the previously developed structures for the safety, efficacy, and quality of medical products might not suffice. Regulatory agencies should ensure that strong protocols exist in using nanotechnology-based products in clinical trial missions, ensuring that safety and effectiveness are achieved.

However, cost-effectiveness and accessibility continue to be major hindrances to the application of wound dressings based on nanotechnology on a large scale. These dressings are quite costly because of their complicated production processes and the specialized materials and advanced technologies required in manufacture. The high cost of nanodressing may dissuade many patients, especially in low-income or developing regions, despite better healing outcomes from such pillowcases. In addition, healthcare systems that are heavily based on minimal-cost, standard solutions may be slow to implement novel, expensive technology if there is no proof of benefits further than just short-term benefits and economic gain. For these innovations to be disseminated globally, manufacturers will have to strike a balance between the price of production and the clinical gains for these high-tech dressings to be budget-friendly and available to all patients across the globe. Lastly, ethical and environmental considerations need to be considered when designing nanotechnology-based wound dressing. The possibility of nanoparticles accumulating in the environment and their long-term effects on ecosystems is an area of concern. If correctly disposed of, then nanoparticles should not contaminate the water supply, the soil, or wildlife, thus wreaking havoc on the environment inadvertently. Moreover, the ethical issues of applying nanomaterials in medical devices, e.g., issues of privacy regarding smart wound dressing, or the use of nanoparticles in vulnerable populations, should be considered. Manufacturers, as well as researchers, should ensure that the benefits are superior to the risks of these technologies and measures, such as disposal, ecological, and appropriate ethical measures, are established.

In summary, though the application of nanotechnology in wound care can cure wound-associated diseases positively, the application is not free from several challenges that must be met to yield its full potential. It will be crucial to address problems in regard to biocompatibility, stability, manufacturing, regulatory approval, cost, and the environmental impact to ensure the widespread adoption and success of the wound dressings based on nanotechnology. With research still progressing, the issues being resolved, nanotechnology offers the capacity to transform the way in which we heal wounds and will provide more efficient, tailored, and effective treatment options for patients across the world.

FUTURE DIRECTIONS AND EMERGING TRENDS

The area of nanotechnology in wound care remains in its infancy, but it promises much in transforming the way we treat wounds, especially chronic and complex wounds. As nanomaterials research and development strive to improve the fabrication techniques of nanotechnology-based wound dressings, the scope and possibilities of the same are likely to increase. Some of the current emerging trends provide a bit of insight into how future innovators will be concentrating not only on the functional aspect of innovations related to such dressings, but also on those that hinder the actual clinical implementation of these innovations as they are.

The most exciting prospects for future development involve combining smart technologies with wound care. As cited before, smart dressings for wounds, which can monitor the environment of the wound and respond in real time, also give an inkling of what could be the future of personalized medicines. In the future years, we will certainly observe even more advanced smart dressings that will be fitted with a kind of biosensor that will be able to score particular biomarkers, specifically those associated with infection, inflammation, or tissue regeneration. For example, the sensors that should have been able to detect the presence of bacterial biofilms resistant to traditionally used modes of therapy should have mobilized the release of antibiotics or antimicrobial peptides in a localized form. Consistent with this, dressings that respond to situations such as changes in wound pH, temperature, or moisture can automatically vary their properties to help produce the optimal conditions for healing, resulting in both shorter healing time and comfort for the patient. Such integration of wireless communication with these dressings may make it possible to collect and monitor real-time data by healthcare providers, thus allowing more accurate and timely interventions.

With an increasing demand for personalized medicine, we can look forward to the creation of individualized wound care solutions according to different particularities of wounds, medical background, and genetic factors of individual patients. Advancements in 3D printing and biofabrication technologies will contribute greatly to the trend in question. The potential of 3D printing to tailor wound care products to an unparalleled level arises from its capacity to produce patient-specific dressings whose shapes, sizes, and types of wounds are apt to each recipient. Such customized dressings could also include nanomaterials tailored for specific therapeutic applications, e.g., delivery of growth factors or antimicrobial or anti-inflammatory agents under control. Moreover, future wound dressings may also promote regeneration of tissue, as a result of being able to combine bioprinting with stem cell therapy or tissue engineering methods.

In the area of drug delivery, it may be that the production of more sophisticated nanocarriers will represent one of the next-generation wound dressings' most significant priorities. Nanoparticles can be engineered to convey a large variety of therapeutic agents, such as antibiotics, anti-inflammatory agents, growth factors, and even genes such as DNA and RNA. Scientists are also paying a lot of attention on the development of nanocarriers that would allow unloading a cargo in the presence of certain stimuli, such as a shift of pH, an overall temperature change, or the presence of some enzyme activity. The stimuli-responsive drug delivery enables a more efficient and controlled release—meaning the appropriate dose is released into the exact location it is intended to be when it is required. Furthermore, better nanoencapsulation technologies will make it possible to deliver vulnerable compounds (biologics or proteins) stably in the body, which would otherwise degrade or fail to work due to rapid clearance.

Another area where tremendous improvements can be achieved is in biodegradable and environmentally friendly nanomaterials. Due to the increased worries about the environmental impact of the synthetic nanomaterials, scientists are striving to invent "green nanotechnology" using sustainable natural materials. For example, nanocellulose, chitosan, and other biodegradable polymers are considered for wound care due to their low toxicity and environmental safety. These materials can be developed into dressings for wounds that not only promote healing, but can also safely degrade in the body, thus eliminating the need for wound dressings made from non-biodegradable materials to be removed and disposed of. This resonates with the emerging trend in sustainable healthcare and minimizes the impact on the environment left by medical instruments.

In the future, regenerative medicine will probably have an ever more prominent place in the treatment of wounds. The combination of nanotechnology to stem cell therapy and tissue engineering will help in expediting the wound healing process and even regenerating lost tissues. For instance, dressings containing nanofibers or nanostructured scaffolds could be developed to promote stem cell proliferation and differentiation and direct new tissue formation at the wound site. In addition, the nano-enabled growth factors and signaling molecules can be used to further promote the regenerative capacity of these dressings and accelerate the complete healing process. In association with other cutting-edge treatments such as gene editing or exosomes treatment, the possibility of regenerating tissues at the molecular level may lead to new opportunities for healing desperately damaged wounds and even chronic ones, unlike anything else.

Additionally, integration of nanotechnology-based wound dressings into conventional clinical practice would increase as clinical trials and real-world data are increasingly gathered. The activity will require collaborative efforts on the part of both academic researchers and medical device manufacturers, as well as healthcare providers, to find solutions to the remaining manufacturing, cost, and regulatory approval issues. With more safety profiles and efficacy data of these dressings, we expect greater utilization at hospitals, outpatient clinics, and home care settings, with improved quality of life for patients with acute and chronic wounds.

CONCLUSION

Nanotechnology has made a significant impact on the field of wound care, providing innovative solutions to challenges that have long hindered effective wound healing. From the ability to deliver controlled therapeutic agents to providing antimicrobial protection and enhancing tissue regeneration, nanotechnology-based wound dressings offer a multifaceted approach to treating both acute and chronic wounds. The integration of nanomaterials, such as nanoparticles, nanofibers, and smart sensors, into wound dressings has transformed them from passive coverings into active systems that engage with the wound environment at the cellular and molecular levels. These advancements hold the potential to accelerate healing, reduce infection, and improve overall patient outcomes.

However, as the field continues to evolve, several challenges must be addressed to ensure the widespread clinical adoption of nanotechnology-based wound dressings. Issues related to biocompatibility, stability, scalability, and regulatory approval must be carefully considered to ensure that these innovative products are both safe and effective for patient use. Moreover, the high cost associated with the production of nanomaterials and the complexity of manufacturing scalable, standardized products remain significant barriers to accessibility, especially in resource-limited settings. As such, addressing these challenges will require collaboration among researchers, manufacturers, regulatory agencies, and healthcare providers to create practical solutions that balance efficacy with cost-effectiveness.

Looking to the future, the continued advancement of nanotechnology, particularly in the areas of smart dressings, personalized medicine, and regenerative therapies, will likely lead to even more sophisticated and targeted treatments. The incorporation of sensors and stimuli-responsive materials into dressings, for example, could offer real-time monitoring and dynamic therapeutic interventions. Additionally, as 3D printing and biofabrication technologies evolve, we can expect the development of personalized wound care solutions that are tailored to individual patient needs. The integration of nanotechnology with regenerative medicine, including stem cell therapy and tissue engineering, holds the potential to heal wounds that are currently difficult or impossible to treat.

In conclusion, nanotechnology has opened up exciting possibilities for the future of wound care, offering the potential for more effective, personalized, and patient-friendly treatments. While several challenges remain, the ongoing research and innovation in this field suggest that nanotechnology-based wound dressings will play an increasingly important role in healthcare in the coming years. As we overcome these hurdles, we can expect these advanced wound dressings to transform the way we treat wounds, ultimately improving the quality of life for patients and providing healthcare professionals with more effective tools for managing complex wound healing scenarios.

REFERENCES

1. A. McNicol and S. Israels, "Beyond Hemostasis: The Role of Platelets in Inflammation, Malignancy and Infection," *Cardiovasc Hematol Disorders-Drug Targets*, vol. 8, no. 2, pp. 99–117, 2008, doi:10.2174/187152908784533739.
2. M. J. E. Kuijpers, J. W. M. Heemskerk, and K. Jurk, "Molecular Mechanisms of Hemostasis, Thrombosis and Thrombo-Inflammation," *Int J Mol Sci*, vol. 23, no. 10, p. 5825, 2022, doi:10.3390/ijms23105825.
3. I. T. Swinehart and S. F. Badylak, "Extracellular Matrix Bioscaffolds in Tissue Remodeling and Morphogenesis," *Develop Dyn*, vol. 245, no. 3, pp. 351–360, 2016, doi:10.1002/dvdy.24379.

4. C. E. Attinger, J. E. Janis, J. Steinberg, J. Schwartz, A. Al-Attar, and K. Couch, "Clinical Approach to Wounds: Debridement and Wound Bed Preparation Including the Use of Dressings and Wound-Healing Adjuvants," *Plast Reconstr Surg*, vol. 117, no. Supplement, pp. 72S–109S, 2006, doi:10.1097/01.prs.0000225470.42514.8f.
5. N. Mammari, E. Lamouroux, A. Boudier, and R. E. Duval, "Current Knowledge on the Oxidative-Stress-Mediated Antimicrobial Properties of Metal-based Nanoparticles," *Microorganisms*, vol. 10, no. 2, p. 437, 2022, doi:10.3390/microorganisms10020437.
6. A. E. Stoica, C. Chircov, and A. M. Grumezescu, "Nanomaterials for Wound Dressings: An Up-to-Date Overview," *Molecules*, vol. 25, no. 11, p. 2699, 2020, doi:10.3390/molecules25112699.
7. M. Divya et al., "Biopolymer Gelatin-Coated Zinc Oxide Nanoparticles Showed High Antibacterial, Antibiofilm and Anti-Angiogenic Activity," *J Photochem Photobiol B*, vol. 178, pp. 211–218, 2018, doi:10.1016/j.jphotobiol.2017.11.008.
8. V. Andreu, G. Mendoza, M. Arruebo, and S. Irusta, "Smart Dressings based on Nanostructured Fibers Containing Natural Origin Antimicrobial, Anti-Inflammatory, and Regenerative Compounds," *Materials*, vol. 8, no. 8, pp. 5154–5193, 2015, doi:10.3390/ma8085154.
9. D. Chenthamara et al., "Therapeutic Efficacy of Nanoparticles and Routes of Administration," *Biomater Res*, vol. 23, no. 1, 2019, doi:10.1186/s40824-019-0166-x.
10. M. M. de Villiers, D. P. Otto, S. J. Strydom, and Y. M. Lvov, "Introduction to Nanocoatings Produced by Layer-by-Layer (LbL) Self-Assembly," *Adv Drug Deliv Rev*, vol. 63, no. 9, pp. 701–715, 2011, doi:10.1016/j.addr.2011.05.011.
11. L. Yang, Q. Yuan, T.-T. Li, C.-W. Lou, C. Hung, and J.-H. Lin, "Exploration and Application Prospect of the Advanced Technology of Time–Temperature Indicators," *Textile Res J*, vol. 95, no. 3–4, pp. 404–428, 2025, doi:10.1177/00405175241266999.
12. J. A. Ataide et al., "Nanotechnology-based Dressings for Wound Management," Pharmaceuticals, vol. 15, no. 10, p. 1286, 2022, doi:10.3390/ph15101286.
13. S. T. Haque, S. K. Saha, Md. E. Haque, and N. Biswas, "Nanotechnology-based Therapeutic Applications: *In Vitro and In Vivo* Clinical Studies for Diabetic Wound Healing," *Biomater Sci*, vol. 9, no. 23, pp. 7705–7747, 2021, doi:10.1039/D1BM01211H.
14. B. Blanco-Fernandez, O. Castaño, M. Á. Mateos-Timoneda, E. Engel, and S. Pérez-Amodio, "Nanotechnology Approaches in Chronic Wound Healing," *Adv Wound Care (New Rochelle)*, vol. 10, no. 5, pp. 234–256, 2021, https://doi.org/10.1089/wound.2019.1094.
15. H. W. Boucher and G. R. Corey, "Epidemiology of Methicillin-Resistant *Staphylococcus aureus*," *Clin Infect Dis*, vol. 46, no. S5, pp. S344–S349, 2008, doi:10.1086/533590.
16. Z. B. Nqakala, N. R. S. Sibuyi, A. O. Fadaka, M. Meyer, M. O. Onani, and A. M. Madiehe, "Advances in Nanotechnology towards Development of Silver Nanoparticle-based Wound-Healing Agents," *Int J Mol Sci*, vol. 22, no. 20, p. 11272, 2021, doi:10.3390/ijms222011272.
17. D. Schmaljohann, "Thermo- and pH-Responsive Polymers in Drug Delivery," *Adv Drug Deliv Rev*, vol. 58, no. 15, pp. 1655–1670, 2006, doi:10.1016/j.addr.2006.09.020.

12 Case Studies and Future Directions

Iqra Zainab, Zohra Naseem, Syeda Rubab Batool, and Muhammad Anwaar Nazeer

INTRODUCTION

The skin helps to protect our bodies from damage, clearly showing that it is the largest organ in the human body. It interacts with the environment through touch and provides the necessary thermal stability and insulation, among other functions. In the trauma due to any injury, the skin starts to heal automatically and in a well-defined sequence of events [1]. This intricate process begins immediately after an injury and can sometimes extend over a long period—even years—depending on the severity of the wound. A wound is essentially any break or damage to the normal structure of the tissue that also causes loss of function. When the outer layer of skin is affected, we call it an open wound, but injuries deeper in the body where the skin remains unbroken are considered closed wounds. The body heals these wounds either by regeneration, where it restores the tissue to its original state, or by repair, where scar tissue takes its place. Skin healing relies on various cells and signals working in harmony [2]. The first step in this process is called hemostasis. It happens right after the injury and is usually completed within a few hours. This stage is all about stopping the bleeding and forming a temporary structure called the wound matrix, which sets the stage for the rest of the healing process. It's also known as the "lag phase" because, during this time, the body starts gathering all the cells and tools it needs to repair the damage, even though the wound itself is still fragile [3]. Blood and lymphatic vessels may be compromised when a wound extends below the skin layer. This results in an outpouring of liquids that irrigate the area, assisting in the elimination of any bacteria or toxic agents. At the same time, the clotting mechanism of the body is activated, and platelet cells, which are specialized blood cells, migrate to the site of injury. They continue to slide onto the wound while firmly adhering to the collagen that has been previously exposed and contributing substances that facilitate the clotting process. This clot serves both as a means of controlling the flow of blood and as a filler in the wound while serving as a building framework for future phases of the recuperation process. In effect, the blood clot works as a temporary dressing to promote healing of the wound. It contains proteins like fibrin and compounds, which prompt diverse sets of cells to migrate into the wound region [4]. These encompass white blood cells that combat infection, keratinocytes that repair skin, fibroblasts that generate new tissue, and endothelial cells that aid in neovascularization. In this phase, however,

DOI: 10.1201/9781003616726-14

the blood vessels undergo constriction for several minutes to reduce blood loss: this in turn results in low oxygen levels in the region, thereby yielding a few alterations to the tissue. Recapturing blood circulation triggers various cell types to move toward the injury site and initiate the healing process. During the recovery phase, platelets and leukocytes play a crucial role [5]. These cells produce a variety of growth factors and cytokines that initiate the repair process. The products of inflammation facilitate collagen synthesis and fibroblast transformation into myofibroblasts that assist in wound closure. New vessels are generated, and the epidermal layer starts to restore. Increased blood supply to the site of tissue damage causes the region to get inflamed, claimed, or reddened, which is the body's response while recovery is in process. The ability of human body to repair tissues is very complex and organized, starting with arresting the bleeding at the site of injury, which is the first and a very important step [6]. Neutrophils are the most traditional first responders to any tissue injury and self-explain through various mechanisms that they are the first line of defense of the human body. Immediately after hemostasis, which is the cessation of blood loss, is the beginning of the inflammatory phase that is important for wound healing according to the article from Thomas et al. [7]. Signals from activated platelets, tissue, and the complement system are the reasons for the recruitment of neutrophils toward the wound. So, in addition to engulfing dead tissue, neutrophils are crucial in bacterial cleanup, which marks them as a critical factor in injury cleaning. They have been shown to have a 2–5-day lifespan under the condition that the wound is not infected. Neutrophils release important cytokines such as TNF-a, IL-1, and IL-6 in addition to debris clearance, which is essential for wound repair since they enhance and modulate the immune response. These cells are also attracted by these molecules, ensuring that the inflammatory response is both effective and adequate. Neutrophils along with macrophages secrete harsh enzymes such as elastase and proteinase, which serve the purpose of eliminating microorganisms [8]. In addition, they regulate the activity of macrophages which manipulate them in a way that ensures this necessary changeover stage in the healing process. Thereafter, macrophages take over around day three after being deployed to the site together with these complementary substances [9]. Like all other cells in the body, they are programmed to perform some functions such as growth factors like VEGF, TGF-b, and FGF, which aid in clearing dead cells and preventing infection [10].

Tissues change and adapt due to these components that are required for cell division, angiogenesis, and extracellular matrix (ECM) synthesis. It has been shown that macrophages are involved in the process of healing, but more importantly, they help control inflammation so that it does not result in significant damage to the tissue. It has been reported that the amount of inflammation present affects the amount of scarring that occur; in particular, a common observation is that the inflammation is less in fetal wounds and there is no scarring [11]. Macrophages serve as the link between the first inflammatory response and the wound undergoing the subsequent healing process, confirming that the wound has been set for tissue growth and reconstruction. This stage is important as it allows the body to efficiently and effectively repair itself. The body's complex process of repair begins after a wound has been locked in place and bleeding has stopped. In general, this phase occurs in three to ten days post-injury period and looks into covering the wound up, building tissue over, and repairing blood vessels. The body's repair crew comes into action, starting with fibroblasts special cells that migrate into the wound along the framework of the fibrin clot [12]. Construction of the connective tissue is accomplished by these fibroblasts through their synthesis of collagen and fibronectin. These layers assist in filling missing structural elements and increasing the strength of the wound area. Keratinocytes, which are skin cells for regeneration, from the edges of the wound, start moving toward the center of the wound. They respond to directions from other cells around them or to growth factors like epithelial growth factors (EGF) and keratinocyte growth factor (KGF), which make them start to disengage from neighboring cells and move. The combination of fibronectin and chemotactic stimulus directs the cells to extend out, change the orientation of their internal structural elements, and crawl toward the centermost part of the wound. This managed migration that is called "shuffling" helps to ensure the coverage of the surface of the wound that occurs gradually. In the increase of such migrating cells coalescing together at the center of the wound, there is a natural zipper effect that closes it [13].

Construction of the connective tissue is accomplished by these fibroblasts through their synthesis of collagen and fibronectin. These layers assist in filling missing structural elements and increasing the strength of the wound area. Keratinocytes, which are skin cells for regeneration, from the edges of the wound, start moving toward the center of the wound. They respond to directions from other cells around them or to growth factors like EGF and KGF, which make them start to disengage from neighboring cells and move. The combination of fibronectin and chemotactic stimulus directs the cells to extend out, change the orientation of their internal structural elements, and crawl toward the centermost part of the wound. This managed migration that is called "shuffling" helps to ensure that the coverage of the surface of the wound occurs gradually. In the increase of such migrating cells coalescing together at the center of the wound, there is a natural zipper effect that closes it [14]. Eventually, the chambers of these vessels become stagnant as other neighboring support cells like pericytes and smooth muscle cells are recruited. This ensures that the wound is continually provided with oxygen and nutrients. Granulation tissue begins to present itself within the wound as the vascular system is being constructed. This type of tissue, which takes the form of immature blood vessels with macrophages and fibroblasts, leads to a brighter red coloration as a result of its vast blood supply [15]. During this stage, fibroblasts heavily aid in the tissue healing, with collagen, glycosaminoglycans, and other matrix components enabling other cells to migrate and better organize the tissue. Although the granulation tissue is weak, it acts as an initial placeholder until the injury site is properly repaired with well-organized tissues. At this stage, myofibroblasts help to complete the healing process, as they contract the wound edges and bring them closer together [16]. Once the edges have approximated, these cells complete their self-destructive process called apoptosis, where many cells simply vanish and a few others aid in modulating the microenvironment, forming a more robust wound region with an intact vascular network. This self-sustaining and very elegant mechanism indicates the transition from the active to passive rehabilitation phase, which is the remodeling phase (Figure 12.1). In this phase, the wound is passively monitored, and the physiological tissue structure is restored. The body has an astonishing and understated ability to heal itself, and its various structures,

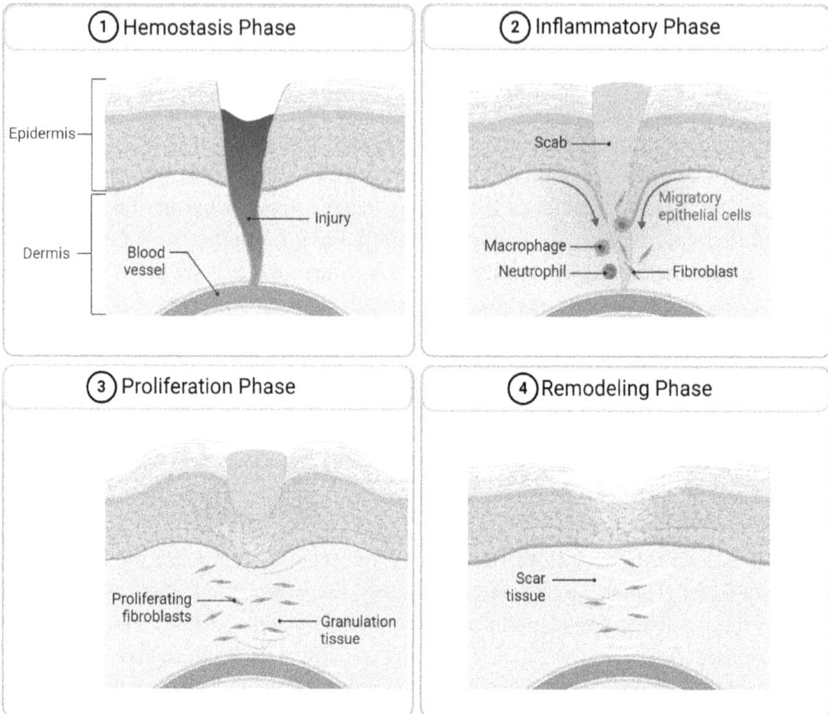

FIGURE 12.1 Steps for wound regeneration process: hemostasis, inflammatory, proliferation, and remodeling phases.

internal and external, are protected and repaired in an orderly manner through this multifaceted process [2]. When a wound starts to heal, the last step is called the remodeling phase. This phase is like the final touch on a project, where everything gets tidied up and strengthened. It usually begins around three weeks after the injury and can last up to a year, depending on how big the wound is. At this stage, the body doesn't need to keep making new tissue, so the cells that helped to create the granulation tissue begin to shut down through a natural process called apoptosis. As a result, the wound area becomes less active and loses its blood vessels and cells, leaving behind a scar that's quieter and less "alive" compared to earlier phases [17]. Inside the wound, collagen, the protein that gives skin its structure, also evolves. Early in the healing process, the wound is filled with collagen type III, which is softer and more flexible. During remodeling, it's replaced with collagen type I, a stronger, more durable version. This new collagen is arranged in tight, parallel bundles, which is different from the looser basket-weave pattern found in normal, healthy skin [18]. One of the stars of this phase is the myofibroblast. These special cells are like tiny ropes, pulling the edges of the wound together, making it smaller and tighter. Once they finish this job, they disappear. Meanwhile, the extra blood vessels that had sprouted during the earlier stages to deliver nutrients and oxygen start to fade away, and the metabolic activity of the wound slows down until it eventually stops.

However, even with all this effort, the skin doesn't fully return to its original state after a major injury. Structures like hair follicles and sweat glands don't grow back in the scarred area, and the new skin lacks the tiny projections called rete pegs that normally anchor the top layer of skin to the lower layers. This makes scarred skin a bit weaker and less stable than uninjured skin [19].

What's truly fascinating is how differently wounds heal in fetuses. When a fetus gets injured in the early stages of development, it heals without leaving a scar. Scientists first discovered this amazing ability in 1979, and since then, it's been observed in humans as well as animals like rats, mice, and monkeys. This scar-free healing only happens up until about 24 weeks of pregnancy in humans. Before this point, the fetal skin has a remarkable ability to not just heal, but to completely regenerate even restoring complex structures like glands and hair follicles. So, what makes fetal wound healing so special? For starters, the inflammation response in fetal wounds is much gentler than in adults. In adult wounds, the body sends an army of immune cells like neutrophils and macrophages to fight off infection and help with repair, but this process can cause damage to surrounding tissue. In fetuses, fewer immune cells are involved, and they don't stick around as long, which creates a more peaceful healing environment [20]. The next contrast resides in the development of the skin's ECM—the material in which skin cells are embedded and fused. For instance, the ECM in fetal tissue is arranged in a manner that favors renewal processes yet in adults it is more like scarring. The concentrations of some growth factors are also influential. Fetal wounds possess lower amounts of TGF-β1 and TGF-β2, which have an association with scarring, and higher amounts of TGF-β3, which aids in fast, smooth, non-scarring repair [21]. Additionally, fetal skin contains large amounts of morphogenetic factors, which are specific molecules that induce the formation and development of tissues. All these factors along with the fast growth of the skin in fetus ensure that all wounds heal within the cover of normal skin without any scars remaining. Unfortunately, as the fetus matures, it loses this extraordinary ability. By the time the baby is born, its skin has become more like adult skin, and wounds begin to heal with scars. The way fetuses heal wounds is a reminder of how powerful and efficient nature can be. Scientists are studying these processes closely, hoping to one day figure out how to replicate them in adults. If they succeed, it could mean a future where scars are a thing of the past [22].

Scarring is a natural part of the healing process that happens after an injury, but sometimes it doesn't go as planned. When you get hurt, your body works hard to repair the damage, and the result of that repair is usually a scar. While scar formation is important for healing, sometimes it can become more than what we expect, leading to excessive or abnormal scarring. One of the main things that affects scarring is inflammation. Inflammation is the body's way of responding to an injury, but it can be a bit of a problem if it's too strong or lasts too long. This is clearly seen in fetal wound healing [23]. In fetuses, wounds heal without forming scars because their bodies don't have the same kind of intense inflammatory response that adults do. When scientists try to trigger inflammation in fetal wounds, scars form, showing just how closely inflammation is linked to scarring. Hormones also play a big role in how scars form. For example, studies have shown that when estrogen levels are low, as seen in some mice, the healing process gets slower and leads to more inflammation and scarring. This proves that our hormone levels are very important for proper healing. Sometimes, wounds don't heal properly and stay stuck in the inflammation stage for too long. This is what happens with chronic wounds, which never move on to the next stages of healing. Instead of healing completely, these wounds stay inflamed, which can cause severe scars like hypertrophic scars or keloids [24]. Hypertrophic scars are different from regular scars. They have thinner collagen fibers, which are grouped into nodules. Keloids, on the other hand, are thick and raised scars with extra collagen fibers. Both types of scars form when the healing process goes off track. They happen because of too much growth factor being released and not enough of the necessary tissue being removed during healing. In these scars, the blood vessels in the area can become more than usual, but they don't work as they should. This happens because of an overproduction of collagen and overactive cells called myofibroblasts, which help close the wound. These cells keep producing collagen, leading to thick, raised scars like hypertrophic scars and keloids [25]. Sometimes, a protein called p53, which normally helps to remove unnecessary cells during healing, gets involved and prevents normal cell death. When this happens, it can contribute to the formation of more scars. Additionally, things like physical irritation, pressure, or friction during the early healing stages can stop the body from properly clearing away extra cells, leading to more scarring. Changes in the structure of the skin and the body's response to the injury also affect scarring. Some researchers believe that nerves in the skin might play a part in scarring [26]. When there's mechanical stress, nerves in the skin release chemicals that impact blood vessels and cells that produce collagen. This disruption can cause too much tissue to form, resulting in scars that go beyond normal healing. So, scarring is a natural part of how our body heals, but sometimes the process gets disrupted. Inflammation, hormones, irritation, and changes in skin structure all contribute to scarring, and understanding how these things work can help us manage and improve the healing process [27].

IMPORTANCE OF WOUND DRESSING

Wound dressing serves as a protective covering as well as acts as a supportive mechanism during the healing process. It is crucial in healing and offers immense value in serving the many functions that wound care encompasses. This includes changes and alterations made to the wound site in a manner that makes it clean and prevents infection to aid in making the healing faster and effective. There are processes that one has to go through before applying the dressing to ensure that the wound has been cleaned and fully prepared. These procedures include cleaning the wound of debris and dead tissue and eliminating any associated microorganisms that pose the risk of infection [28]. Cleaning plastics and cotton may work with traditional surgical dressings, but cleaning them for traumatic injuries involves more complex procedures such as irrigation or debridement. This ensures that the contaminants are fully removed. After cleaning the area, the scrubs are changed to applying dressings to the wound to protect it from environmental exposures. Maintaining the right level of moisture in the wound is essential. Softening and damaging the healthy skin that surrounds the wound is referred to as maceration, something that happens if there is too much moisture present. Wounds that are overly dry are problematic as they result in tissue desiccation, which inhibits healing [29]. Most modern dressings perform this function by encouraging the fluid balance of wounds by absorbing the exudates while keeping the injury moist enough to promote cellular activities and tissue formation. Alongside cell activity, proper oxygen exchange further simplifies tissue recovery. Oxygen-permeable dressings facilitate cell regeneration since they allow carbon dioxide and other gases to leave the wound area. Moreover, the best dressings not only allow these gases to pass freely, but they also aid in preventing other complications such as effusion, hematoma, or abscess by filling spaces in tissues and applying light pressure in some regions [30].

Wound dressings typically consist of two primary layers: the contact layer and the secondary layer. The contact layer, as its name suggests, is the part of the dressing that directly touches the wound. This layer plays a significant role in how the dressing functions. Since no single type of dressing works for every kind of wound or healing stage, selecting the right material for the contact layer is critical. The choice depends on factors like the wound's size, depth, amount of fluid it produces, and whether there is an infection or not. Regular evaluation of the wound ensures that the dressing continues to meet its needs as healing progresses. The secondary layer usually provides additional protection and helps secure the contact layer in place. Often made of gauze or other absorbent materials, this layer works in tandem with the contact layer to create an optimal healing environment [31].

TYPES OF WOUND DRESSINGS

Over the years, various types of dressings have been developed, each tailored to address specific wound conditions and healing requirements, as shown in Table 12.1. These range from traditional options like gauze to advanced solutions incorporating bioactive materials and therapeutic agents. Transparent film dressings are thin, self-adhesive sheets made of polyurethane. They allow oxygen to enter the wound while preventing fluid and bacteria from escaping. These dressings are ideal for dry wounds that need to retain moisture but are unsuitable for wounds with heavy fluid, as they can cause maceration [32]. Hydrogel dressings, which are made of a soft, jelly-like material, are considered the best dressings for dry or lightly draining wounds. The moisture they supply to the wound speeds up the healing process greatly. They are also easy to remove as they are not adhesive; thus, they do not cause any pain when taking them off. Impregnated gauzes are gauze pads coated in substances like petrolatum or antiseptics. This reduces the adherence of the gauze to the wounded area because it causes less pain during the changing of the dressing. They find application more in surgical wounds, abrasions, and even in draining wounds where a secondary gauze is used to soak up the extra liquid. Hydrocolloid dressings usually have two sides. The inner one sticks onto the wound, while the outer one acts as a waterproof cover preventing contamination. These types of dressings promote healing by maintaining a moist environment and minimizing the need for replacements. However, it is not the best option for infected wounds [33]. Dressings made from calcium alginate, which is derived from seaweed, turn into gel upon contact with the wound fluid. They are ideal for high exudate wounds as the gel takes the shape of the wound. Such dressings may require a secondary layer for extra protection and

TABLE 12.1
Various Types of Wound Dressings and Their Applications

Type of Wound Dressing	Applications
Transparent film dressings	• Made of self-adhesive polyurethane films • Allow gas exchange but prevent fluid loss • Suitable for dry wounds needing moisture retention • Should not be used for heavily exudative wounds to avoid maceration [36]
Hydrogel dressings	• Made from gelatinous sheets or amorphous fillers • Non-adhesive and gas permeable • Ideal for dry or minimally exuding wounds • Maintain a moist environment to promote tissue regeneration [36]
Impregnated gauzes	• Gauze treated with petrolatum, antiseptics, or other substances • Non-adhesive, minimizing discomfort during dressing changes • Often used for surgical wounds, abrasions, and draining wounds • Usually combined with an absorptive secondary dressing [37]
Hydrocolloids	• Contain a gum-like inner layer that adheres to the wound • Feature a water-resistant outer layer to shield against contaminants • Help maintain moisture but are not recommended for infected wounds • Cost-effective, with fewer dressing changes required [38]
Calcium alginates	• Derived from seaweed and form a gel upon absorbing exudate • Conform well to the wound surface • Manage heavy exudates effectively • Require a secondary dressing for additional absorption [39]
Exudate absorbers	• Include calcium alginates, powders, and starches • Absorb significant fluid amounts and aid in removing necrotic tissue (autolytic debridement) [40]

fluid absorption. Exudate absorbers are materials that include alginates, powders, and starch-based dressings to soak up the extra liquid from a wound. These types of dressing aids are meant to soak in large quantities of fluid while aiding the body to get rid of devitalized tissue on its own. Such dressings are of a particular value in heavily draining wounds [34].

The approach to dress a wound should be specific to the requirements of the wound. To illustrate, film dressings are appropriate for dry wounds, while calcium alginate dressings are suitable for moist wounds. Hydrocolloids are ideal for moisture retention but do not suit infected ulcers. Change of dressings is also determined by the dressing technique used and the state of the wound. For example, hydrocolloid dressings are semipermeable and can be left in place for one week. This is economically advantageous as gauze dressings have to be changed more often, and in some cases, every day. Dressings for some wounds for sure are not mere bandages. They are sophisticated instruments that cover the wound, assist healing, and respond to the needs of the wound. With correct selection of the dressing and competent application of the prop, one can speed up the healing and improve the final results of treatment [35].

CURRENT CHALLENGES IN WOUND REGENERATION

Chronic wounds are different from regular wounds because they don't heal like they should. While normal wounds go through stages of healing, chronic wounds get stuck, especially in the inflammation phase. No matter what the cause, chronic wounds share some common problems. These wounds tend to have too many harmful molecules like cytokines, proteases, and reactive oxygen species (ROS) that keep the healing process from moving forward. On top of that, there's often an infection that just won't go away, and the stem cells needed to fix the tissue aren't working properly. In these wounds, tissue keeps getting damaged, and this invites more immune cells to the area. This causes the body's natural healing process to get stuck in overdrive, leading to an endless cycle of inflammation [41]. When wounds first happen, they trigger the release of helpful substances like transforming growth factor-beta (TGF-β) and others that should promote healing. In chronic wounds, these substances don't help healing, but instead, they contribute to the cycle of inflammation and tissue damage. There's also a buildup of proteases, which break down the skin's structure. In healthy wounds, these proteases are controlled, but in chronic wounds, they overpower the natural inhibitors. This destruction of the skin's support structure (extracellular matrix or ECM) prevents the wound from moving to the next stage of healing. Worse, it attracts more immune cells, keeping the inflammation going and preventing healing from progressing [42]. In specific cases like venous leg ulcers, instead of healing tissue, there are tiny blood vessels surrounded by a thick layer of fibrin. This is a sign that the healing process is disrupted. The body's immune system tries to fight off infection, but the immune cells involved are not doing their job correctly. They become stuck in an unusual state, causing the wound to stay stuck in the inflammation stage. At the same time, the skin cells (keratinocytes) that are supposed to help rebuild the tissue are overactive but not really helping. They're hyper-proliferative, meaning they're multiplying too much but not creating new, healthy tissue [43]. Similarly, the fibroblasts in the wound, which are the cells that should help rebuild the tissue, become senescent and stop responding to growth signals. All of this shows that chronic wounds have deeply changed the way the body's cells behave, making it harder for the wound to heal. This complexity means there's no one simple cause of chronic wounds, and it's difficult to pinpoint a single solution. Trying to fix these wounds in animals is also hard because their wounds don't behave in the same way as human wounds. So, treating chronic wounds in humans is even more challenging, and doctors need to address many different factors at once [44]. For instance, patients with venous leg ulcers need compression therapy to help improve blood flow, while those with diabetic foot ulcers need offloading to relieve pressure on the foot. Doctors also need to clean the wound and remove any dead tissue, which is called debridement. And since chronic wounds often have biofilm (a layer of bacteria that is hard to treat), they need to manage infections carefully. A key part of treating chronic wounds is managing the patient's overall health. Many people with chronic wounds also have other health problems, such as kidney or heart disease, which must be controlled to help the wound heal. For example, if a person with a diabetic foot ulcer also has kidney disease, their treatment options may be limited. This means wound care isn't just about the wound itself; it's about managing a patient's overall health. Because of all these factors—both biological and clinical—it's no wonder that finding effective treatments for chronic wounds has been so difficult. Despite much research, many studies haven't shown the hoped-for results, as the problem is much more complicated than it appears at first glance [45].

INFECTION CONTROL AND ANTIMICROBIAL RESISTANCE

Wound infections are one of the biggest obstacles to proper healing, often worsening a patient's condition and affecting their overall quality of life. When the skin's surface gets damaged, it opens the door for all kinds of microorganisms to enter and take hold. Normally, the skin has a natural defense system, with its own bacterial community acting like a shield, keeping harmful microbes out and protecting the underlying tissues. But when that barrier is broken, wounds become vulnerable, and infections can set in. These infections are rarely caused by just one microorganism; they often involve a mix of bacteria and sometimes fungi, making treatment even trickier [46]. Every wound carries some risk of infection, but when infections do occur, they can spiral into a much bigger problem. For instance, bacteria from the air, the skin's surface, or even the gastrointestinal tract can invade a wound. Complications like dead tissue, restricted blood flow (ischemia), or blood pooling (hematoma formation) create the perfect breeding ground for these invaders. Unfortunately, the rise in antimicrobial resistance—where bacteria and fungi become immune to the drugs we use to fight them—has made treating infections much harder than it used to be. Both Gram-positive and Gram-negative bacteria play a big role in wound infections. Gram-negative bacteria, such as *Pseudomonas aeruginosa*, *Klebsiella pneumoniae*, and *Escherichia coli*, are particularly troublesome and are commonly found in burn wounds and other infected injuries. Studies have shown that while some bacteria, like *E. coli*, still respond to certain antibiotics like gentamicin, they've become much less sensitive to others, such as cloxacillin. On top of that, fungi can also cause infections in wounds. These fungal infections are less common than bacterial ones, but when they do occur, they can be just as dangerous [47].

Many bacteria and fungi are constantly evolving as they adapt, mutate, and develop resistance to the drugs designed to kill them. This means that antibiotics that once worked perfectly can suddenly become useless. Chronic wounds, in particular, are difficult to treat because they're already stuck in a cycle of inflammation and delayed healing, and infections only make things worse. Not only does this prolong the healing process, but it also increases treatment costs and, in severe cases, can lead to life-threatening complications. Typical treatment of infection in the wound has to incorporate multifaceted measures. To control an infection, physicians routinely employ a mix of systemic antibiotics, topical antiseptics, and other sophisticated wound dressings. Nevertheless, owing to the issue of increasing antibiotic resistance, new approaches are imperative. The extended use of certain antibiotics makes some strains of bacteria resistant, which prompts the search for other treatments, next-generation antibiotics being one. The focus cannot only be on the wound healing process; prevention of severe infections, systemic complications such as sepsis, and amputation need to be addressed. Antimicrobial resistance is a challenge to tackle, but further investigations and enhanced treatment plans can deliver more successful outcomes in the management of problematic and complex wounds for the patients [48].

SCAR FORMATION AND KELOID MANAGEMENT

Scars pose a significant concern to several individuals in dermatology and their physical as well as mental health. The process that leads to scarring is quite multifaceted as it entails an understanding and processing of inflammation, tissue growth, and remodeling. The perception of scars is usually negative in our societies, and their formation is influenced by several factors, which range from genetics to skin tension or surrounding factors like Sun exposure. Recently, there have been attempts to develop a wide spectrum of technologies that provide options from surgery to lasers, or even biological treatments like cytokines. In our everyday lives, skin injuries are almost inevitable. When the deeper layer of the skin, the dermis, is damaged, the body repairs it with connective tissue, often leaving a scar [49]. In surgeries, for example, skin incisions are unavoidable, so it's important to use techniques that minimize scarring. Burns are another common cause of scarring that can sometimes cover large areas of the body. Acne scars, especially those on the face, can leave lasting marks that deeply affect self-confidence. Even activities like getting piercings, tattoos, or removing tattoos with lasers can lead to scars if proper precautions aren't taken [50].

Non-surgical treatments like chemical peels, lasers, and injections are increasingly popular for treating scars. However, these methods can disrupt the skin and require recovery time, during which good post-procedure care is essential to prevent unwanted marks. Scars that are raised, sunken, wide, or red often cause discomfort, itching, or even pain, adding to the emotional and physical challenges for the person affected [51]. There are three main types of scars: hypertrophic, keloid, and atrophic scars. Hypertrophic scars are often the result of burns that take a long time to heal. They appear as firm, raised, and red tissue that stands out from the skin. Keloid scars, on the other hand, are caused by an overproduction of collagen and are often itchy, invasive, and difficult to treat. They tend to come back even after being removed. Atrophic scars are the most common and noticeable form of scars due to collagen deficit in skin tissues. These types of scars may appear as shallow contours, such as those seen in acne, chickenpox, or with stretching of skin, and they are easily distinguished. Effective prevention and treatment of scars is achievable with proper skin preparation and adequate post-treatment care. Scars may also improve significantly with the use of restorative, anti-inflammatory, and restorative dressings. Also, scarring may be improved by incorporating antioxidants, anti-aging, and whitening agents into the skincare regimen. This suggests that a high degree of reduction in scarring, enhanced healing, and other patient outcomes are possible with proper care and follow-up [52].

LIMITED ACCESS TO ADVANCED TREATMENTS

Wound healing is an intrinsic and multifaceted process that relies on several considerations. An appropriate dressing for the wound is of great importance as it minimizes the chances of infection occurrence while also helping the wound to heal.

An ideal dressing should eliminate excessive fluids, maintain a moist environment without drying the tissue, enable natural ventilation, and possess sufficient strength. Furthermore, it should be non-toxic, comfortable, painless upon removal, and inhibition to bacterial or fungal growth. Also, it must be more efficient than traditional ones with scarring reduction properties. One of the most difficult problems with conventional dressings is that they are painful to take off. If a dressing is securely affixed to the wound, removing it is likely to injure the wound, result in inflammation, and hinder healing. To address these problems, newer dressings have been constructed that possess the ability to monitor the healing process and minimize these difficulties [53].

The optimal choice of dressing for chronic wounds is determined by their size and shape, as well as by the quantity and quality of the fluid that the wounds exude. High exudate wounds require special dressings that cope with this steep challenge. If the exuded fluid is not adequately dealt with, it has the potential to encourage the growth of bacteria and slow the recovery progress. Furthermore, excessive leakage of fluid, which leads to the need for dressing changes and leakage of the dressing inflow interface, needs to be controlled at all times in order to maintain homeostasis within the wound, as it can also cause problems [54]. Recent technological development in wound management has centered on the production of materials that mimic the properties of skin, such as the ability to maintain moisture while blocking bacterial infiltration. One such example is asymmetric polymeric membranes, which are composites of layers designed to perform different functions. These novel dressings are produced by advanced methods such as electrospinning, bioprinting, and other construction methods, which makes these advanced dressings to aid in effective wound care. However, these sophisticated therapies are not always an option due to lack of availability, their complexity, and cost [55].

ADVANCEMENTS IN WOUND DRESSING TECHNOLOGIES

Wound dressings have significantly changed from simple covers that protect the wound to complex materials that promote wound healing. Advances in the textile industry have introduced a variety of woven and nonwoven gauze dressings made from both natural and synthetic fibers, broadening their application in wound care. Traditional dressings are effective for managing dry or mildly exuding wounds, but they often fail to meet the needs of chronic wounds. Chronic wounds need dressings that accommodate changing conditions, which traditional options cannot cope with. These conventional dressings generally don't drain well, requiring frequent, painful changes of dressing. In addition, their mechanical strength, adhesive properties, and bioactivity are suboptimal to bring inadequate control of infection as well as poor tissue regeneration, leading to chronic inflammatory conditions [56]. In response to these challenges, bioactive dressing is one of the latest developments in wound management. This contemporary dressing entails the integration of either natural or synthetic polymers incorporating bioactive components such as antimicrobial agents, anti-inflammatory drugs, and regenerative agents. Antimicrobial agents (antibiotics and anti-fungal nanoparticles) play an important role in infection control, while anti-inflammatory agents (corticosteroids and NSAIDs) reduce pain and inflammation. Regenerative agents, including growth factors, PRP (Platelet-Rich Plasma), and stem cells, work to enhance recovery and the generation of new tissue [57]. Technological advancements have revolutionized the production of wound dressings. For instance, electrospun nanofiber-based dressings mimic the ECM, which provides an optimal healing environment. Bioactive glass-based dressings release ions such as silver, copper, and zinc, which enhance tissue regeneration and angiogenesis, and fight infection. New technologies including 3D bioprinting make it possible to design and build bioactive dressings that contain living cells using cell-laden bioinks, which can add precision and customization to wound care products. Despite these advances, bioactive dressings still have limitations as one of the major challenges is ensuring the appropriate interaction between biomaterials and wound tissue along with standardized manufacturing and storage practices. Nevertheless, the ongoing research on advanced biomaterials and smart dressings is opening new opportunities for the wound care management of complex wounds such as diabetic ulcers and pressure sores [58].

BIOACTIVE DRESSINGS AND THEIR IMPACT

Bioactive materials can be defined as substances that assist in healing or repairing body tissues or organs. These materials can be completely organic, fully artificial, or a composite of the two and can work without adding any other drug. These characteristics make bioactive materials potential candidates for wound dressing applications. They are biocompatible, meaning there are no foreign immune reactions when applied to a wound, and engage in primary activities that are core to healing a wound, including cell adhesion and proliferation, exudate control, antimicrobial activity, gas exchange, drug delivery, and conformability. Bioactive dressings are wound coverings that are designed to modify the wound environment by releasing active compounds to the site of injury in response to specific conditions, especially when disruptive cytokine levels increase. Additionally, these dressings actively interact with the wound environment and adapt in response to certain chemical or environmental factors [59].

An important component of bioactive dressings is the use of natural biopolymers that are derived from plants, animals, fungi, bacteria, and algae. Polymers formed from peptides and polysaccharides consist of long chains of amino acids or sugars that are linked together and have many benefits including biocompatibility, biodegradability, and the ability to enhance cell growth and tissue healing. The incorporation of agents like antimicrobials and anti-inflammatory drugs alongside regenerative compounds like growth factors, PRP, platelet-rich fibrin (PRF), and even stem cells is a great milestone in the field of regenerative medicine. Modern techniques such as electrospinning, sol-gel processing, and 3D bioprinting are used to fabricate bioactive dressings. Electrospinning involves the use of high voltage to draw polymer solutions into fine, fibrous mats that have a high surface area, while sol-gel methods form porous, bioactive coatings. On the other hand, 3D bioprinting enables the construction of precise, customizable, and patient-specific dressings through layer-by-layer deposition [60].

ADVANCED MATERIALS: HYDROGELS, NANOFIBERS, AND BIODEGRADABLE POLYMERS

As new technologies have emerged, promising new materials have started to present intriguing opportunities for enhancing wound care. One such area of interest is multifunctional hydrogels that are emerging as versatile dressings for wounds. Such materials provide excellent biocompatibility, permeability, and other beneficial characteristics, making them suitable for active wounds [61]. In addition, hydrogels form soft and transparent films over wounds, which maintain moisture over the wound site, ensuring rapid tissue regeneration and healing. Their antioxidant properties can also decrease oxidative stress in and around the wound area, which will allow for better recovery. Furthermore, hydrogels can help control bleeding by sealing the wound rapidly, which reduces blood loss. They can be adapted to the wound condition, allowing the treatment to be more effective as the wound changes. Nanocomposite hydrogels take it a step further by allowing the dynamic real-time control of the environment around the wound. They can monitor and control the pH, temperature, amount of drained fluid, and even the position of the wound, adjusting the wound environment dynamically to improve healing [62].

Another promising material is electrospun nanofibers that are used in wound care. They have a range of diameters starting from the nanoscale to the microscale, while simultaneously providing a high surface-to-volume ratio along with pores at the microscale. Electrospun nanofibers are used in scaffolds, drug delivery, supporting tissue engineering, and wound healing. These fibers replicate the structure of an ECM, which gives support to growing tissues. Their combination of strength from synthetic polymers and biocompatibility from natural polymers allows for the controlled release of active ingredients, enhancing their effectiveness. In addition, these nanofibers are biodegradable, so they are designed to be compatible and support the body's healing processes without any further interventions. Whether natural or synthetic, biodegradable polymers are essential in contemporary wound management [63]. Natural polymers such as hyaluronic acid, collagen, and chitosan, along with synthetic alternatives like polylactic acid and polyglycolic acid, have shown tremendous potential in promoting wound healing. They can be used to deliver therapeutic agents such as drugs, bioactive substances, and even metallic elements while modulating their release to enhance the healing process. In addition, new materials are being employed such as nanoparticles-loaded hydrogels, nanofibrous scaffolds, and nanocomposites to improve healing. These materials accelerate tissue regeneration, stimulate the formation of blood vessels, and enhance cell growth [64].

EXAMPLES OF ADVANCED WOUND DRESSINGS

New wound care advancements have led to the development of novel dressings that aim to enhance the treatment process. These dressings not only speed up the healing process but also reduce the chances of infections and help in tissue regeneration. They possess advanced elements and medical technologies that allow the dressings to be more effective at treating wounds than traditional approaches.

UrgoStart Contact

The Urgo medical laboratories have created a special contact dressing known as UrgoStart contact that is specifically designed for the treatment of diabetic wounds. This contact dressing was infused with a colloid matrix, which consists of a sucrose octasulfate potassium salt to make the dressing soft and non-adhering. The effectiveness of UrgoStart contact dressing was evaluated in a comparative study against standard dressing on 240 patients suffering from diabetic foot ulcers in 43 hospitals throughout Europe. The results showed that the developed dressing significantly improved wound healing, with 48% of patients in the sucrose octasulfate group experiencing wound closure, compared to only 30% in the control group using the standard dressing [65].

Soy Protein-Based Nanofiber Wound Dressing

A wound dressing using soy-based nanofibers was developed, enriched with estrogen-like molecules. Estrogen is known to aid in wound healing, particularly in pregnant women. In vitro, the dressing stimulated the growth and movement of fibroblasts, which are essential for wound healing. In vivo, the dressing accelerated the process of skin regeneration and minimized scarring [66].

Eggshell Membrane Dressing

The company Biovotec developed a unique wound dressing made from eggshell membranes, which are believed to have healing properties similar to the human placenta. The key advantage of this approach is that it utilizes a high volume of discarded eggshells, making it a sustainable and cost-effective solution. In trials with rats, this dressing led to 21% faster healing in the early stages of wound recovery compared to the control group. However, the difference became less pronounced after five days [67].

MicroMend™

MicroMend™ is an innovative wound closure bandage that replaces the need for traditional stitches or staples. It is easy to apply, less painful, and provides a more efficient way to close wounds. Clinical studies show that both patients and surgeons preferred MicroMend™ because it is quicker and more convenient than suturing, with less risk of infection and better wound closure results [68].

XSTAT®

XSTAT® is an FDA-approved life-saving hemostatic device used primarily in military settings to control severe bleeding in traumatic injuries. The device consists of a syringe containing absorbent cellulose sponges. When injected into a wound, the sponges expand and create a temporary seal, which helps to stop bleeding for up to four hours. This gives injured individuals valuable time to reach medical care in trauma situations [69].

Wound Dressings to Manage Exudate

Exudate, or excessive fluid, is a common issue for chronic wounds that pose added difficulty to proper healing. Effective management of this exudate is vital to avoid skin maceration and bacterial infection while promoting adequate wound healing. Traditional dressings like medical gauze absorb the exudate, but they also get stuck to the wound and dry out the healing tissue which is not ideal. Novel dressings are being developed to absorb excess fluid and create a moist environment that promotes better healing so that these issues can be mitigated [70].

AQUACEL Ag Extra™

AQUACEL is an innovative type of wound dressing made of hydrofiber and foam that are combined to form a three-layered dressing. The outer layer is waterproof, which prevents external bacteria from entering the wound site as well as stopping exudate from leaking out. The innermost layer is sodium carboxymethylcellulose (NaCMC) fiber, which creates a gel upon contact with exudate, keeping the wound site moist. It also contains silver ions, enabling it with potent antimicrobial properties. Studies have shown that this dressing helps to manage wound exudate effectively while reducing the chances of infection, thus accelerating the healing process [71].

Vliwasorb® Pro

Vliwasorb® is a specifically designed non-adherent dressing that absorbs wound exudate at a controlled rate. It contains sodium polyacrylate, a material known for absorbing liquids in huge quantities without leaking. It possesses good tolerance, in terms of human skin, to absorb exudate while causing no irritation or discomfort during the painful dressing change processes. Furthermore, the superabsorbent dressing minimizes complications caused by excessive exudate, increases the healing rate of the tissue, and decreases the cost of wound care by providing effective treatment [72].

Konjac Glucomannan/Silver Nanoparticle Composite Sponge

Chen et al. developed a wound dressing with a naturally occurring plant-derived material called konjac and silver nanoparticles that provided healing properties and bacterial protection. In vivo, this dressing was found to enhance healing and protect against bacterial infection. Its absorbent sponge-like structure also draws away excess fluid from the wound, ensuring the optimal environment for healing. Moreover, this dressing can promote neovascularization and fibroblast proliferation, which is important for repairing tissue. All these factors make this dressing ideal for wound care, especially for wounds with infections and excessive exudate [73].

Dressings to Control Wound Infection

Modern wound dressings have been developed to control infections and promote healing at the same time. These advanced dressings incorporate antibacterial agents, biofilm-disrupting technologies, or controlled drug-release systems to control the sterile wound environment and promote healing.

Bamboo Leaf-Based Cellulose Crystal Dressing

Singla et al. fabricated an advanced form of wound dressings by using cellulose nanocrystals (NC) sourced from bamboo leaves and infused with silver nanoparticles. This new material can be used to create strong antibacterial dressings. In vivo showed that this dressing greatly reduced inflammation, enhanced angiogenesis, increased fibroblast activity, and new skin cell formation, thereby enabling faster skin regeneration. It also enhanced tissue regeneration and kept the environment moist around the wound, both of which are essential for healing. In diabetic wound studies, complete healing occurred within 18 days, aided by the regulation of growth factors and inflammation-related markers. These results suggest that this dressing is an excellent option for promoting quick and effective wound healing, especially in diabetic patients [74].

Procellera®

Bark et al. developed a cutting-edge wound dressing called Procellera®, which uses weak electric fields to prevent bacterial infections and accelerate healing. This dressing is made with silver and zinc, which becomes active when it gets wet, producing an electric field that disrupts bacterial biofilms. It interferes with bacterial communication systems (quorum sensing) and helps to restore proteins like E-cadherin, which bacterial biofilms may damage. In vivo has been shown to improve faster wound closure and effectively fight antibiotic-resistant bacteria. This makes it a unique and innovative approach to preventing infections and supporting the healing process [75].

Silverlon®

The Silverlon is a unique antimicrobial dressing, formulated to prevent surgical site infections (SSIs) from occurring. Clinical studies demonstrate that the use of Silverlon dressing reduces the chances of infection following surgical operations like joint and colorectal surgeries. It prevents both surface and internal infections, which eventually minimizes complications and the overall cost of treatment. Extensive researches intend to reaffirm the importance of this dressing, enabling it to be utilized in a broader spectrum of surgical procedures [76].

Multidrug Releasing Self-Assembled Film

A team from MIT's Hammond Lab has created an advanced bandage to deal with two major challenges of wound care: bleeding and infection. This innovation is composed of two layers of dressings that serve different purposes. First, the dressing releases thrombin, a compound that helps to stop blood flow. Second, the antibiotic vancomycin is released slowly over the next 24 hours. This innovative bandage improves the quality of treatment by addressing both severe bleeding and bacterial contamination during and after surgery [77].

Smart Dressings and Sensors

Significant advancements have been achieved in the design of smart dressings over time. The most recent version of these dressings employs multiplexed sensing technology, which can monitor several biomarkers in the wound area, putting these dressings a step closer to practical use. These smart dressings not only monitor the conditions but can also provide therapeutic treatment of the wound, thus having a combined diagnostic and treatment function [78]. Certain smart materials that respond to changes in temperature, pH, and enzymatic activity have also entered the field of wound care. These responsive materials allow the wound dressings to adjust to the changing environment of the wound. Different kinds of these materials have been developed and tested, such as those that are activated by ROS, temperature, pH levels, and enzymes that interact with fluctuating conditions during healing. Different ROS such as hydrogen peroxide, superoxide, and peroxynitrite are very important in several biological processes including healing wounds. Another advancement in smart wound care is the invention of shape memory polymers (SMPs). These materials have a temporary shape at room temperature, but when exposed to a particular external stimulus like heat, light, pH, or moisture, they return to their original form. This technology has also been employed to make dressings that can control drug release or monitor wound conditions over time. The smart microsensors incorporated within smart bandages can identify and measure wound exudate to assess the healing stage. These sensors focus on specific markers residing in the wound's environment, providing helpful information regarding the wound and its healing process [18].

Multi-Parameter Sensing Dressing

Jankowska et al. developed a novel wound dressing based on fluorescent sensors for monitoring pH and glucose concentrations within wounds during the healing process. Monitoring these biomarkers is essential because raised glucose levels in wounds are often associated with poor healing. This novel wound dressing has a pH-sensitive dye called carboxynaphthofluorescein, which works between pH 6 and 8, and a metabolite-sensing enzymatic system for glucose detection. The enzymatic system is based on the sequential reaction of glucose oxidase and horseradish peroxidase where the changes in fluorescent signals are proportional to the glucose concentration. Furthermore, this technology could be expanded toward the detection of other metabolites, such as lactate and uric acid, presenting a multifaceted approach to assess the wound healing process [79].

Stretchable Hydrogel Dressing

Lin et al. made an innovative development in the form of an adaptable hydrogel bandage, which includes components such as temperature sensors, LED lights, conductive wires, semiconductor chips, and drug-delivery systems. This electronic hydrogel bandage can respond to temperature changes in the wound and releasing drugs when they are required. Furthermore, it activates the LEDs when the drug supply is too low to signal a need for a resupply. These electrical elements maintain the flexibility of the bandage so that they can work during body movements. Subsequently, this technology can be modified for internal usage, such as monitoring glucose levels or even as neural probes [80].

Color-Changing Microbe-Sensitive Dressing

Thet et al. introduced a novel wound dressing that changes color in response to bacterial infection, facilitating early detection and treatment. The dressing is made from agarose film, embedded with a fluorescent dye that is released from nanocapsules when exposed to bacterial toxins. This release causes a color change in the dressing, which occurs within 4 hours, and varies depending on the type of bacteria present [81].

EMERGING THERAPIES AND INNOVATIONS

Wound regeneration and dressing technologies have seen considerable advancements with new therapeutic approaches providing creative solutions to promote healing and enhance patient outcomes [82]. Skin wound treatments are typically divided into two categories: conventional and regenerative. In traditional wound care, cotton wool or dry gauze were frequently used to make wound dressings because they are sticky and enable the absorption of wound exudates. Therefore, these dressings needed frequent changes due to their ability to absorb significant amounts of fluid. Moreover, as the gauze dressings get wet from absorption, they tend to stick to the wound, causing wound damage and pain to the patient when the dressing is frequently changed [83]. In the conventional method, split-thickness autographs are one of the standard treatment options for large or full-thickness skin defects. Despite their critical role in patient survival, these procedures are associated with numerous limitations, including the need for multiple surgical interventions, limited availability of donor sites, hypertrophic scarring, and the risk of functional impairments. Consequently, none of these treatment strategies is adequate for full wound healing as different types of wounds have varied molecular and cellular mechanisms [84].

Recent advances in wound healing research have substantially broadened the understanding of therapeutic interventions. The shift from traditional dry dressings to advanced moist wound dressings, stimuli-responsive materials, tissue-engineered skin constructs, and bioengineered substitutes has revolutionized the field. Additionally, therapies with growth factors, gene editing, nanotechnology, or stem cells have opened new avenues of treatment. Newer technologies like three-dimensional bioprinting along with PRP therapy strongly advocate the promise of customizable and multifunctional options for wound care. These developments highlight a new era in wound management that combines biological insights with the latest technological inventions to tackle different aspects of the wound healing process [85] (Figure 12.2).

STEM CELL THERAPY

Stem cell therapy has emerged as a viable treatment option for previously untreatable conditions. Focusing on the potential of stem cells, regenerative medicine has evolved as a completely new discipline that offers different therapeutic solutions for enhancing wound healing and restoring the skin structure. Stem cells have tissue self-renewal abilities, which allow for their expanded use in multiple areas of

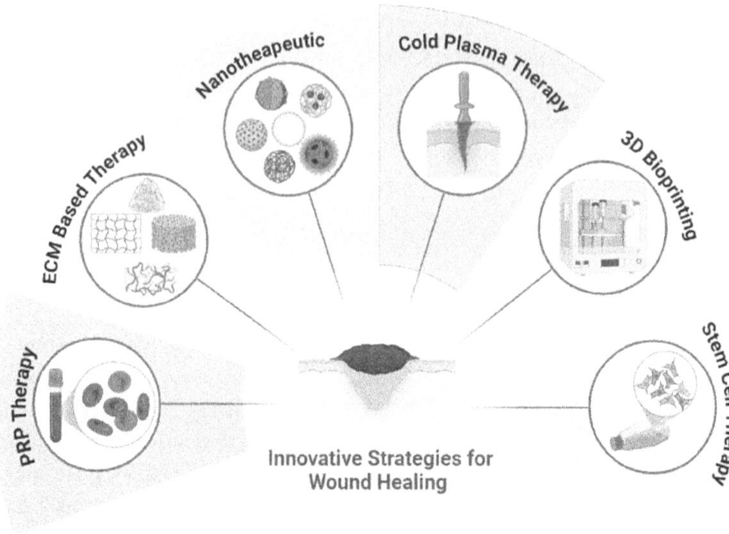

FIGURE 12.2 Emerging therapies, innovations, and strategies to promote wound regeneration process.

medicine including oncology, immunology, and wound treatment [86]. The increased focus and attention toward stem cell-based therapies for skin regeneration and wound healing is mainly due to the unique properties of stem cells such as their ability for continuous self-renewal and to differentiate into diverse cell types. Also, this therapy has been reported to be effective in patients with chronic wounds that do not heal with traditional approaches [87]. In the management of chronic wounds, the stem cell therapies approach combines the use of different growth factors with the regulation of inflammation, immune response, and tissue vascularization. Furthermore, its capacity to release growth factors and cytokines enables skin regeneration that promotes wound healing [88]. Autologous stem cells are advantageous because of their high differentiation capacity and ability to promote new blood vessel formation while having minimal adverse effects. These properties make stem cells a viable candidate for promoting cell proliferation and accelerating the recovery process [89].

Stem cells are thought to have a positive effect on wound healing due to their capacity to activate resident skin cells, secrete bioactive molecules, control inflammation, and remodel the ECM specific to the injury site. These properties enhance the quality of the wound healing process, restrict tissue damage while creating a scar, and encourage the growth of new tissue. By far, the most common stem cells used for skin healing and regeneration are adult mesenchymal stem cells (MSCs), embryonic stem cells (ESCs), and induced pluripotent stem cells (iPSCs) [90]. ESCs have large potential but are not frequently used because of ethical constraints. On the other hand, MSCs are more accepted because they can participate in all stages of wound healing, including inflammation control, blood vessel formation, and fibroblast activation [91]. MSCs can be derived from blood, bone marrow, adipose tissue, umbilical cord, and amniotic fluid. Clinical studies have reported successful outcomes with MSC treatment for chronic, non-healing wounds, and burns with significant improvements in angiogenesis and reduced scar formation [92].

Recent advances in regenerative medicine include scaffold-based treatments, which have been demonstrated to improve the lifespan and functioning of transplanted stem cells. These scaffold systems provide an optimal microenvironment for stem cells at the wound site, increasing cell viability and speeding up the healing process. In addition to MSCs, there has been growing interest in the therapeutic application of MSC-derived exosomes. These small extracellular vesicles are enriched with growth factors that may help in tissue repair and regeneration. Out of all the types of MSCs, adipose-derived MSCs have attracted greater attention as they are readily available, do not pose ethical challenges, and have great potential to improve chronic wound healing. Furthermore, iPSCs can be raised ethically, and recent advancements have shown their stem cell-like properties that provide the closest alternative to ESCs. Additionally, iPSCs have opened new avenues in the formation of skin substitutes. Alongside, they may aid in novel methods of accelerated wound healing [85]. Stem cell therapies have made remarkable advances, yet they have numerous obstacles to overcome. One of the main issues is the lack of comprehensive clinical trials to assess the effectiveness, practicality, and optimal delivery methods for these therapies over extended periods. Further research and observation at all levels must be maintained so that stem cell therapy is integrated into medical practice in the right way. If these problems are solved, stem cells can offer a revolution in therapeutic possibilities and, to a great extent, enhance the well-being of people suffering from various diseases [93].

GENE THERAPY

Gene therapy is one of the latest technologies in biomedical science, as it can improve the overall wound healing and skin regeneration. It involves the process of adding particular genes to the target cell making it perform desired biological functions. Initially, this therapy was aimed at treating inherited metabolic disorders along with certain types of cancers. However, recent studies have shown that it can also be used to facilitate the natural processes of wound repair. Gene therapy helps in repairing tissue damage and speeding up the healing process by altering the biological functions of specific cells, even if only for a short period. The incorporation of various cellular components and growth factors has enabled researchers to use gene therapy as a more efficient and accurate method to target and correct disruptions in the healing process, providing a more efficient and precise approach to tissue regeneration [94].

The current research evaluates the efficiency of viral and non-viral vectors for gene transfer using in vivo and ex vivo methods. In vivo refers to the technique in which genetic material is delivered directly into the target tissue of a living organism. In contrast, ex vivo involves removing relevant cells from the host, growing and modifying them in the lab, and then reintroducing them into the host. In both approaches, its progress relies heavily on the selection of a suitable vector to ensure proper and exact gene alteration [95].

Viral Vectors, Their Types, and Applications

In gene therapy, viral vectors play an important role because they use the virus's inherent capability to deliver genetic material to the host cells. To assure safety and efficacy, the viral genes responsible for replication and assembly are removed and replaced with therapeutic genes. This is done with the help of packaging cells that permit the creation of the recombinant viruses needed for gene delivery. Various viruses are employed as vectors, each one having distinct features that make it appropriate for a specific therapeutic application [96].

Retroviruses and Lentiviruses

Retroviruses and lentiviruses are classified as non-lytic since they can replicate without harming a host cell. Retroviruses are effective for lytic infecting cells that divide. Retroviruses are exceptionally advantageous when the intention is to target proliferating cells, commonly involved in wound healing, as many cells in this process are actively dividing. Major drawbacks that retroviruses possess are their high instability and low gene transfer efficiency [95]. Some of the disadvantages of these viruses can be overcome by using lentiviruses, a subtype of retroviruses because they can transduce non-dividing cells, thus making them more versatile. Studies have indicated that some genes (including PDGF and IGF-I) have been incorporated into keratinocytes via retroviral vectors, which aid in tissue growth and effective wound healing. In addition, the combination of lentiviral and retroviral vectors is being investigated for greater efficiency in targeting non-dividing cells [96,97].

Adenoviruses

Adenoviruses, known for their double-stranded DNA composition, are commonly utilized in gene therapy due to their easy availability, safety, and high transfection efficiency, which can reach up to 95% in skin cells. Unlike retroviruses, they are incapable of integrating their genetic material into the host's genome. As a result, the gene expression exhibited by adenoviruses is only temporary [98]. For example, the recombination of the adenovirus with the PDGF-B gene accelerated wound healing in an ischemic rabbit ear. However, the approach gave rise to acute inflammation, which is attributed to the viral capsid protein. This indicates both the pros and cons associated with the use of adenoviruses in medical treatments [99].

Adeno-Associated Viruses (AAVs)

Adeno-associated viruses (AAVs) are safe and non-pathogenic single-stranded DNA viruses that have been used for gene therapies. AAVs have been aimed at healing surgical and burn wounds by delivering vascular endothelial growth factor-A (VEGF-A). This greatly enhanced the healing, blood vessel formation, and epithelial tissue regeneration. Advanced research is currently being conducted on utilizing different AAV serotypes to improve gene delivery efficiency as well as targeting the genes more efficiently in wound healing treatments [100].

Herpes Simplex Viruses (HSVs)

HSVs function as lytic vectors, generating new viral particles through the destruction of the host cell. Although these vectors are not frequently mentioned in wound healing, they stand out for their high transfection rates and significant capacity for genetic payload [101].

NON-VIRAL VECTORS

Non-viral gene delivery methods have gained more attention since they are safer and carry a lower risk of infection and inflammation than viral vectors. Additionally, these methods are cost-effective and easier to implement. They provide transient gene expression, which makes them appropriate in wound healing applications. Nevertheless, non-viral approaches frequently demonstrate a lack of cell selectivity and variability in gene expression levels. These methods are mainly divided into two categories: naked DNA transfection and liposomal transfection [102].

Naked DNA Transfection

Several methods are used to introduce naked DNA into the skin, including direct injection, topical application, gene gun technology, microseeding, and electroporation.

Direct injection and microseeding: The direct injection technique, first introduced in 1995, entails the direct injection of DNA into the skin. Although it demonstrated certain efficacy, such as the recruitment of dermal neutrophils, it is considered ineffective due to the inherent fragility, size, and rapid degradation of DNA in the extracellular environment, which restricts its capacity to effectively penetrate cellular membranes [103]. To address this, Eriksson et al. developed "microseeding," which involves injecting DNA directly into cells using solid microneedles in a modified tattooing machine. This method facilitates transient gene expression in the upper layers of the skin while causing minimal damage to the surrounding tissue [104].

Topical application: Applying naked DNA topically has shown that it can permeate the layers of the skin, resulting in gene expression in the dermis, epidermis, and follicular keratinocytes. Nonetheless, the hydrophobic nature of the stratum corneum is a considerable barrier, and further research into its effectiveness remains limited [96].

Gene gun technology: Gene gun technology uses physical force to introduce DNA-coated particles, such as tungsten or gold, into skin cells. This approach facilitates transient gene expression, with optimal activity observed within 1–3 days. It has demonstrated efficacy in enhancing wound healing, promoting re-epithelialization, and increasing tensile strength in wounds treated with PDGF and EGF. However, this technique primarily affects the epidermis, exhibiting limited penetration into deeper tissue layers and achieving a transfection rate of around 10%. Recent advancements in gene gun technology have improved gene expression in both the epidermis and dermis while reducing tissue damage, thereby expanding its potential applications in wound healing [105].

Electroporation: Electroporation is a technique that uses electric fields to enhance gene transfer into cells. When combined with growth factor genes like transforming growth factor-beta 1 (TGF-β1) or KGF, this technique enhances wound healing by stimulating angiogenesis, collagen production, and re-epithelialization. This method has proven to be successful in promoting the closure of diabetic and chronic wounds [106].

Liposomal Gene Therapy

Cationic liposomes are synthetic vesicles that carry a positive charge that forms complexes with DNA, shielding it from degradation and facilitating its uptake into cells through endocytosis. These liposomal formulations can be administered both topically and via direct injections. The latter is more effective as it allows for deeper penetration into the skin [107]. Studies have shown that using cationic liposomes, which contain gene delivery factors such as insulin-like growth factor I (IGF-I) and acidic fibroblast growth factor (aFGF) can enhance healing of diabetic and chronic burn wounds. This method improves collagenous synthesis, promotes cell proliferation, and also inhibits inflammation [108,109]. The liposomal delivery of IGF-I resulted in high transfection efficiency of 70%–90% in dermal cells, which subsequently accelerated re-epithelialization and improved skin cell survival when compared to other treatments. Furthermore, combining multiple growth factors such as KGF and IGF-I yielded better results such as improved skin regeneration, increased skin cell proliferation, and decreased apoptosis, which truly underlines the capabilities of liposomal gene therapy in revolutionizing healing through advanced wound care technologies [95].

NANOTHERAPEUTICS

The treatment of chronic wounds poses multifarious challenges when compared to the treatment of acute ones. This is due to the vast complexities and the many complications that arise during the healing process. Traditional treatment methods such as systemic antibiotics and topical medications are not very effective. The lack of satisfactory results from those methods can be linked to poor drug penetration into the deeper tissues and the constantly growing problem of bacterial resistance [110]. As a result, there has been a change in focus toward new therapeutic approaches. Treatments based on nanotechnology have shown a lot of promise when it comes to wound care. Such treatments, also called nanotherapeutics, use materials at a nanoscale including nanoparticles, nanofibers, nanogels, and nanoemulsions. These materials are used to deliver therapeutic agents such as antimicrobial compounds, growth factors, and peptides directly to the wound. This specific approach tackles slow healing, inadequate drug absorption, as well as persistent bacterial infections. Nanotherapeutics strengthen the stability of treatments and enhance the drug's availability at the wound site [111]. Furthermore, these therapies aid in maintaining a moist wound environment, which is essential for faster healing. Another key advantage of nanotechnology is its ability to penetrate bacterial biofilms and tissue barriers, enabling treatments to target the underlying infection more effectively [112]. Nanomaterials used in wound care are generally categorized into two types:

Organic Nanomaterials

This category includes polymer-derived materials such as nanogels, nanofibers, micelles, liposomes, and solid lipid nanoparticles. Biodegradable materials such as chitosan and polysaccharides are often used because of their natural biocompatibility with biological systems [113].

Inorganic Nanomaterials

This category includes metal-based nanoparticles that contain silver, gold, zinc, and titanium dioxide. These materials are capable of combating bacteria by producing ROS, which can target bacterial DNA and break down their biofilms. Concerns about toxicity do exist, but these risks can be mitigated by carefully managing the size and properties of the nanoparticles [114]. In addition to infection control, nanotherapeutics can improve cellular regeneration, inflammation control, and precise delivery of therapeutic compounds. In particular, polymeric nanoparticles can incorporate antibiotics and growth factors, which enhance healing. Despite their advantages, certain challenges still need to be addressed such as the toxicity of metal-based nanoparticles and regulating the inflammatory phase during wound healing [115]. Due to these factors, there is a need to develop nanomaterials with improved anti-inflammatory effects to improve the immune response and overall healing process [116].

Platelet-Rich Plasma (PRP)

PRP is being incorporated into practice, with a lot of focus on its application in wound healing. PRP is derived from a patient's blood and processed through centrifugation to enhance the maximum level of platelets beyond the ordinary range. These platelets contain numerous growth factors, including PDGF, EGF, FGF, VEGF, and TGF-β1, which are useful in a variety of biological functions such as the migration, proliferation of cells, remodeling, and angiogenesis, which are essential in the wound healing process [117]. One of the primary benefits of PRP is the patient's own blood is used, which decreases allergic or infection risk. It is also less expensive and easier to prepare. The activation and centrifugation techniques allow the alteration of PRP growth factors to personal preference, making it exceptionally useful for chronic wounds like diabetic foot ulcers. Furthermore, its application may lower the expense put toward wound healing as PRP has shown antibacterial properties that help the wound heal faster [118]. Many clinical trials have confirmed PRP's efficacy in the treatment of various wounds such as chronic ulcers, burns, acute injuries, or wounds, followed by cosmetic or plastic surgeries. PRP speeds the healing process, enhances tissue regeneration, and alleviates pain and inflammation while having almost no negative side effects. Furthermore, PRP is exceptional in promoting new blood vessel formation, stimulating fibroblast activity, and supporting mesenchymal stem cell migration, all of which increase the wound healing process [119].

Cold Atmospheric Plasma (CAP) Therapy

Cold atmospheric plasma (CAP) therapy has developed into a viable treatment strategy over the last twenty years, particularly for healing wounds and treating cancer. Plasma, which is often referred to as the fourth state of matter, can be divided into two primary types: cold and thermal. The latter requires very high temperatures to function, while cold plasma, which is also known as non-thermal plasma, operates at temperatures lower than 40°C, making it suitable for medical applications. CAP can be described as an ionized gas, consisting of a complex mixture of reactively charged particles such as electrons, reactive oxygen and nitrogen species, neutral atoms, molecules, UV radiation, and electric fields. This type of plasma is produced when gaseous atoms and molecules are exposed to high-energy electrons and photons [120]. There are two common sources of CAP:

i. Dielectric Barrier Discharge (DBD)
ii. Atmospheric Pressure Plasma Jet (APPJ)

Additional devices have been developed to deliver CAP, particularly in wound management. One such device is the kINPen® MED, a small pen-like instrument that was initially designed for laboratory use but later adapted for clinical applications. This device is widely used for the management of acute and chronic wounds such as diabetic foot ulcers [121]. Other machines such as PlasmaDerm® VU-2010 and SteriPlas are used for wound care with underlying conditions as the design of these units is such that they minimize bacterial contamination while facilitating the healing process. These devices are approved and certified for their therapeutic benefits [122].

CAP has been demonstrated to reduce the bacterial load in the wound, increase wound closure, and promote early-phase cell migration, all of which are needed for optimal wound healing. The primary action of CAP lies in its capability to form reactive species, such as ROS and reactive nitrogen species (RNS), which activate tissue regeneration. Both preclinical and clinical trials have reported that CAP therapy can safely treat chronic wounds without causing damage to healthy tissues [85]. One study indicated that the CAP treatment assists in inducing cell proliferation, neovascularization, and skin regeneration by controlling inflammation and promoting the secretion of growth factors, particularly TGF-β1. There is enormous potential in CAP therapy for the treatment of both acute and chronic wounds considering its abilities to improve healing processes, reduce the risk of infections, and offer improved treatment options for future clinical applications [123].

THREE-DIMENSIONAL (3D) BIOPRINTING

Several conventional procedures are performed to treat acute or chronic wounds via manual interventions, which are often inefficient and very lengthy while at the same time, unable to treat large or complicated wounds such as burns. To facilitate these procedures, 3D bioprinting has surfaced as an improved automated technique that has potential in regenerative medicine, particularly in wound healing. It is a

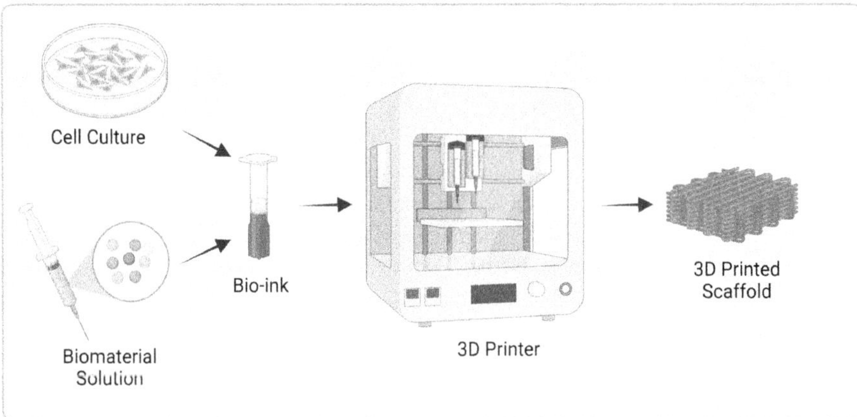

FIGURE 12.3 3D bioprinting process to construct a 3D scaffold by using cells and biomaterials.

process within additive manufacturing that layers cells, biomaterials, growth factors, and other biomolecules to form a skin substitute that is suitable for the human body (Figure 12.3). This approach has many advantages over traditional methods because it utilizes computer-aided design (CAD) technology to efficiently construct intricate, 3D tissue-like structures in a single step, thus overcoming many pre-existing challenges [124].

The first step of 3D bioprinting involves extracting cells from the patient, growing them, and then combining them with other materials to form a substance, referred to as bioink. Bioink has to satisfy certain conditions such as being compatible with the human body, biodegradable, and structurally stable to maintain its shape after printing. One of the most important considerations when working with living cells in bioinks is the possibility of an immunological response after implantation. Therefore, the selection of cells to be used is of absolute importance. In addition to stem cells, 3D bioprinting for skin also involves primary cultured skin cells such as fibroblasts, melanocytes, or keratinocytes. The physical properties of bioinks, particularly their elasticity and viscosity, play an important role in cell migration, expansion, and ECM remodeling. Bioprinting can achieve personalized custom structures through medical imaging data like MRI or CT scans [125]. A novel approach in 3D bioprinting is the drop-on-demand technique. This gives bioink the ability to be deposited precisely where it is required with the flexibility to change the cell density and design. Solid freeform fabrication is another important feature of bioprinting that makes it possible to create structures with no restrictions on consistency or shape. This technology can create intricate 3D structures that closely mimic the microscopic and macroscopic characteristics of natural tissues owing to the integration of CAD and computer-aided manufacturing technologies [126,127]. There are many advantages of using 3D bioprinting technology in the wound healing process. It not only offers rapid and cost-effective manufacturing but also enables the incorporation of various cell types and biomolecules to promote tissue regeneration and enhance features like vascularization, pigmentation, and innervation. Moreover, bioprinted large-scale skin substitutes are extremely pliable and stretchable, which makes them suitable for diverse clinical applications [128].

To treat a wound adequately, bioprinted skin must have some functional properties, such as the capability to transfer nutrients as well as wound exudate, deposit various skin cell types in a specific order, and have a porosity, degradation rate, and mechanical strength that are similar to natural skin. The constructs must also be strong, biocompatible, biodegradable, and non-soluble at the external pressures in the body. In recent advancements, 3D bioprinting has also led to the development of in vitro 3D disease models and high-throughput screening systems for testing medical treatments. To create personalized therapies for various wound types, it is essential to take a comprehensive approach that combines autologous cells with bioprinting techniques tailored to each patient's unique needs [129].

Various bioprinting techniques are currently used for skin tissue regeneration, including extrusion, inkjet, laser, and stereolithography methods. Among these, extrusion-based bioprinting is the most often utilized method due to its rapid printing capabilities, low cost, and ability to mimic complex tissue structures. However, this technique has limitations including nozzle blockage, necessitating advancements in both device design and methodology [130]. So, other alternative innovative strategies, including continuous liquid interface production (CLIP), multi-material multi-nozzle 3D printing (MM3D), and computed axial lithography (CAL), present promising solutions. For instance, CLIP facilitates considerably faster printing rates and supports the large-scale production of multilayered skin constructs [131]. Meanwhile, MM3D printing improves rigidity and material diversity within layers, and CAL offers versatility by employing visible light for volumetric construction [132,133]. Skin bioprinting can be performed by ex vivo or in situ methods. The ex vivo technique involves maturing bioprinted constructs in vitro before grafting them onto the patient, while in situ bioprinting entails the direct application of bioinks into the wound site using handheld extrusion bioprinters [134]. Considerable advancements in this domain have resulted in the creation of several bioprinting techniques and bioink compositions. Initial strategies including the bioprinting of skin constructs from collagen hydrogel and fiber-based bioinks opened the way for more sophisticated technologies that now enable the production of full-thickness human skin equivalents. These constructs possess organized structure and mechanical properties resembling the native skin and have been used in the treatment of chronic ulcers, burns, and other injuries. 3D bioprinting is developing due to ongoing developments in cell biology, bioink formulations, and bioprinter designs, presenting potential options for skin regeneration and wound healing [135,125]. One recent development is the integration of angiogenic peptides into bioinks to improve vascularization and promote wound healing. Researchers have successfully created vascularized human skin grafts by combining bioinks loaded with keratinocytes, endothelial cells, and dermal fibroblasts to form dermis and epidermis layers [136]. In another study, decellularized ECM derived from pig dermis combined with human dermal fibroblasts was used to formulate a bioink, creating a natural environment for cell survival and proliferation [137].

IN SITU FORMING INJECTABLE HYDROGELS AND BIOADHESIVES

There has been growing interest in in situ forming hydrogels and injectable systems for wound repair and regeneration. These systems include thermosensitive and pH-responsive gels, which remain in liquid form at room temperature but transition into hydrogels when exposed to body temperature (37°C) and specific pH levels. This property enables these gels to conform to the wound's outline easily without requiring sutures or extra adhesives. They also promote crosslinking with the native tissue at the wound site, thus forming a healing environment. Another significant advantage of injectable hydrogels is their ability to incorporate autologous stem cells or other tissue-specific cells at the wound site, forming a cellular matrix that hastens the healing process. Such systems have been used successfully in the management of severe wounds like third-degree burns and chronic diabetic ulcers [138].

In a study, a crosslinker-free method was used to develop an injectable silk fibroin (SF) hydrogel. This hydrogel was able to self-assemble within 10 minutes when placed on rat burn wounds, promoting wound hydration and skin regeneration [139]. In another study, pH and glucose-responsive hydrogels were developed for the treatment of diabetic wounds. These hydrogels were synthesized by using chemical crosslinking methods and included more regulated and efficient healing outcomes using polyvinyl alcohol (PVA) and modified chitosan [140]. The adhesive properties of these injectable systems are also under investigation. Inspired by the natural adhesive properties of plant tannins, researchers have developed cost-effective bioadhesives made from gelatin, which are crosslinked with silver nitrate to improve their performance. These adhesives, irrespective of the gelatin source, have demonstrated potential as tissue sealants, hemostats, or drug or cell delivery systems [141]. Another new development is light-responsive, mussel protein-derived bioadhesives, which replicate the adhesive and crosslinking processes seen in mussels. These hydrogels, activated by blue light, have shown remarkable hemostatic properties and can serve as water-resistant sealants for critical injuries [142]. Additionally, nanocomposite hydrogels have been developed to promote enhanced wound healing. For example, the natural polysaccharide kappa-carrageenan has been modified with nanosilicates, leading to the development of injectable hydrogels that enhance cell adhesion, facilitate platelet binding, and decrease blood clotting time, making them effective hemostatic agents [143]. Furthermore, microfluidic technology has provided advanced ways for creating injectable microspheres. In a study, microgel building blocks made of annealed hydrogels were used to create an injectable scaffold, facilitating tissue regrowth and regeneration [144]. Another strategy was used for the synthesis of hollow bacterial cellulose microspheres using the microfluidic technique. These microspheres have alginate cores and agarose shells, which offer an optimal environment for the secretion of bacterial cellulose. After assembly, they resulted in injectable scaffolds that effectively supported cell proliferation, tissue ingrowth, and enhanced healing [145].

CONCLUSION AND OUTLOOK

Wound dressings have come a long way from simple coverings to highly advanced tools that actively aid the body in healing. This chapter has outlined the critical challenges faced in wound care, such as chronic wounds, infections, and scarring, while also highlighting the strides made in addressing these issues through innovation. Modern dressings and therapies now offer more targeted, effective, and sustainable solutions, significantly improving patient care. The emerging therapies discussed, such as stem cell applications and tissue engineering, hold the potential to redefine wound treatment entirely. Additionally, the focus on sustainability and the integration of artificial intelligence (AI) into personalized wound care represents the future direction of this field.

The future of wound dressing development is likely to see a significant shift toward sustainability using natural materials. Substances such as EGCG, curcumin, cellulose, aloe vera, ascorbic acid, quercetin, and tannic acid have been used as main active agents or supporting elements in wound dressings, offering an environmentally friendly alternative to synthetic options. Since these natural substances are readily available, biodegradable, and can be regenerated within a human lifetime, they provide an easily accessible and sustainable solution. Incorporating these natural agents into wound dressings not only benefits the environment but also supports the well-being of both consumers and manufacturers by reducing reliance on harmful chemicals and improving the ecological footprint of the product. The incorporation of renewable materials such as corn protein (zein), shellac, and keratin in novel wound dressings is another promising area for sustainable wound care. These materials have shown potential for enhancing the mechanical properties of dressings, promoting cell proliferation, and improving tissue adhesion. This direction in research could pave the way for creating smarter, more efficient wound dressings that are not only eco-friendly but also highly effective in supporting the healing process [146].

In addition to the development of smart and sustainable wound dressings, a critical topic for future study is the incorporation of AI into wound care procedures, which has enormous promise in wound healing. One key area is developing AI algorithms that would target the problem of high wound care costs. For example, AI could aid in determining the most cost-effective treatments depending on a patient's insurance plan, which would save money in the short and long term of the insurance holder. Additionally, the integration of AI-enabled mobile applications into regular clinical settings has to be done. This would enable real-time wound analysis and remote wound management in places where there is no access to a hospital. AI technology has the potential to improve the wound healing process by preventing complications like infections or other serious conditions such as sepsis and necrotizing fasciitis. While research in this area has not been fully explored, it has great promise for the future of wound healing. AI could also assist in identifying the conditions of the wound environment, such as the type of bacteria present, exudates, or even the degree of swelling. With the integration of nanotechnology, AI may one day enable the identification and monitoring of bacterial infections in wounds, which would result in great improvements in treatment selection. Moreover, exploring genetic factors associated with wound healing could allow AI to offer more tailored treatment by forecasting potential complications based on an individual's unique genetic profile [147].

ACKNOWLEDGMENTS

The schematics are made by using the paid version of BioRender® (https://BioRender.com). The authors acknowledge the funding from the Higher Education Commission of Pakistan under Grant No. TTSF-195 for completing this work.

REFERENCES

1. H. Sorg and J. Tilkorn, "Skin Wound Healing: An Update on the Current Knowledge and Concepts," *Eur. Surg. Res.*, vol. 1–2, pp. 81–94, 2017, doi:10.1159/000454919.
2. M. Rodrigues et al., "Wound Healing: A Cellular Perspective," *Am. Physiol. Soc.*, pp. 665–706, 2025, doi:10.1152/physrev.00067.2017.
3. B. Transfusion, "An Overview of Hemostasis," *Congenit. Bleeding Disord.*, 2018, doi:10.1007/978-3-319-76723-9.
4. A. Malik, S. Qaisar, and K. U. Shah, "Hemostatic Strategies for Uncontrolled Bleeding : A Comprehensive Update," *J. Biomed. Mater.*, pp. 1465–1477, 2021, doi:10.1002/jbm.b.34806.
5. A. Tsepkolenko et al., "The Regenerative Potential of Skin and the Immune System: The Regenerative Potential of Skin and the Immune System," 2019, doi:10.2147/CCID.S196364.
6. J. J. Haddad, "Cytokines and Related Receptor-Mediated Signaling Pathways," vol. 297, pp. 700–713, 2002, doi:10.1016/S0006-291X(02)02287-8.
7. S. Ellis, E. J. Lin, and D. Tartar, "Immunology of Wound Healing," pp. 350–358, 2018.
8. N. J. Hallab and J. J. Jacobs, "Chemokines Associated with Pathologic Responses to Orthopedic implant Debris," vol. 8, no. January, pp. 1–10, 2017, doi:10.3389/fendo.2017.00005.
9. T. A. Wilgus, S. Roy, and J. C. Mcdaniel, "Neutrophils and Wound Repair : Positive Actions and Negative Reactions," vol. 2, no. 7, pp. 379–388, 2013, doi:10.1089/wound.2012.0383.
10. M. A. Nazeer, I. C. Karaoglu, O. Ozer, C. Albayrak, and S. Kizilel, "Neovascularization of Engineered Tissues for Clinical Translation: Where We Are, Where We Should Be?" *APL Bioeng.*, vol. 5, no. 2, 2021.
11. D. Miricescu, S. C. Badoiu, A. R. Totan, C. Stefani, and M. Greabu, "Growth Factors, Reactive Oxygen Species, and Metformin: Promoters of the Wound Healing Process in Burns ?" 2021.
12. Y. Oishi and I. Manabe, "Macrophages in Inflammation, Repair and Regeneration," vol. 30, no. 11, pp. 511–528, 2018, doi:10.1093/intimm/dxy054.
13. X. Shi-wen et al., "Fibroblast Matrix Gene Expression and Connective Tissue Remodeling: Role of Endothelin-1," pp. 417–425, 2001, doi:10.1046/j.1523-1747.2001.01256.x.
14. A. R. Pries and T. W. Secomb, "Making Microvascular Networks Work ," pp. 446–455, 2025, doi:10.1152/physiol.00012.2014.
15. A. C. Finney, A. W. Orr, and A. W. Orr, "Guidance Molecules in Vascular Smooth Muscle," vol. 9, no. September, pp. 1–18, 2018, doi:10.3389/fphys.2018.01311.
16. L. E. Tracy, R. A. Minasian, and E. J. Caterson, "Extracellular Matrix and Dermal Fibroblast Function in the Healing Wound," vol. 5, no. 3, pp. 119–136, 2016, doi:10.1089/wound.2014.0561.

17. S. Enoch and D. J. Leaper, "Basic Science of Wound Healing," 2007.
18. M. Farahani and A. Shafiee, "Wound Healing : From Passive to Smart Dressings," vol. 2100477, pp. 1–32, 2021, doi:10.1002/adhm.202100477.
19. L. Yao et al., "Temporal Control of PDGFR a Regulates the Fibro-Blast-to-Myofibroblast Transition in Wound Healing," *CellReports*, vol. 40, no. 7, p. 111192, 2022, doi:10.1016/j.celrep.2022.111192.
20. M. T. Longaker, "Special Topic," pp. 1172–1180, doi:10.1097/PRS.0b013e3181eae781.
21. A. L. Moore, C. D. Marshall, L. A. Barnes, M. P. Murphy, R. C. Ransom, and M. T. Longaker, "Scarless Wound Healing : Transitioning from Fetal Research to Regenerative Healing,"pp. 1–19, 2018, doi:10.1002/wdev.309.
22. X. Fu, "Regenerative medicine in China."
23. M. W. J. Ferguson and S. O. Kane, "Scar-Free Healing : From Embryonic Mechanisms to Adult Therapeutic Intervention," pp. 839–850, 2004, doi:10.1098/rstb.2004.1475.
24. R. G. Rosique, M. J. Rosique, and J. A. F. Junior, "Curbing Inflammation in Skin Wound Healing : A Review," vol. 2015, no. iv, 2015, doi:10.1155/2015/316235.
25. L. I. Nares, K. I. Sc, H. E. R. Ph, and M. Dobrkovsky, "The Histiotypi C Organization of the Hypertrophic Scar in Humans," pp. 323–331, 1972, doi:10.1111/1523-1747.ep12627386.
26. A. J. Levine, "p53: 800 Million Years of Evolution and 40 Years of Discovery," *Nat. Rev. Cancer*, vol. 53, doi:10.1038/s41568-020-0262-1.
27. S. Ud-din, S. W. Volk, and A. Bayat, "Regenerative Healing, Scar-Free Healing and Scar Formation across the Species : Current Concepts and Future Perspectives," pp. 615–619, 2014, doi:10.1111/exd.12457.
28. P. G. Bowler, "Wound Pathophysiology, Infection and Therapeutic Options," vol. 3890, 2009, doi:10.1080/07853890232101 2360.
29. A. N. Epidemic, "Wound Care: Getting to the Depth of the Tissue," 2016.
30. Z. Obagi, G. Damiani, A. Grada, and V. Falanga, "Principles of Wound Dressings: A Review," 2019.
31. K. Vowden and P. Vowden, "Wound Dressings: Principles and Practice," *Surg. (United Kingdom)*, vol. 35, no. 9, pp. 489–494, 2017, doi:10.1016/j.mpsur.2017.06.005.
32. A. E. Stoica, C. Chircov, and Grumezescu, "Nanomaterials for Wound Dressings: An Up-to-Date Overview," 2020.
33. B. Harshavardhan and V. Pawar, "Development and Characterisation of Medicated Wound Dressings for Chronic Wound," 2013.
34. S. Kim, Wound Dressings from Algal Polymers. 2015.
35. A. M. Cybulska, K. S.- Zydecka, K. Augustyniuk, and B. Karakiewicz, "Effectiveness of Hydrocolloid Dressings for Treating Pressure Ulcers in Adult Patients : A Systematic Review and Meta-Analysis," pp. 1–19, 2020, doi:10.3390/ijerph17217881.
36. S. F. Bernatchez, "Care of Peripheral Venous Catheter Sites," *J. Vasc. Access*, vol. 19, no. 4, pp. 256–261, 2014, doi:10.1016/j.java.2014.09.001.
37. J. M. Souza, M. Henriques, P. Teixeira, M. M. Fernandes, R. Fangueiro, and A. Zille, "Comfort and Infection Control of Chitosan-impregnated Cotton Gauze as Wound Dressing," vol. 20, no. 5, pp. 922–932, 2019, doi:10.1007/s12221-019-9053-2.
38. A. Finnie, "Hydrocolloids in Wound Management : Pros and Cons," vol. 7, no. 7, 2002.
39. W. Paul and C. P. Sharma, "Chitosan and Alginate Wound Dressings : A Short Review," pp. 17–23, 2015.
40. C. Morris, "Flivasorb® and the Management," vol. 5, no. 2, pp. 63–66, 2009.
41. T. Bjarnsholt et al., "Why Chronic Wounds Will Not Heal : A Novel Hypothesis," vol. 16, no. 1, pp. 2–10, 2008, doi:10.1111/j.1524-475X.2007.00283.x.
42. K. W. Finnson, S. Mclean, G. M. Di Guglielmo, and A. Philip, "Dynamics of Transforming Growth Factor Beta Signaling in Wound Healing and Scarring," vol. 2, no. 5, pp. 195–214, 2013, doi:10.1089/wound.2013.0429.

43. T. Glaser et al., "Perspectives of Purinergic Signaling in Stem Cell Differentiation and Tissue Regeneration," no. 8, pp. 523–537, 2012, doi:10.1007/s11302-011-9282-3.
44. P. Bainbridge, W. Healing, and T. Repair, "Wound Healing and the Role of Fibroblasts," vol. 22, no. 8, p. 407, 2013, doi:10.12968/jowc.2013.22.8.407.
45. J. Dissemond et al., "Compression Therapy in Patients with Venous Leg Ulcers," vol. 14, no. 11, pp. 1072–1087, 2016, doi:10.1111/ddg.13091.
46. S. Kapp, V. Academic, and C. Miller, "The Quality of Life of People Who Have Chronic Wounds and Who Self-Treat," pp. 182–192, 2018, doi:10.1111/jocn.13870.
47. E. A. Azzopardi et al., "Gram Negative Wound Infection in Hospitalised Adult Burn Patients-Systematic Review and Metanalysis," vol. 9, no. 4, 2014, doi:10.1371/journal.pone.0095042.
48. B. A. Lipsky and C. Hoey, "Topical Antimicrobial Therapy for Treating Chronic Wounds," vol. 49, pp. 1541–1549, 2009, doi:10.1086/644732.
49. B. C. Brown, S. P. Mckenna, K. Siddhi, D. A. Mcgrouther, and A. Bayat, "The Hidden Cost of Skin Scars : Quality of Life After Skin Scarring," vol. 44, no. December 2006, 2008, doi:10.1016/j.bjps.2008.03.020.
50. D. Son and A. Harijan, "Overview of Surgical Scar Prevention and Management," pp. 751–757, 2014.
51. E. Behrangi, A. Goodarzi, M. Roohaninasab, and A. Sadeghzadeh-bazargan, "Review Article A Review of Scar Treatment Related to Acne and Burn," vol. 7, no. 4, pp. 714–722, 2020.
52. G. Road, "International Journal of Clinical Dermatology & Research (IJCDR) Skin Aging & Modern Age Anti-Aging Strategies," vol. 7, no. 4, pp. 209–240, 2019. ISSN 2332-2977
53. E. R. Ghomi, S. Khalili, S. N. Khorasani, and R. E. Neisiany, "Wound Dressings : Current Advances and Future Directions," vol. 47738, pp. 1–12, 2019, doi:10.1002/app.47738.
54. M. Miraftab and G. Collyer, "A Critical Review of Modern and Emerging Absorbent Dressings Used to Treat Exuding Wounds," pp. 601–612, 2012, doi:10.1111/j.1742-481X.2011.00923.x.
55. X. Deng and M. A. Ali, "A Review of Current Advancements for Wound Healing : Biomaterial Applications and Medical Devices," no. July, pp. 2542–2573, 2022, doi:10.1002/jbm.b.35086.
56. B. S. Atiyeh, J. Ioannovich, C. A. Al-amm, and K. A. El-musa, "Management of Acute and Chronic Open Wounds : The Importance of Moist Environment in Optimal Wound Healing," pp. 179–195, 2010.
57. G. Schoukens, *Bioactive Dressings to Promote Wound Healing*, 2nd ed., Elsevier, 2019. doi:10.1016/b978-0-08-102192-7.00005-9.
58. E. Umur, E. Bayrak, F. Arslan, S. B. Bulut, and E. Baysoy, "applied sciences Advances in Three Dimensional Bioprinting for Wound Healing : A Comprehensive Review," 2023.
59. R. Li et al., "Bioactive Materials Promote Wound Healing through Modulation of Cell Behaviors," vol. 2105152, pp. 1–22, 2022, doi:10.1002/advs.202105152.
60. F. Prospects, "Sulfated Polysaccharides from Marine Algae as a Basis of Modern Biotechnologies for Creating Wound Dressings : Current Achievements and Future Prospects".
61. O. C. Onder, S. R. Batool, and M. A. Nazeer, "Self-Assembled Silk Fibroin Hydrogels: From Preparation to Biomedical Applications," *Mater. Adv.*, vol. 3, no. 18, pp. 6920–6949, 2022, doi:10.1039/d2ma00568a.
62. M. Farokhi, F. Mottaghitalab, M. Babaluei, Y. Mojarab, and S. C. Kundu, "Advanced Multifunctional Wound Dressing Hydrogels as Drug Carriers," vol. 2200111, pp. 1–20, 2022, doi:10.1002/mabi.202200111.

63. M. Abrigo, S. L. Mcarthur, and P. Kingshott, "Electrospun Nanofibers as Dressings for Chronic Wound Care : Advances, Challenges, and Future Prospects," pp. 772–792, 2014, doi:10.1002/mabi.201300561.
64. M. Mir, M. Najabat, A. Afifa, B. Ayesha, G. Munam, and A. Shizza, "Synthetic Polymeric Biomaterials for Wound Healing : A Review," *Prog. Biomater.*, vol. 7, no. 1, pp. 1–21, 2018, https://doi.org/10.1007/s40204-018-0083-4.
65. M. Edmonds et al., "Sucrose Octasulfate Dressing Versus Control Dressing in Patients with Neuroischaemic Diabetic Foot Ulcers (Explorer): an International, Multicentre, Double-Blind, Randomised, Controlled Trial," *Lancet Diabetes Endocrinol.*, vol. 6, no. 3, pp. 186–196, 2018, doi:10.1016/S2213-8587(17)30438-2.
66. S. Ahn et al., "Soy Protein/Cellulose Nanofiber Scaffolds Mimicking Skin Extracellular Matrix for Enhanced Wound Healing," *Adv. Healthc. Mater.*, vol. 7, no. 9, pp. 1–13, 2018, doi:10.1002/adhm.201701175.
67. A. Aggarwal and M. K. Sah, "Eggshell Membrane in Skin Tissue Engineering and Wound Healing," *Nat. Polym. Wound Heal. Repair From Basic Concepts to Emerg. Trends*, pp. 417–435, 2022, https://doi.org/10.1016/B978-0-323-90514-5.00007-9.
68. T. Nizami, F. Beaudoin, S. Suner, A. Aluisio, R. A. Bhatt, and G. D. Jay, "Evaluation of microMend Wound Closure Device in Repairing Skin Lacerations," *Emerg. Med. J.*, vol. 40, no. 8, pp. 564–568, 2023, doi:10.1136/emermed-2022-212667.
69. J. Dilday and J. B. Holcomb, "Strategies to Control Hemorrhage in the Trauma Patient," *High-Risk Surg. Patient*, pp. 867–881, 2023, doi:10.1007/978-3-031-17273-1_78.
70. F. Feng, Z. Zhao, J. Li, Y. Huang, and W. Chen, "Multifunctional Dressings for Wound Exudate Management," *Prog. Mater. Sci.*, vol. 146, p. 101328, 2024, doi:10.1016/J.PMATSCI.2024.101328.
71. Y. Zhang, E. Holland, M. Chun, M. O'brien, A. Nguyen, and L. Sun, "Just a Flesh Wound? A Detailed Review of Modern Dressings," *Heal. Sci. J.*, vol. 14, no. 4, pp. 1–11, 2020.
72. K. C. Münter, S. De Lange, T. Eberlein, A. Andriessen, and M. Abel, "Handling Properties of a Superabsorbent Dressing in the Management of Patients with Moderate-to-Very High Exuding Wounds," vol. 27, no. 4, pp. 246–253, 2018, doi:10.12968/JOWC.2018.27.4.246.
73. H. Chen et al., "A novel Wound Dressing based on a Konjac Glucomannan/Silver Nanoparticle Composite Sponge Effectively Kills Bacteria and Accelerates Wound Healing," *Carbohydr. Polym.*, vol. 183, pp. 70–80, 2018, doi:10.1016/j.carbpol.2017.11.029.
74. R. Singla et al., "In Situ Functionalized Nanobiocomposites Dressings of Bamboo Cellulose Nanocrystals and Silver Nanoparticles for Accelerated Wound Healing," *Carbohydr. Polym.*, vol. 155, pp. 152–162, 2017, doi:10.1016/j.carbpol.2016.08.065.
75. K. G. Barki et al., "Electric Field Based Dressing Disrupts Mixed-Species Bacterial Biofilm Infection and Restores Functional Wound Healing," *Ann. Surg.*, vol. 269, no. 4, pp. 756–766, 2019, doi:10.1097/SLA.0000000000002504.
76. A. Dhyani et al., "Antimicrobial Wound Dressings for Full-Thickness Infected Burn Wounds," *Shock*, vol. 62, no. 4, 2024, doi:10.1097/SHK.0000000000002426.
77. B. B. Hsu et al., "Multifunctional Self-Assembled Films for Rapid Hemostat and Sustained Anti-infective Delivery," *ACS Biomater. Sci. Eng.*, vol. 1, no. 3, pp. 148–156, 2015, doi:10.1021/ab500050m.
78. M. A. Weigelt et al., "Advanced Wound Diagnostics : Toward Transforming Wound Care into Precision Medicine," vol. 11, no. 6, pp. 330–359, 2022, doi:10.1089/wound.2020.1319.
79. D. A. Jankowska et al., "Simultaneous Detection of pH Value and Glucose Concentrations for Wound Monitoring Applications," *Biosens. Bioelectron.*, vol. 87, no. January, pp. 312–319, 2017, doi:10.1016/j.bios.2016.08.072.

80. S. Lin et al., "Stretchable Hydrogel Electronics and Devices," *Adv Mater*, vol. 28, no. 22, pp. 4497–4505, 2016, doi:10.1002/adma.201504152.
81. N. T. Thet et al., "Prototype Development of the Intelligent Hydrogel Wound Dressing and Its Efficacy in the Detection of Model Pathogenic Wound Biofilms," *ACS Appl. Mater. Interfaces*, vol. 8, no. 24, pp. 14909–14919, 2016, https://doi.org/10.1021/acsami.5b07372.
82. R. Ghosh, P. Singh, A. H. Pandit, U. Tariq, B. K. Bhunia, and A. Kumar, "Emerging Technological Advancement for Chronic Wound Treatment and Their Role in Accelerating Wound Healing," *ACS Appl. Bio Mater.*, 2024, https://doi.org/10.1021/acsabm.4c01064.
83. M. E. Aljghami, S. Saboor, and S. Amini-Nik, "Emerging Innovative Wound Dressings," *Ann. Biomed. Eng.*, vol. 47, no. 3, pp. 659–675, 2019, doi:10.1007/s10439-018-02186-w.
84. A. Alsaif, M. Karam, A. Hayre, A. Abul, A. Aldubaikhi, and N. Kahlar, "Full Thickness Skin Graft Versus Split Thickness Skin Graft in Paediatric Patients with Hand Burns: Systematic Review and Meta-Analysis," *Burns*, vol. 49, no. 5, pp. 1017–1027, 2023, doi:10.1016/j.burns.2022.09.010.
85. P. Kolimi, S. Narala, D. Nyavanandi, A. A. A. Youssef, and N. Dudhipala, "Innovative Treatment Strategies to Accelerate Wound Healing: Trajectory and Recent Advancements," *Cells*, vol. 11, no. 15, 2022, doi:10.3390/cells11152439.
86. B. M. Hussen, M. Taheri, R. K. Yashooa, and G. H. Abdullah, "Revolutionizing Medicine : Recent Developments and Future Prospects in Stem-Cell Therapy," pp. 10–12, 2007.
87. S. Kanji and H. Das, "Advances of Stem Cell Therapeutics in Cutaneous Wound Healing and Regeneration," *Mediators Inflamm.*, vol. 2017, 2017, doi:10.1155/2017/5217967.
88. P. Sharma, A. Kumar, A. D. Dey, T. Behl, and S. Chadha, "Stem Cells and Growth Factors-based Delivery Approaches for Chronic Wound Repair and Regeneration: A Promise to Heal from Within," *Life Sci.*, vol. 268, p. 118932, 2021, doi:10.1016/j.lfs.2020.118932.
89. B. Farabi, K. Roster, R. Hirani, K. Tepper, M. F. Atak, and B. Safai, "The Efficacy of Stem Cells in Wound Healing: A Systematic Review," *Int. J. Mol. Sci.*, vol. 25, no. 5, pp. 1–17, 2024, doi:10.3390/ijms25053006.
90. A. Garg, S. Garg, P. Adlak, M. L. Kori, and S. Lodhi, "Stem Cells and Regenerative Strategies for Wound Healing: Therapeutic and Clinical Implications," *Curr. Pharmacol.* Rep., vol. 10, no. 2, pp. 121–144, 2024, doi:10.1007/s40495-024-00352-4.
91. S. Zhidu, T. Ying, J. Rui, and Z. Chao, "Translational Potential of Mesenchymal Stem Cells in Regenerative Therapies for Human Diseases: Challenges and Opportunities," *Stem Cell Res. Ther.*, vol. 15, no. 1, 2024, doi:10.1186/s13287-024-03885-z.
92. S. Wu, S. Sun, W. Fu, Z. Yang, H. Yao, and Z. Zhang, "The Role and Prospects of Mesenchymal Stem Cells in Skin Repair and Regeneration," *Biomedicines*, vol. 12, no. 4, 2024, doi:10.3390/biomedicines12040743.
93. R. Mei et al., "Advances and Clinical Challenges of Mesenchymal Stem Cell Therapy," *Front. Immunol.*, vol. 15, no. July, pp. 1–14, 2024, doi:10.3389/fimmu.2024.1421854.
94. C. Pang, K. S. Fan, L. Wei, and M. K. Kolar, "Gene Therapy in Wound Healing Using Nanotechnology," *Wound Repair Regen.*, vol. 29, no. 2, pp. 225–239, 2021, doi:10.1111/wrr.12881.
95. L. K. Branski, C. T. Pereira, D. N. Herndon, and M. G. Jeschke, "Gene Therapy in Wound Healing: Present Status and Future Directions," *Gene Ther.*, vol. 14, no. 1, pp. 1–10, 2007, doi:10.1038/sj.gt.3302837.
96. L. K. Branski, G. G. Gauglitz, D. N. Herndon, and M. G. Jeschke, "A Review of Gene and Stem Cell Therapy in Cutaneous Wound Healing," *Burns*, vol. 35, no. 2, pp. 171–180, 2009, doi:10.1016/j.burns.2008.03.009.

97. J. A. Lee et al., "Lentiviral Transfection with the PDGF-B Gene Improves Diabetic Wound Healing," *Plast. Reconstr. Surg.*, vol. 116, no. 2, pp. 532–538, 2005, doi:10.1097/01.PRS.0000172892.78964.49.
98. G. Romano, P. Micheli, C. Pacilio, and A. Giordano, "Latest Developments in Gene Transfer Technology: Achievements, Perspectives, and Controversies over Therapeutic Applications," *Stem Cells*, vol. 18, no. 1, pp. 19–39, 2000, doi:10.1634/stemcells.18-1-19.
99. J. Dwivedi et al., "Gene Augmentation Techniques to Stimulate Wound Healing Process: Progress and Prospects," *Curr. Gene Ther.*, vol. 25, 2024, doi:10.2174/011566 5232316799241008073042.
100. M. Galeano et al., "Adeno-Associated Viral Vector-Mediated Human Vascular Endothelial Growth Factor Gene Transfer Stimulates Angiogenesis and Wound Healing in the Genetically Diabetic Mouse," *Diabetologia*, vol. 46, no. 4, pp. 546–555, 2003, https://doi.org/10.1007/s00125-003-1064-1.
101. E. A. Burton, D. J. Fink, and J. C. Glorioso, "Gene Delivery Using Herpes Simplex Virus Vectors," *DNA Cell Biol.*, vol. 21, no. 12, pp. 915–936, 2002, doi:10.1089/104454902762053864.
102. M. Ramamoorth and A. Narvekar, "Non Viral Vectors in Gene Therapy: An overview," *J. Clin. Diagnostic Res.*, vol. 9, no. 1, pp. GE01–GE06, 2015, doi:10.7860/JCDR/2015/10443.5394.
103. M. H. Butt et al., "Appraisal for the Potential of Viral and Nonviral Vectors in Gene Therapy: A Review," *Genes (*Basel*)*, vol. 13, no. 8, 2022, doi:10.3390/genes13081370.
104. E. Eriksson et al., "In Vivo Gene Transfer to Skin and Wound by Microseeding," *J. Surg. Res.*, vol. 78, no. 2, pp. 85–91, 1998, doi:10.1006/jsre.1998.5325.
105. S. M. Alnasser, "Review on Mechanistic Strategy of Gene Therapy in the Treatment of Disease," *Gene*, vol. 769, p. 145246, 2021, doi:10.1016/j.gene.2020.145246.
106. N. Sayed et al., "Gene Therapy: Comprehensive Overview and Therapeutic Applications," *Life Sci.*, vol. 294, p. 120375, 2022, doi:10.1016/J.LFS.2022.120375.
107. N. Sindhu, S. Kumar, and R. Kumar, "Nanotechnology in Wound Healing," pp. 587–613, 2024, doi:10.1007/978-981-16-1610-5_25.
108. J. P. Yadav, D. K. Patel, A. Verma, and P. Pathak, "Revolutionizing Diabetic Wound Healing: Targeted Therapeutic Strategies based on Growth Factors," *Obes. Med.*, vol. 47, p. 100535, May 2024, doi:10.1016/J.OBMED.2024.100535.
109. Y. Liu, Y. Liu, J. Deng, W. Li, and X. Nie, "Fibroblast Growth Factor in Diabetic Foot Ulcer: Progress and Therapeutic Prospects," *Front. Endocrinol. (*Lausanne*).*, vol. 12, no. October, pp. 1–14, 2021, doi:10.3389/fendo.2021.744868.
110. P. Kaiser, J. Wächter, and M. Windbergs, "Therapy of Infected Wounds: Overcoming Clinical Challenges by Advanced Drug Delivery Systems," *Drug Deliv. Transl.* Res., vol. 11, no. 4, pp. 1545–1567, 2021, doi:10.1007/s13346-021-00932-7.
111. R. Huang, J. Hu, W. Qian, L. Chen, and D. Zhang, "Recent Advances in Nanotherapeutics for the Treatment of Burn Wounds," *Burn. Trauma*, vol. 9, 2021, doi:10.1093/burnst/tkab026.
112. D. Medina-Cruz, B. Saleh, A. Vernet-Crua, A. Ajo, A. K. Roy, and T. J. Webster, *Drug-Delivery Nanocarriers for Skin Wound-Healing Applications*, Elsevier, 2020. doi:10.1016/B978-0-12-816413-6.00022-8.
113. Z. Niknam, F. Hossein Zadeh, S. Toosi, N. K. Haji Shoreh, Y. Rasmi, and I. Saleem, "Organic-based Nanomaterials for Regenerative Medicine," *Handb. Nanomater. Vol.* 2 *Biomed. Environ. Food, Agric.*, pp. 359–400, 2024, doi:10.1016/B978-0-323-95513-3.00003-4.
114. E. Sánchez-López et al., "Metal-based Nanoparticles as Antimicrobial Agents: An Overview," *Nanomaterials*, vol. 10, no. 2, pp. 1–39, 2020, doi:10.3390/nano10020292.

115. S. Das and A. B. Baker, "Biomaterials and Nanotherapeutics for Enhancing Skin Wound Healing," *Front. Bioeng. Biotechnol.*, vol. 4, no. Oct, pp. 1–20, 2016, doi:10.3389/fbioe.2016.00082.
116. J. P. Yadav et al., "Phytoconstituents as Modulators of NF-κB Signalling: Investigating Therapeutic Potential for Diabetic Wound Healing," *Biomed. Pharmacother.*, vol. 177, p. 117058, 2024, doi:10.1016/j.biopha.2024.117058.
117. I. Hasan and P. Kumar, "Platelet Rich Plasma (P.R.P) Treatment: A View," *Int. J. Clin. Nurs.*, vol. 1, no. 1, pp. 34–47, 2020.
118. H. Patel, A. Pundkar, S. Shrivastava, R. Chandanwale, and A. M. Jaiswal, "A Comprehensive Review on Platelet-Rich Plasma Activation: A Key Player in Accelerating Skin Wound Healing," *Cureus*, vol. 15, no. 11, 2023, doi:10.7759/cureus.48943.
119. R. Verma, S. Kumar, P. Garg, and Y. K. Verma, "Platelet-Rich Plasma: A Comparative and Economical Therapy for Wound Healing and Tissue Regeneration," *Cell Tissue Bank.*, vol. 24, no. 2, pp. 285–306, 2023, doi:10.1007/s10561-022-10039-z.
120. S. Emmert et al., "Combining Biocompatible and Biodegradable Scaffolds and Cold Atmospheric Plasma for Chronic Wound Regeneration," *Int. J. Mol. Sci.*, vol. 22, no. 17, 2021, doi:10.3390/ijms22179199.
121. M. S. Mann et al., "Introduction to DIN-Specification 91315 based on the Characterization of the Plasma Jet kINPen® MED," *Clin. Plasma Med.*, vol. 4, no. 2, pp. 35–45, 2016, doi:10.1016/j.cpme.2016.06.001.
122. T. Bernhardt, M. L. Semmler, M. Schäfer, S. Bekeschus, S. Emmert, and L. Boeckmann, "Plasma Medicine: Applications of Cold Atmospheric Pressure Plasma in Dermatology," *Oxid. Med. Cell. Lo*ngev., vol. 2019, pp. 10–13, 2019, doi:10.1155/2019/3873928.
123. S. Fathollah et al., "Investigation on the Effects of the Atmospheric Pressure Plasma on Wound Healing in Diabetic Rats," *Sci. Rep.*, vol. 6, pp. 1–9, 2016, doi:10.1038/srep19144.
124. K. Y. Pradhan and M. Pradhan (Eds.), *3D Printing and Microfluidics in Dermatology: Innovations in Drug Delivery*. CRC Press.
125. S. Masri, M. Zawani, I. Zulkiflee, A. Salleh, and N. I. Fadilah, "Cellular Interaction of Human Skin Cells towards Natural Bioink via 3D-Bioprinting Technologies for Chronic Wound: A Comprehensive Review," 2022.
126. D. Singh, D. Singh, and S. S. Han, "3D Printing of Scaffold for Cells Delivery: Advances in Skin Tissue Engineering," *Polymers (*Basel*)*, vol. 8, no. 1, pp. 1–17, 2016, doi:10.3390/polym8010019.
127. P. Fomby et al., "Stem Cells and Cell Therapies in Lung Biology and Diseases: Conference Report," *Ann. Am. Thorac. Soc.*, vol. 12, no. 3, pp. 181–204, 2010.
128. I. D. Derman et al., "Advancements in 3D Skin Bioprinting: Processes, Bioinks, Applications and Sensor Integration," *Int. J. Extrem. Manuf.*, vol. 7, no. 1, p. 012009, 2024, doi:10.1088/2631-7990/ad878c.
129. A. Mazzocchi, S. Soker, and A. Skardal, "3D Bioprinting for High-Throughput Screening: Drug Screening, Disease Modeling, and Precision Medicine Applications," *Appl. Phys. Rev.*, vol. 6, no. 1, 2019, https://doi.org/10.1063/1.5056188.
130. I. T. Ozbolat and M. Hospodiuk, "Current Advances and Future Perspectives in Extrusion-based Bioprinting," *Biomaterials*, vol. 76, pp. 321–343, 2016, doi:10.1016/j.biomaterials.2015.10.076.
131. J. Tumbleston, Tumbleston, and John, "Continuous Liquid Interface Production (CLIP)," *APS*, vol. 2016, p. X4.001, 2016.
132. Z. Gao et al., "Simultaneous Multi-Material Embedded Printing for 3D Heterogeneous Structures," *Int. J. Extrem. Manuf.*, vol. 5, no. 3, 2023, doi:10.1088/2631-7990/acd285.

133. D. J. Whyte, E. H. Doeven, A. Sutti, A. Z. Kouzani, and S. D. Adams, "Volumetric Additive Manufacturing: A New Frontier in Layer-Less 3D Printing," *Addit. Manuf.*, vol. 84, no. March, p. 104094, 2024, doi:10.1016/j.addma.2024.104094.
134. P. Jain, H. Kathuria, S. Ramakrishna, S. Parab, M. M. Pandey, and N. Dubey, "In Situ Bioprinting: Process, Bioinks, and Applications," *ACS Appl. Bio Mater.*, 2023, https://doi.org/10.1021/acsabm.3c01303.
135. W. Park, G. Gao, and D. W. Cho, "Tissue-Specific Decellularized Extracellular Matrix Bioinks for Musculoskeletal Tissue Regeneration and Modeling Using 3d Bioprinting Technology," *Int. J. Mol. Sci.*, vol. 22, no. 15, 2021, doi:10.3390/ijms22157837.
136. T. Baltazar et al., "Three Dimensional Bioprinting of a Vascularized and Perfusable Skin Graft Using Human Keratinocytes, Fibroblasts, Pericytes, and Endothelial Cells," *Tissue Eng. A*, vol. 26, no. 5–6, pp. 227–238, 2020, doi:10.1089/ten.tea.2019.0201.
137. J. Y. Won et al., "A potential Dermal Substitute Using Decellularized Dermis Extracellular Matrix Derived Bio-Ink," *Artif. Cells, Nanomedicine Biotechnol.*, vol. 47, no. 1, pp. 644–649, 2019, doi:10.1080/21691401.2019.1575842.
138. D. Chouhan, N. Dey, N. Bhardwaj, and B. B. Mandal, "Emerging and Innovative Approaches for Wound Healing and Skin Regeneration: Current Status and Advances," *Biomaterials*, vol. 216, no. June, p. 119267, 2019, doi:10.1016/j.biomaterials.2019.119267.
139. D. Chouhan, T. u. Lohe, P. K. Samudrala, and B. B. Mandal, "In Situ Forming Injectable Silk Fibroin Hydrogel Promotes Skin Regeneration in Full Thickness Burn Wounds," *Adv. Healthc. Mater.*, vol. 7, no. 24, pp. 1–15, 2018, doi:10.1002/adhm.201801092.
140. L. Zhao, L. Niu, H. Liang, H. Tan, C. Liu, and F. Zhu, "PH and Glucose Dual-Responsive Injectable Hydrogels with Insulin and Fibroblasts as Bioactive Dressings for Diabetic Wound Healing," *ACS Appl. Mater. Interfaces*, vol. 9, no. 43, pp. 37563–37574, 2017, https://doi.org/10.1021/acsami.7b09395.
141. J. Guo et al., "Development of Tannin-Inspired Antimicrobial Bioadhesives," *Acta Biomater.*, vol. 72, pp. 35–44, 2018, doi:10.1016/j.actbio.2018.03.008.
142. E. Y. Jeon et al., "Rapidly Light-Activated Surgical Protein Glue Inspired by Mussel Adhesion and Insect Structural Crosslinking," *Biomaterials*, vol. 67, pp. 11–19, 2015, doi:10.1016/j.biomaterials.2015.07.014.
143. G. Lokhande et al., "Nanoengineered Injectable Hydrogels from kappa-Carrageenan and Two-dimensional Nanosilicates for Wound Healing Application," *Acta Biomater.*, vol. 70, pp. 35–47, 2018, doi:10.1016/j.actbio.2018.01.045.
144. D. R. Griffin, W. M. Weaver, P. O. Scumpia, D. Di Carlo, and T. Segura, "Accelerated Wound Healing by Injectable Microporous Gel Scaffolds Assembled from Annealed Building Blocks," *Nat. Mater.* $_{2014}$ 147, vol. 14, no. 7, pp. 737–744, 2015, doi:10.1038/nmat4294.
145. J. Yu et al., "Production of Hollow Bacterial Cellulose Microspheres Using Microfluidics to Form an Injectable Porous Scaffold for Wound Healing," *Adv. Healthc. Mater.*, vol. 5, no. 23, pp. 2983–2992, 2016, doi:10.1002/adhm.201600898.
146. H. Supriya, S. Tripathi, and S. Bose, "A Review of Past Promises, Present Realities and a Vibrant Future for Wound Dressing from Naturally Occurring to Sustainable Materials," *RSC Sustain.*, vol. 1, no. 4, pp. 763–787, 2023, doi:10.1039/d3su00065f.
147. M. P. Jairam and R. Ha, "A Review of Artificial Intelligence in Mammography," *Clin. Imaging*, vol. 88, pp. 36–44, 2022, doi:10.1016/j.clinimag.2022.05.005.

Index

N

O

P

R

S

T

W

For Product Safety Concerns and Information please contact our EU
representative GPSR@taylorandfrancis.com
Taylor & Francis Verlag GmbH, Kaufingerstraße 24, 80331 München, Germany

www.ingramcontent.com/pod-product-compliance
Ingram Content Group UK Ltd.
Pitfield, Milton Keynes, MK11 3LW, UK
UKHW022215190926
475702UK00003B/367
9781041018711